Contraception

A Casebook from Menarche to Menopause

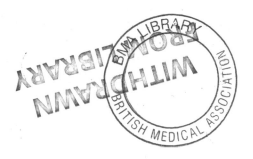

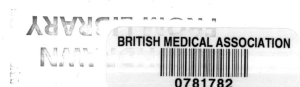

Contraception

A Casebook from Menarche to Menopause

Edited by

Paula Briggs
Contraceptive Lead, Southport and Ormskirk Hospital NHS Trust, Southport, UK

Gabor Kovacs
Professor of Obstetrics and Gynaecology, Monash University;
Honorary Consultant to Family Planning Victoria, Melbourne, Victoria, Australia

John Guillebaud
Emeritus Professor of Family Planning and Reproductive Health, University College London, London, UK

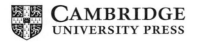
CAMBRIDGE
UNIVERSITY PRESS

CAMBRIDGE
UNIVERSITY PRESS

University Printing House, Cambridge CB2 8BS, United Kingdom

Published in the United States of America by Cambridge University Press, New York

Cambridge University Press is part of the University of Cambridge.

It furthers the University's mission by disseminating knowledge in the pursuit of education, learning and research at the highest international levels of excellence.

www.cambridge.org
Information on this title: www.cambridge.org/9781107614666

First published 2013

Printed in the United Kingdom by Bell and Bain Ltd

A catalog record for this publication is available from the British Library

Library of Congress Cataloging in Publication data
Contraception : a casebook from menarche to menopause / edited by Paula Briggs, contraceptive lead, Southport and Ormskirk Hospital NHS Trust, Southport, UK, Gabor Kovacs, professor of Obstetrics & Gynaecology, Monash University, and honorary consultant to Family Planning Victoria, Melbourne, Victoria, Australia, John Guillebaud, emeritus professor of Family Planning & Reproductive Health, University College London, London, UK.
    pages   cm
Includes bibliographical references and index.
ISBN 978-1-107-61466-6 (pbk.)
1. Contraception.   2. Contraceptives – Side effects.   3. Reproductive health.   4. Women – Health risk assessment.   I. Briggs, Paula, 1964–editor of compilation.   II. Kovács, Gábor, editor of compilation.
III. Guillebaud, John, editor of compilation.
RG136.C5325   2013
618.1'82 – dc23   2013017354

ISBN 978-1-107-61466-6 Paperback

....

Contents

Contributors

Mike Abbott, MB ChB, FRCP, Dp Bact, Dp Ven, Dip Psychosex Ther
Consultant in Sexual Health and HIV Medicine, Department of Genitourinary Medicine, Southport and Formby District General Hospital, Southport, UK

Jean-Jacques Amy, MD, DTM
Emeritus Professor of Obstetrics and Gynaecology, Vrije Universiteit, Brussels, Belgium

Deborah J. Bateson, MA(Oxon), MSc, MB\BS
Medical Director, Family Planning New South Wales, Ashfield, New South Wales, Australia

Johannes Bitzer, MD
Chairman, Department of Obstetrics and Gynaecology, University Hospital Basel, President of the European Society of Contraception, Basel, Switzerland

Paula Briggs, MB ChB, MRCGP, FFSRH, Dip Ven, DMJ(Clin), Dip Gynaecology
Contraceptive Lead, Southport and Ormskirk Hospital NHS Trust, Southport, UK

Anne Connolly, MB ChB Bham, DRCOG, MRCGP, DFSRH, Dip Gynae, GPSI Gynae
The Ridge Medical Practice, Bradford, UK

David Crook, PhD
Senior Research Fellow, University of Brighton, Brighton, UK

Tony Feltbower, MB BChir, DRCOG, AFOM, CUEWcert
Westminster Road Medical Services Ltd, Coventry, UK

Kathy French, RN, BSc Hons, PhD, MPhil, PG Dip IP, Cert Ed
Nurse Advisor, London Sexual Health Programme, London Specialized Commissioning, London, UK

Lynne Garforth, BSc Hons PG Dip IP
Primary Care Pharmacist, Medicines Management Service, Liverpool Community Health NHS Trust, Liverpool, UK

Ailsa E. Gebbie, MB ChB, FRCOG, FFSRH, FRCP(Ed)
Consultant Gynaecologist, Chalmers Centre, Edinburgh, UK

Kristina Gemzell-Danielsson, MD, PhD
Professor of Obstetrics and Gynaecology, Karolinska Institutet and Karolinska University Hospital, Stockholm, Sweden

Marie-Odile Gerval, MB BS
Clinical Research Fellow, Imperial College London, London, UK

John Guillebaud MA, FRCSE, FRCOG, MFFP
Emeritus Professor of Family Planning and Reproductive Health, University College London, London, UK

Sunanda Gupta, FRCOG, FFSRH
Consultant in Contraception and Reproductive Health Care, Royal Wolverhampton NHS Trust, Wolverhampton, UK

Kate Guthrie, MD, FRCOG, FFSRH
Clinical Director, Hull and East Riding Sexual and Reproductive Health Care Partnership, Hull, UK

Susanna Hall, MB ChB, MRCOG, DFSRH
Speciality Trainee in Sexual and
Reproductive Health Care, Bristol Sexual
Health Services, Bristol, UK

Philip C. Hannaford, MD, FRCGP
Professor of Primary Care, Centre of
Academic Primary Care, University of
Aberdeen, Aberdeen, UK

Caroline Harvey, MB BS(Hons), MPM
Medical Director, Family Planning
Queensland, Brisbane, Queensland,
Australia

Mary Hernon, BSc, MB ChB, MRCOG,
DFSRH Dip
Paediatric and Adolescent Gynaecologist,
Alder Hey Hospital, Liverpool, UK

Lisa Iversen, BSc, MSc, PhD
Research Fellow, Centre of Academic
Primary Care, University of Aberdeen,
Aberdeen, UK

Gabor Kovacs, MB BS (Hons), MD,
FRCOG, FRANZCOG, CREI
Professor of Obstetrics and Gynaecology,
Monash University and Honorary
Consultant to Family Planning Victoria,
Melbourne, Victoria, Australia

Ali A. Kubba, MB ChB, FRCOG, FFSRH
Consultant Community Gynaecologist,
Guy's and St Thomas' NHS Foundation
Trust, London, UK

Kathleen McNamee, MB BS, FRACGP,
Dip Ven, Grad Dip Epi Bio, MEpi
Medical Director, Family Planning Victoria
and Adjunct Senior Lecturer, Department
of Obstetrics and Gynaecology, Monash
University, Melbourne, Victoria, Australia

Nicholas Panay, BSc, MRCOG, MFFP
Consultant Gynaecologist, Queen
Charlotte's and Chelsea and Westminster

Hospitals and Honorary Senior Lecturer,
Imperial College London, London, UK

Tina Peers, MB BS, DRCOG, DFSRH,
FFSRH, BCAM
Consultant in Sexual Health and
Reproductive Health Care and Clinical
Director of Sexual Health Services, Surrey,
UK

Victoria Sephton, MRCOG
Consultant Obstetrician and
Gynaecologist, Warrington and Halton
NHS Trust and Clinical Director, Brook,
Liverpool, UK

Sven O. Skouby, MD, DMSc
Director of the Endocrinological and
Reproductive Unit, Department of
Obstetrics and Gynaecology, Herlev
Hospital, University of Copenhagen,
Denmark, and Department of Thrombosis
Research, Esbjerg, University of Southern
Denmark

Lesley Smith
Curator of Tutbury Castle, Staffordshire,
UK

Anne Szarewski, MB BS, DRCOG, PhD,
FFSRH
Clinical Senior Lecturer, Queen Mary
University of London and Associate
Specialist, Margaret Pyke Centre, London,
UK

Rik H. W. van Lunsen, MD, PhD
Head of Department of Sexology and
Psychosomatic Obstetrics and
Gynaecology, Academic Medical Centre,
University of Amsterdam, Amsterdam, The
Netherlands

Catherine White, MB ChB, FFFLM,
MRCGP, DMJ, DRCOG, DCH, DFFP
Clinical Director, St Mary's Sexual Assault
Referral Centre, Manchester, UK

Foreword

When scanning the shelves for a new and interesting 'contraceptive' book I am looking for a text that is comprehensive yet to the point, factually correct but written so as to hold the reader's attention, and for it to have something new to say. *Contraception: A Casebook from Menarche to Menopause* fills this gap.

The authors of each chapter read like a 'Who's Who' list of experts in global contraception, ensuring a good read. As you would expect from the book's title there are sections focusing on the different contraceptive methods available in the twenty-first century. But the editors have not shied away from tackling the more difficult scenarios facing us each day and there are thought-provoking chapters covering sexual assault and psychological issues associated with sex.

Healthcare professionals working in primary, community and secondary care seeing couples requesting contraceptive advice will find the case-based scenario approach refreshing with the chapters devoted to unplanned pregnancy and abortion helping to explain why over 40% of pregnancies worldwide are still unintended and accounting for almost 100 million pregnancies each year.

We have seen great advances in the field of hormonal contraception yet couples still find it difficult to choose the best method that suits their lifestyle. Requests to 'go on the pill' are common but hide the public's ignorance of contraceptive choice and the myths surrounding lower user-dependent contraceptive methods. As we have children our needs change, yet a recent survey suggests that women spend more time choosing a pair of shoes than they do their contraceptive method. Women are now often having their first child in their late 20s and will need contraception for at least 30 years of their lives. Knowing the facts are vital and dispelling the myths essential to selecting the ideal option and helping to make every child a wanted child.

The editors need to be congratulated on producing a book with such a practical approach to contraception from the menarche to the menopause. This is a book we can dip into for help and, armed with the latest facts, provide quality sexual health care.

Diana Mansour, MB BCh, FRCOG, FFSRH, DIPM
Consultant in Community Gynaecology and Reproductive Health Care, Head of Sexual Health Services, Newcastle Hospitals Community Health, New Croft Centre, Newcastle upon Tyne, UK

Preface

This book was written to provide practitioners working in all areas of reproductive medicine with a comprehensive, up-to-date review of current management options. The book covers the history of contraception, currently available methods as well as abortion, the primary care of subfertility, diagnosis and management of sexually transmitted infections and dealing with sexual assault.

This book is unique in two ways: first, it considers women in their various life stages and, secondly, most chapters commence with a case history to which the reader can easily relate.

Although there are many excellent texts on contraception available, the editors' aim with this book was to provide a resource to engage not only specialists but also the main providers of sexual health advice, general practitioners and practice nurses. The book is also very suitable for medical students who are looking for a broad understanding of reproductive and sexual health.

The book could easily be read from cover to cover or the reader can dip into the various chapters as required.

All three editors are keen and experienced teachers and with this book they wanted to share their enthusiasm and knowledge, but most importantly, they wanted to produce a book that the reader would enjoy.

The success of this book is due to the outstanding talent of the chapter authors, who represent the leading experts in reproductive health in Europe and Australia.

Chapter

1

What women want from their contraceptives … and what we can offer

Johannes Bitzer

The basic 'universal' wish underlying any contraceptive activity is to separate sexuality from reproduction and thus provide protection against unwanted pregnancies. The second wish which is also universally found is that the use of contraceptive methods is safe, meaning that the individual health of the woman practising contraception is preserved and not threatened [1, 2]. Apart from the fact that these two wishes have the potential of getting into a conflict-laden relationship (highest efficacy may be in conflict with highest safety) there is a lot of individual 'prioritizing' between the two major motives and there are a lot of other wishes of women around contraception as some case vignettes may exemplify:

Dorothy is 17 years old. She has recently fallen in love with Robert, a school mate. In his presence she feels butterflies in her stomach and at a party they had been dancing with very close body contact and they had kissed each other evoking a feeling she had never experienced before. She wants him and she knows that he wants her. Becoming pregnant would be a horror with her being at school and her dreams of becoming a doctor or a teacher would be threatened or destroyed. She wants contraception in which she can completely trust. This is her only and dominant wish.

Her girlfriend Lisa has already had intercourse with John. Lisa is very much concerned about her skin and her attractiveness since John had terminated their relationship quite abruptly. She wants to get rid of all these little pimples and look sexy again. Of course she does not want to get pregnant but more important is looking good and maybe getting John back.

Liz is the same age as Lisa, living in another country. Just recently it has been on the news: a girl of her age who had taken the same pill as her had suffered a blood clot, collapsed and had to be resuscitated, which was successful but had resulted in a severe handicap for the girl. Liz is horrified by the news. She stops taking that pill immediately and she wants contraception that does not have the risk of such a disease or better no risk at all.

Lesley is 33 years old. She has been married to Frank for 10 years and they have two children. They have a good relationship. Sex has become a bit of a routine. She has increased in weight, which is a big concern for her. Her mother has recently been diagnosed with breast cancer. She does not want to become pregnant but more important for her is that she does not increase weight and that she does not develop breast cancer like her mother. She would also like to feel more sexual desire again and be more responsive to her husband's advances like it was before.

Sefira is now 35 years old. She has four children and wants to get some rest from procreation. She is a Muslim and leads a life quite strictly according to the rules of Islam. Her biggest concern is that her menstrual cycle would change and she wishes by all means a contraceptive method that has no impact on her natural cycle especially no unexpected bleeding or spotting, which would keep her from praying and keep her from fulfilling her duties towards her husband.

Contraception, eds Paula Briggs, Gabor Kovacs and John Guillebaud. Published by Cambridge University Press. © Cambridge University Press 2013.

Yvonne is a very successful single business woman. She is also very active in long distance running and has even started with the women's triathlon. Menstruation is a nuisance to her, which keeps her from activities she likes. She feels bothered by this 'bloody business' and has read in a magazine that menstruation is a relic of former times.

Carla is 17 years old. She has to stay at home when these horrible pain attacks at the beginning of her menstrual bleed start. This is not good for her performance at school and she withdraws from all her physical activities and stays in bed with pain killers and a hot water bottle.

As can be seen by these case illustrations there is no simple answer to the question 'What do women want from contraceptives?' because women are so different and so different in their wishes, or even in the same woman across her life cycle.

Looking at this question from a population-based view and trying to understand the literature about these issues it appears that women's wishes can be subdivided into two major groups.

General wishes of (almost) all women

Efficacy

As mentioned above efficacy seems to be the most important and most general request or wish of women regarding contraceptive methods. They want 100% effectiveness. It seems an inherent wish and a logical request when practising contraception.

This wish can almost be fulfilled because modern contraceptive methods have an efficacy that approaches 100%. To have this high efficacy, modern methods interfere with the normal reproductive physiology (by inhibiting ovulation, destroying sperm capacity to fertilize, interfering with endometrial maturation, etc.) and thus these methods are basically 'unnatural'. Some women want a high efficacy with little or no interference with nature – a wish which until now has not been fulfilled. It is important to take into consideration these wishes when it comes to counselling and explaining the mechanisms of action.

Regarding efficacy, an unknown number of women may not want an absolutely effective method to keep some risk or chance of becoming pregnant alive [3, 4]. This is a possible conflict between the cognitive wish for contraception and the emotional wish to feel the potency to get pregnant. We do not have empirical studies about the frequency of this internal conflict, but for practical reasons it seems important to keep this possible ambivalence towards efficacy in mind [5, 6].

Safety

We can assume and this is confirmed by studies, that all women want to be safe and run no health risks when practising contraception [1, 2, 4, 5]. This is the same across countries and cultures.

There are, however, very large individual differences regarding the acceptability of some risks with respect to the character of the risk and relative height or intensity of the risk.

Examples

- There seems to be a higher acceptability of cardiovascular risks compared to breast cancer risk. Women, especially in Western industrialized countries, seem to be more afraid of cancer than of cardiovascular disease, although the mortality of the latter is higher. This has to do with social images of diseases and the emotional attribution to

these conditions, which vary across different ages, educational and socioeconomic levels [7].
• Women (and doctors) seem to have difficulty differentiating between 'relative risk' and 'absolute risk' and there is in general no understanding of more complex risk parameters like 'number to treat' or 'number to harm'. If a contraceptive method increases the thromboembolic cases among 10 000 users compared to non-users from 3 cases (non-users) to 6 cases (users) per 10 000 women this can be described and communicated as a 'relative risk' increase of 2 (doubling the risk) or as a 100% increase.

Depending on how these numbers are communicated the emotional response to this statistical information may be very different. Risks described in absolute numbers usually better reflect real-life conditions [8].

Taking these facts into account, it is understandable that safety perception of a method in a specific country and society is very much influenced by the sources of information and the way risks are described. Contraceptive methods have social images or social stereotypes which may vary over time and may be strongly influenced by single events like a serious complication in a young woman.

The basic problem regarding the wish for safety lies in the fact that there is no effective method without any risk and that methods without any risk lack effectiveness and increase the risk of unwanted pregnancies with its specific risks.

This means for contraceptive counselling that the wish for safety cannot be fulfilled completely and that an important part of contraceptive counselling is what has been called risk counselling. This means informing women in a patient centred way and therefore empowering them to make a decision in their individual interest. It means also that healthcare providers try to understand the individual risk perception and where this perception comes from to increase knowledge and educate women [8].

Side effects and quality of life

Another universal wish is to have no unwanted side effects while using a contraceptive method. These side effects include changes in menstrual pattern, period pain, weight gain, skin and hair changes, mood changes, sexual problems, etc. [9–12].

Here again the tolerability and acceptability of side effects varies to a large extent depending on the individual cultural and educational background. It is noticeable that studies done several years ago have shown that the profile and frequency of side effects when using contraceptives is comparable to those observed among placebo users [9, 10].

Weight gain has a very low acceptability in Western industrialized countries whilst amenorrhoea may be well accepted. In other countries weight gain is considered much less of a problem, but amenorrhoea may not be acceptable or irregular unexpected bleeding is considered an unacceptable side effect [13].

Changes in sexual function may be viewed as a minor problem in middle-aged women, while this 'side effect' may be experienced as very disturbing in adolescents.

Several studies have shown that side effects seem to be the most frequent reason for discontinuing a method and becoming exposed to the risk of an unwanted pregnancy.

Again, it is therefore very important during contraceptive counselling to understand the individual importance given to specific side effects to better adapt the decision to the individual wishes and concerns [14, 15].

Wishes and needs with larger inter-individual and intra-individual variability

Relation to sexual activity

Some women want to practise contraception on demand meaning that contraception is practised in the context of sexual activity only. These women want a method that acts specifically and exclusively on the sexual encounter by inhibiting the 'individual' act of fertilization. They do not want methods that need continuous application beyond the sexual act.

This seems to be especially true in countries where modern contraceptives have just recently been introduced.

Other women want to be protected explicitly independent of the sexual act. They find disturbing the direct interaction between a contraceptive method and sexual activity and believe it has a negative impact on the quality of their sexual life. They prefer contraception as a continuous preventive behaviour, which may become a habit and also give more security for unplanned and unexpected sexual encounters [14, 15].

Duration of action

Many women seem to prefer a method that acts for a longer period of time without needing regular daily intervention by the woman. This daily routine can become stressful and lead to failures as studies have shown [16, 17].

Other women, however, feel safer and more autonomous and somehow freer in their decisions if they use a short-acting method.

These wishes seem to be determined by social learning, social class and education.

Control

Women may want control over their contraceptive method (like daily, weekly or monthly self applications). This is often combined with the wish to be independent of others like healthcare professionals, pharmacists, etc.).

Other women want a method that acts without having to think about it. They are not interested in having control but are relieved if the method is applied by a healthcare professional in whom they trust. These women prefer to be put in a state of reversible infertility until the moment when they want to become pregnant [1, 16, 17].

Physical properties, mechanism of action and mode of application

Fertility can be controlled by various properties of methods (hormones, rubber, copper, etc.), by various mechanisms (ovulation inhibition, changes in cervical mucus, endometrial changes, spermicidal action, etc.) and by various routes of administration (oral, transdermal, intravaginal, transnasal, intrauterine, etc.). Fertility can also be controlled by specific sexual behaviour (avoiding sexual intercourse during the fertile days of the cycle).

Women may have very variable wishes regarding the properties, the ways of administration and even the mechanism of action, although the latter seems to be of less practical interest [16, 17].

These variable wishes correspond to intra-familiar learning processes, individual body image, general concepts about nature and are also influenced by the sociocultural environment (religion, media, etc.).

This internal representation of a method is important to understand because this will, among other factors, determine the acceptability and continuation.

Independence/involvement of partner or other family members

Wishes regarding the role and/or involvement of the partner vary largely. Many women especially from Western industrialized countries want to be independent of their partner's decisions or behaviour. Self determination in sexual and reproductive health has become a highly valued issue. Other women still in the same countries would want male partners to be more involved in contraception and to share the responsibility and the load of fertility control. In some countries the involvement of partners or other family members is imposed on the woman due to rules specific to this culture.

In contraceptive counselling we have to try to understand these wishes and sometimes constraints to increase the acceptability of methods.

Costs

The wish for a low cost contraceptive method depends very much on the socioeconomic condition of the woman herself and the country in which she lives. This wish may be especially strong and important in young unemployed women. The wish for free contraceptives is fulfilled in some countries and for some special age groups. The focus is generally on adolescent women. On one hand it seems that providing free contraceptives to adolescents increases uptake and continuation, as has been shown in the USA. On the other hand, it remains an interesting fact that in the UK where contraceptives are free, the rate of unwanted pregnancies is still very high.

Elucidation of the wishes and concerns regarding costs is, however, an important part of the dialogue between the healthcare provider and the woman.

Additional benefits

Additional benefits of contraception refer mainly to hormonal methods. The benefits include a reduction in heavy menstrual bleeding and dysmenorrhoea, an improvement in premenstrual symptoms, acne and hirsuitism. Women affected by these conditions wish to profit from these non-contraceptive positive effects and may use the method mainly because of these benefits.

Some women may want protective effects with respect to diseases they have experienced in members of their family or in people they know, such as osteoporosis, ovarian cancer and iron deficiency anaemia.

For healthy women not suffering from any of these conditions potentially positive side effects are of no or minor importance.

Condoms have the very important additional benefit of protecting against the majority of sexually transmitted infections (STIs) and as such respond to the wishes of women feeling at risk of STIs. It is interesting to note that the protection against STIs seems to be of less importance for young women compared to the protection against unwanted pregnancies.

Conclusion

The knowledge and understanding of what the individual woman wants is an important part of contraceptive counselling. This part of the contraceptive dialogue is often forgotten in the limited space of time of a contraceptive consultation. Healthcare professionals seem to be very focused on the objective characteristics of the woman seeking advice, rather than what the woman actually wants and is comfortable with. The medical history is certainly important for safety reasons, but it is equally important to take a woman's personal feelings into account. 'Subjectivity' includes wishes, motives, values, priorities, etc., and in this domain the woman is her own expert.

Studies have shown that if healthcare providers do not listen to 'what women want', the discontinuation rate of methods is quite high, whilst in those situations in which women's views and wishes are integrated there is a positive impact on satisfaction and continuation.

One way of assessing the subjectivity of the woman is asking, either during the dialogue in the consultation room or by using a questionnaire in the waiting room, about her expectations and experiences regarding the criteria mentioned above, like efficacy, safety, side effects, relation to sexual activity, duration of action, control, cost, involvement of partner or other family members and additional health benefits.

In our model of structured contraceptive counselling, we recommend that the assessment of the individual needs and wishes of women regarding family planning and contraceptive methods is the first step to a shared decision-making process, in which the healthcare professional acts as an expert in assessing the risk profile of the woman and as a provider of evidence-based information whilst the woman contributes to the process by expressing her wishes and values and by attributing her individual weight to the information given.

References

1. Edwards JE, Oldman A, Smith L, McQuay HJ, Moore A. Women's knowledge of, and attitudes to, contraceptive effectiveness and adverse health effects. *Br J Fam Plann* 2000; 26(2): 73–80.

2. Glasier A, Scorer J, Bigrigg A. Attitudes of women in Scotland to contraception: a qualitative study to explore the acceptability of long-acting methods. *J Fam Plann Reprod Health Care* 2008; 34(4): 213–17.

3. Bruckner H, Martin A, Bearman PS. Ambivalence and pregnancy: adolescents' attitudes, contraceptive use and pregnancy. *Perspect Sex Reprod Health* 2004; 36(6): 248–57.

4. Schwarz EB, Lohr PA, Gold MA, Gerbert B. Prevalence and correlates of ambivalence towards pregnancy among non-pregnant women. *Contraception* 2007; 75(4): 305–10.

5. Frost JJ, Darroch JE. Factors associated with contraceptive choice and inconsistent method use, United States, 2004. *Perspect Sex Reprod Health* 2008; 40(2): 94–104.

6. Frost JJ, Lindberg LD, Finer LB. Young adults' contraceptive knowledge, norms and attitudes: associations with risk of unintended pregnancy. *Perspect Sex Reprod Health* 2012; 44(2): 107–16.

7. Westoff CL. Breast cancer risk: perception versus reality. *Contraception* 1999; 51: 25–8.

8. Gigerenzer G, Gaissmaier W, Kurz-Milke E, Schwartz ML, Woloshin S. Helping doctors and patients make sense of health statistics. *Psychol Sci Public Interest* 2007; 8(2): 53–96.

9. Rosenberg MJ, Long SC. Oral contraceptives and cycle control: a critical review of the literature. *Adv Contracept* 1992; 8 (Suppl 1): 35–45.

10. Redmond G, Godwin AJ, Olson W, Lippman JS. Use of placebo controls in an oral contraceptive trial: methodological issues and adverse event incidence. *Contraception* 1999; 60: 81–5.

11. Goldzieher JW, Moses LE, Averkin E, Scheel C, Taber BZ. A placebo controlled double-blind crossover investigation of the

side effects attributed to oral contraceptives. *Fertil Steril* 1971; 22: 609–23.

12. Westhoff CL, Heartwell S, Edwards S, *et al.* Oral contraceptive discontinuation: do side effects matter? *Am J Obstet Gynecol* 2007; 196(4): 412–18.

13. Szarewski A, von Stenglin A, Rybowski S. Women's attitudes towards monthly bleeding: results of a global population-based survey. *Eur J Contracept Reprod Health Care* 2012; 17(4): 270–83.

14. Lopez-del Burgo C, Mikolajczyk RT, Osorio A, *et al.* Knowledge and beliefs about mechanism of action of birth control methods among European women. *Contraception* 2012; 85(1): 69–77.

15. Baxter S, Blank L, Guillaume L, Squires H, Payne N. Views regarding the use of

contraception amongst young people in the UK: a systematic review and thematic synthesis. *Eur J Contracept Reprod Health Care* 2011; 16(3): 149–60.

16. Asker C, Stokes-Lampard H, Beavan J, Wilson S. What is it about intrauterine devices that women find unacceptable? Factors that make women non-users: a qualitative study. *J Fam Plan Reprod Health Care* 2006; 32: 89–94.

17. Bharadwaj P, Akintomide H, Brima N, Copas A, D'Souza R. Determinants of long-acting reversible contraceptive (LARC) use by adolescent girls and young women. *Eur J Contracept Reprod Health Care* 2012; 17(4): 298–306.

Chapter 2

Myths and misconceptions about sex and con(tra)ception

Rik H. W. van Lunsen

Introduction

Sexuality in all times has been surrounded by myths and misconceptions that reflect sexual norms and values of that specific time and culture. These myths and misconceptions therefore evolved over time in pace with societal changes. The majority of these myths and misconceptions stem from norms, values and beliefs aimed at controlling sexuality, women's sexuality in particular. Some of these myths even today have their influences on misconceptions in daily medical practice and are remnants of the anti-sexual history of Western medicine. One of the results of this anti-sexual history was that doctors, as the famous advocate of sex education for medical students and physicians Harold Lief stated in the 1970s, were 'woefully ignorant about sex' because of the absence of sex education in medical schools. Although sexual medicine courses in most current medical curricula are obligatory, several recent studies continue to find that the knowledge and skills of doctors concerning sexual health are poor, that questions about sexual functioning are not usual when patients are asking for contraceptive advice and that patients experiencing sexual problems are reluctant to put these concerns forward because they fear judgemental and normative reactions [1–3].

The historical case of masturbatory myths

The history of masturbation is only one of the striking examples of changing health beliefs regarding sexuality. Although in several religions masturbation is seen as a vice, masturbation nowadays is generally seen as part of a healthy sex life. Various medical and psychological benefits have been attributed to masturbation, and there is no evidence for a causal relationship between masturbation and any form of mental or physical disorder. In the Western world before 1700, masturbation was not really an issue and an artist, for instance Rembrandt, without any problem could publish a series of paintings of masturbating adolescents. Around 1700 a book by the title *Onania* appeared anonymously, in which masturbation was held responsible for many mental and physical diseases. *Onania* was joined in 1758 by Tissot's *Onanism; or a Treatise upon the Disorders Produced by Masturbation*, that circulated in many editions for more than a century. By the late nineteenth century medical journals in Europe and the USA were attributing almost every conceivable medical condition to this 'secret vice'.

In the case of males, the assumption that the loss of semen endangered the brain and nervous system was prevailing. In 1848 the superintendent of the Massachusetts Lunatic Asylum gave credence to this belief when in his annual report he asserted that 32% of admissions

Contraception, eds Paula Briggs, Gabor Kovacs and John Guillebaud. Published by Cambridge University Press. © Cambridge University Press 2013.

were for 'self pollution'. Since loss of semen was considered a real danger, nocturnal 'pollutions' were equally hazardous. To prevent masturbation and nocturnal ejaculations, an array of mechanical devices were constructed, such as straitjackets, genital cages and penis rings with sharp points on the inside. Men driven by guilt, who confessed to masturbation, were treated with, for instance, blistering agents, acid solutions, blood letting, circumcision or even castration.

Masturbation in women was regarded as an even graver problem, mainly because from the Middle Ages onwards women were seen as 'raging volcanos of desire' because of the semen sucking capacities of their uteri. The point of much brutal male sexual behaviour was to control the dangerous sexuality of women, who were seen as 'furnaces of carnality, who time and again will lead men to perdition, if given a chance' [4]. On the other hand Victorian women, especially from the middle and upper classes, were viewed as delicate, sensitive, frail and emotional creatures (*'dégénérés supérieurs'*) and many of their diseases, especially those involving the genitals and the brain, were either the result of masturbation or were aggravated by it. A British physician, Isaac Baker Brown, claimed success in treating epilepsy and other nervous disorders in female patients – by clitoridectomy. In medical thinking at the end of the nineteenth century, a hysterectomy was the treatment of choice to cure such 'perversions' as masturbation and promiscuity that were seen as the core symptoms of 'hysteria'.

In the USA, the last recorded clitoridectomy – on a five-year-old girl – for curing masturbation was performed in 1948 [5]. Although Havelock Ellis as early as in 1897 questioned Tissot's premise, a survey in Philadelphia in 1959 found around half of graduating future doctors still believed 'that masturbation is a common cause of insanity'. Warnings that masturbation may lead to blindness, stunted growth or hairy hands persist as myths even today. In 1994, when the Surgeon General of the USA, Dr Joycelyn Elders, said that it should be mentioned in sexual health education that masturbation was safe and healthy, she was forced to resign. As recently as 2009, a leaflet published in Britain, in order to make workers more aware of the necessity of raising the issue of sexual pleasure in sexual health education and to discuss masturbation as a healthy habit, created uproar in the lay press and amongst conservatives and certain religious groups [6].

'Libido' as a myth

During the twentieth century, sexology and sexual medicine were heavily influenced by the ideas of Sigmund Freud at the beginning of the century, the work of Masters and Johnson in the 1960s, the second feminist wave in the 1970s, the medicalization of sexuality and 'disease mongering' by the pharmaceutical industry in the 1990s and in the new millennium.

Freud's ideas about sexuality, influenced by repressive Christian views on sexuality, are mainly based on the concept of male 'libido' as a powerful instinctive energy or force, a constant drive comparative to hunger and thirst. This drive seeks satisfaction, but on the other hand can conflict with the conventions of civilized behaviour. The function of upbringing and socialization is to learn to moderate, control and fence off this drive without frustrating it too much. If the untameable energy of libido does not find a way out, if necessary in other activities such as sports or study, this will result in frustrations, neuroses or even lunacy. In other words: lust has to be oppressed in order to protect society from chaos, but too much oppression will lead to mental disease [7]. For women other mechanisms were applicable. Healthy female sexuality was receptive and passive and too much female sexual arousal continued to be dangerous and the cause of hysteria and other disasters. Freud, therefore, was not in favour of masturbation in adulthood, he regarded it as an infantile transition to mature sexuality.

Masters and Johnson were scientists who described the physiological changes during the sexual response by means of direct observation of men and women who were asked in their laboratory to engage themselves in auto-erotic or copulatory activity. In their description of the human sexual response cycle, consisting of four phases – excitement phase, plateau phase, orgasm and resolution phase – there simply was no place for sexual desire because in their experiments sexual activity was 'on command' [8]. Helen Singer Kaplan pointed out that in women the most prevalent sexual problems are related to (a lack) of desire [9]. Since her work another phase was added to the sexual response cycle, the phase of desire, suggesting a linear process in which sexual desire or libido precedes sexual arousal. As a result of the ideas of Freud and Kaplan lasting more than 100 years, it was believed that 'libido' is a biological entity that spontaneously generates sexual desire and precedes sexual arousal.

More recently, however, psychophysiological research on the interaction between central and peripheral processes during sexual arousal has shown that sexual responses are similar to any other emotional response. As with other emotions, sexual emotions involve altered central and peripheral physiology (e.g., motor preparation, vasocongestion), as well as feelings [10]. Cumulative experimental research using for instance vaginal photoplethysmography has shown that with any competent sexual stimulus, genital responses invariably start within a few heart beats, whether one is aware of these responses taking place or not [11]. Thus sexual responses start automatically when a stimulus is recognized as being sexual. Sexual desire is the result of a positive cognitive elaboration (disinhibition) of preconsciously perceived starting responses. Ongoing sexual responses are related to motivated behaviour based on appraisal of context, stimulation and expected outcome (sexual memory). In this incentive motivation model, sexual arousal and desire both result from a sensitive sexual response system interacting with sexually competent stimuli [12–14].

The sensitivity, receptivity (arousability) of the sexual system for sexual stimuli is mediated by neurotransmitters such as dopamine and by hormones – with androgens being the most important. These mediators are not the source of sexual desire or arousal, but only determine how responsive the sexual system is to sexual stimuli both on a central and a peripheral level. Sexual desire itself is the result of starting arousal and the 'decision' to act upon it. Sexual desire does not come out of the blue and libido does not exist.

Myths about male sexual desire

Although there are differences between men's and women's sexuality, these differences in popular and scientific literature are frequently exaggerated. Men's sexuality is often depicted in a simplified way as if men always have desire, are easily aroused, only want 'one thing' and don't appreciate the more relational aspects of sexuality as much as women do. There is no reason to believe that sexual desire in men is 'spontaneous' and in women 'responsive'. Scientific research indicates that in both genders the incentive motivation model is applicable and that sexual desire is the result of sexually competent stimuli. Possible differences between women and men in intensity of sexual desire might be explained by differences in receptivity for sexual stimuli, both because of hormonal differences and societal factors. The differences in sexual behaviour and in attitudes, however, are much smaller than often is presumed in popular media and similarities are more prominent than disparities. Moreover the differences tend to be smaller in those situations where gender disparity is smaller and there is more social equality between women and men [15]. One of the effects of oversimplifying male sexuality by society is a one-sided emphasis on performance instead of pleasure. This is probably the reason why problems resulting from a lack of desire in men are rarely recognized as such and in most cases are presented and being treated like erectile problems [16].

Myth: androgens are not relevant for women's sexual functioning

As stated before, androgens in general do not influence the sexual response itself, but modulate the responsivity to sexual stimuli of 'the sexual system' both on a central and a peripheral level. Moreover, there is evidence that some women are more sensitive to changes in testosterone levels than others [17]. These are the two most important reasons for the fact that the literature on how androgens influence sexuality shows inconsistencies, and that in non-selected populations the differences in sexual functioning between normo-androgenic and androgen-depleted women are small. Whereas some studies found androgens to enhance sexual motivation, the frequency of sexual fantasies and some aspects of sexual arousal in women, other studies did not.

Women's androgen insufficiency has been defined as consisting of a pattern of clinical symptoms – sexual problems, persistent unexplained fatigue and a decreased sense of well-being – in the presence of decreased bio-available testosterone and normal oestrogen status [18]. Nevertheless some experts recommend against making a diagnosis of androgen insufficiency and treatment of women based on the absence of a clear correlation between androgen plasma levels and sexual disorders [19]. Others disagree strongly with these negative recommendations and argue that androgen insufficiency is a clinically relevant condition that deserves more attention [20].

A similar discussion is ongoing about the possible negative effects of the combined oral contraceptive (COC) on sexuality in a minority of users. Use of COCs has been shown to decrease androgen levels, but has not consistently been shown to be associated with decreased sexual functioning. Some studies have demonstrated a negative effect of COCs on women's sexuality, some studies have found no difference and some studies have demonstrated positive effects [21]. In general every contraceptive method has positive effects on sexuality because the objective of using contraceptives is to improve sexual life. Therefore, studies that compare sexual functioning between users and non-users and studies assessing sexual functioning before and after first use of a contraceptive are confounded by the psychological advantages of using contraception.

On review of the literature, there is no doubt that COCs decrease levels of bio-available androgens, that this decrease is the result of both a decrease in androgen production and a decrease in bio-availability due to increases in sex hormone binding globulin (SHBG) levels. There is also accumulating evidence that for a minority of COC users these effects on androgens have discrete but clinically relevant negative effects on sexual arousability, e.g., receptivity to sexual stimuli. The increase in the level of SHBG is oestrogen dose dependent and dependent on the differential anti-androgenicity of the progestagen used. Therefore COCs with higher oestrogen doses and anti-androgenic progestogens such as cyproterone acetate may affect libido.

Myths about dangers of sex education and liberalization of sexuality

One of the remnants of the idea that sexuality is intrinsically dangerous and has to be regulated is that children have to be kept away from information about sexuality as long as possible. This is why sex education in schools in many countries is still a controversial subject and why promoting chastity until marriage often seems the only educational message. Underlying fears are related to the misconception that knowing 'too much too early' will result in teenage pregnancies, abortions, sexually transmitted infections (STIs) and promiscuity. The striking fact, however, is that it has been shown over and over again that in countries where the goal of sex education is not to prevent adolescents from having sex, but to educate them and thereby empower them to make responsible decisions, sexual debut is not at a younger age, teenage pregnancy and abortion rates are lower, reliable contraceptive use is more prevalent and all other indicators of sexual health are more favourable [22, 23].

A similar mythical 'stepping stone' theory is that free availability of pornography and its accessibility on the Internet leads to both an increase of 'instrumental sex' and increasing numbers of sexual assaults. A recent study in the Netherlands showed that the only variable related to sexual behaviour without an affective component is a lack of affection in childhood. Moreover several studies have shown that rape and other sex crimes do not increase when pornography becomes freely available. In countries where in a certain epoch the possession of child pornography was not illegal, during that period these countries showed a significant decrease in the incidence of child sex abuse [24].

Myths about virginity and the hymen

In many religions and cultures virginity until marriage is regarded as an essential virtue. In some of these cultures blood loss at first sexual intercourse is seen as the ultimate proof of virginity. The fact that approximately 50% of all women do not have any blood loss at first sexual intercourse does not seem to alter the importance attached to staining the nuptial bed. Virginity is supposed to be characterized by an 'intact' hymen, and girls therefore are often raised with constant warnings about activities that might cause harm to the hymen: use of tampons, ballet, gymnastics, sports, jumping up and down, horseback riding, carrying heavy loads and masturbating. Even in societies where virginity is not that much of an issue, there are still healthcare professionals who claim to be able to establish the virginity of women by assessing the condition of their hymen. Virginity, however, is not diagnosable by genital examination. In many sexually active female adolescents the hymen shows no tears, clefts or notches and many virgins have hymens that seem to be not 'intact'. In most women, the hymen is a very stretchable elastic fold. The shape of this fold is very variable and it may be more circumferential (hymen annulare) or more like half a moon (hymen lunare). Because the aspect of the hymen does not reveal whether or not a woman has had coital experience, terminology referring to a hymen as being 'intact' should be abandoned. Blood loss and pain at first intercourse probably are more related to a lack of (pelvic floor) relaxation and a lack of arousal and lubrication than to the morphology of the hymen.

Because of the expected blood loss and pain 'the first time' many women fear this moment. Not only is the myth that virginity can be assessed by inspecting the hymen widespread, many women also think that a doctor or a sexual partner is able to discriminate virgins and non-virgins by their 'tightness' and therefore fear that a future husband will notice. Men, on the other hand, often think that force is needed to 'break' the hymen and fear they will not be able to maintain a rigid erection long enough to succeed [25].

Misconception: the objective of contraception is the prevention of pregnancy

In general there are two categories of motives for sex: procreation and recreation (pleasure and leisure). At least 95% of all human sexual activity is not aimed at procreation. As a consequence, every couple that does want to have heterosexual intercourse and does not want to conceive has to rely on methods that make this possible. Nevertheless, in most articles and textbooks on contraception, contraception is simply defined as the instrument to prevent unwanted pregnancy. This definition is denying that prevention of pregnancy is not the primary goal of contraceptive use. If that were the case, abstinence as a contraceptive method would be suitable and popular. In an ideal world, where abuse and coercion do not exist, the only objective of using contraception is to be able to enjoy pleasurable heterosexual coital activity without the risk of an unplanned or unwanted pregnancy. From this pro-sexual perspective, contraception is a tool to improve sexual health and sexual wellbeing instead of a way to prevent disasters. From the pro-sexual perspective, the ideal contraceptive method has positive effects on sexual functioning by reducing the fear of pregnancy and does not interfere with sexual functioning or sexual activity in any other way.

Due to the fact that contraception is used for sexual reasons and because anticipated effects of contraceptive use on sexuality are a major determinant of contraceptive choices, it is imperative that in contraceptive counselling individual wishes and lifestyles with regard to sexuality are discussed explicitly in order to tailor the method of choice according to these individual variables [26].

Myths about con(tra)ception

Especially in countries where sexual health education is limited and as a consequence young people lack knowledge, a bizarre range of myths on how to reduce risks of pregnancy can be found. A survey among pregnant teenagers in the USA revealed that one third of them conceived as a result of unprotected sexual intercourse because they thought they could not get pregnant, owing to a range of mythical ideas [27]. A personally performed survey on the Internet on myths circulating amongst youngsters revealed some of the most frequently encountered myths – *A woman can't get pregnant:*

- If you have sex standing up
- If the woman is on top
- If you have sex in a hot tub or a swimming pool
- If you jump up and down immediately after sex
- If the girl douches, takes a bath, or urinates immediately after sex
- If it's your first time
- Unless you have sex every night
- If the man pulls out before he ejaculates
- If a man doesn't go all the way in
- If the woman doesn't have an orgasm

- If the man and the woman don't orgasm at the same time
- If the woman pushes really hard on her belly button after sex
- If the woman sneezes for 15 minutes after sex

And even more bizarre are myths such as:

- Putting a watch around your penis before sex means the radioactivity of the dial kills off sperm
- You can't get pregnant on a boat
- You can't get pregnant if you drink a lot of milk
- Keeping your eyes closed stops you getting pregnant
- A man is only fertile if his testicles feel cold
- There's no risk if you're standing on a telephone directory
- If the man drinks a lot of alcohol the woman won't get pregnant
- Coke douches work
- You can use crisp bags as condoms

In this chapter we will not address the many myths surrounding the various methods of contraception except for those that have to be busted in daily practice because of their persistent and confusing effects on contraceptive choices, compliance and correct use. In many cases these myths prevent couples from choosing the most suitable contraceptive method matching their individual needs and preferences.

With regard to COCs, the most important myth is that there are serious health risks associated with long-term use and that, therefore, one should not take 'the pill' for too long a period. However, recently the American College of Obstetricians and Gynecologists stated that weighing the risks versus the benefits based on currently available data, COCs should be available over the counter [28]. Women should self-screen for most contraindications to COCs using checklists. Moreover screening for cervical cancer or STIs is not medically required to provide hormonal contraception.

Another myth is that monthly withdrawal bleeding mimicking menstruation is necessary to 'clean' the uterus. Women should be informed more in depth that the main reason for adding oestrogens to combined methods (pill, ring and patches) is to regulate bleeding in order to make it predictable and that this principle (only in monophasic formulations!) can be used to tailor bleeding to personal needs. If less frequent bleeding is desired an extended pill-taking regimen can be used (see Chapter 12).

Another myth about COCs is that they reduce fertility and that after stopping using them the woman should wait a few months before trying to conceive. Fertility is not affected by hormonal contraceptives irrespective of the duration of use. Furthermore, pill-free 'breaks' are unnecessary; in fact the first month after stopping the pill the chance of getting pregnant is even slightly higher than in any other month during the fertile life-cycle. The myth of 'post-pill amenorrhoea' stems from the fact that women with intrinsic cycle irregularities experience regular withdrawal bleeds whilst on COCs but return to their pattern of amenorrhoea or oligomenorrhoea after discontinuation.

With regard to intrauterine devices, the most frequently encountered myths are that they can cause pelvic inflammatory disease, increase the risk for extra-uterine pregnancy, are less reliable than hormonal methods and should not be used in nulliparous women.

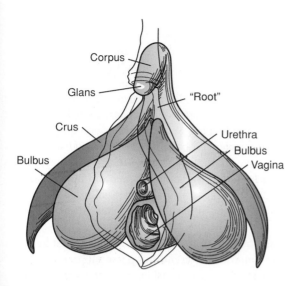

Corpus

Glans

Crus

Bulbus

"Root"

Urethra

Bulbus

Vagina

Figure 2.1 The anatomy of the clitoris. Illustration by Amphis [29] based on O'Connell [30], adapted by Rik H. W. van Lunsen.

Myths and misconceptions about the clitoris, the G-spot, orgasm and dyspareunia

The most striking myths and misconceptions about sexuality are remnants of the long-lasting denial of the importance of arousal for sexual functioning of women and of bizarre post-Freudian concepts of infantile and adult sexual functioning. Even today women, their sexual partners and healthcare professionals are often not aware that for sexual intercourse to be really pleasurable sufficient genital arousal and lubrication is necessary before penetration is attempted. The underlying misconception that women are always available for sexual inter-course is one of the reasons that some women may experience pain during sex. This com-mon belief does not take into account knowledge about the physiological aspects of women's sexual arousal and the recently rediscovered functional anatomy of the clitoris [29, 30] (Figure 2.1).

The clitoris consists of three parts. The first part, in lay language often erroneously called the clitoris, is the glans clitoridis that continues into the externally perceptible corpus. The corpus, suspended by the ligamentum suspensorium clitoridis to the os pubis, bends in an angle of 90° and forms the second part of the clitoris – the clitoral root. When engorged the clitoral root is closely related to the anterior vestibule and the anterior vaginal wall. The base of the clitoral root is located where the so called G-spot is supposed to be [31]. The G-spot therefore is probably nothing more than the vaginally reachable back-side of the clitoris, which might end fruitless and senseless discussions about clitoral versus vaginal orgasms. The clitoral root splits into the third part of the organ – the two crurae that equal the cor-pus spongiosum in men. Each of the two crurae extends 8–10 cm from the lower edge of the pubic arch along the ramus inferior of the pubic bone. In the middle of the two crurae are the two large bulbi vestibuli, similar to the corpora cavernosa in men that fill with blood during sexual arousal. These bulbi vestibuli form, as it were, a kind of air-bags, a pad or buffer that enclose and protect the engorged urethral and vaginal wall. Lubrication during sexual arousal is the result of plasma seepage out of the capillaries of the engorged vaginal wall, which is not covered by 'mucosa' but by stratified squamous epithelium. The functional anatomy of the 'clitoral complex' shows that the female reproductive organ needs to be filled with blood, equal to the male reproductive organ, in order to experience pain-free and pleasurable sex. A lack of arousal and engorgement of the clitoral complex upon penetration is the major explanation for the remarkably high incidence of dyspareunia, especially in young women. According to a Dutch study, only 43% of women under the age of 25 reports to always engage in pain-free intercourse [32]. According to Swedish studies, the prevalence of pain and discomfort associated with sexual intercourse is high even when women characterize their ideal sexual situation in a heterosexual relationship as achieving sexual pleasure on equal terms. Of the participants of these studies, 49% had experienced coital pain or vulvar discomfort during the preceding month [33, 34]. For just over half of these women, those experiences constituted a problem. Remarkably, the other half of these young women did not consider this sexual pain to be a problem, either because they regarded painful sexual intercourse as being normal or perhaps because they obtained other, non-pleasure related rewards from coital activity.

Since sex is only pleasurable for a woman when she is sufficiently aroused, sexual health education should be aimed more at the development of awareness of personal prerequisites for sufficient arousal. Self efficacy to communicate these prerequisites and gaining more control over timing of penetration are necessary for women to experience pleasurable sexual encounters. The myth that women are always able to have intercourse and the misconception that pain is normal are probably the most prominent ones to be busted.

References

1. Fayers T, Crawley T, Jenkins JM, Cahill DJ. Medical student awareness of sexual health is poor. *Int J STD AIDS* 2003; 14: 386–9.
2. Sobecki JN, Curlin FA, Rasinski KA, Lindau ST. What we don't talk about when we don't talk about sex: results of a national survey of US obstetricians/gynecologists. *J Sex Med* 2012; 9: 1285–94.
3. Moreira ED, Glasser DB, Nicolosi A, Duarte FG, Gingell C. Sexual problems and help seeking behaviour in adults in the United Kingdom and continental Europe. *BJU Int* 2008; 101: 1005–11.
4. Shorter E. *A History of Women's Bodies*. New York, NY: Basic Book Inc., 1982: pp. 12–13.
5. Duffy J. Masturbation and clitoridectomy: a nineteenth-century view. *JAMA* 1963; 19: 246–8.
6. The Centre for HIV and Sexual Health NHS. *Pleasure: a booklet for workers on why and how to raise the issue of sexual pleasure in sexual health work with young people*. Sheffield, UK: The Centre for HIV and Sexual Health NHS, 2009.
7. Freud S. *Drei Abhandlungen zur Sexualtheorie*. Wien, Germany: Verlag Franz Deuticke, 1905.
8. Masters WH, Johnson VE. *The Human Sexual Response*. Boston, MA: Little and Brown, 1966.
9. Kaplan HS. *The New Sex Therapy*. New York, NY: Brunner/Mazel, 1974.
10. Damasio A. *Looking for Spinoza: joy, sorrow, and the feeling brain*. Orlando, FL: Harcourt Inc., 2003.
11. Laan E, Van Driel E, van Lunsen RHW. Genital responsiveness in healthy women with and without sexual arousal disorder. *J Sex Med* 2008; 5: 1424–35.
12. Janssen E, Bancroft J. The dual control model: the role of sexual inhibition and excitation in sexual arousal and behavior. In Janssen E. (ed.) *The Psychophysiology of Sex*. Bloomington, IN: Indiana University Press, 2007: pp. 197–222.
13. Both S, Everaerd W, Laan E. Desire emerges from excitement. A psychophysiological perspective on sexual motivation. In Janssen E. (ed.) *The Psychophysiology of Sex*. Bloomington, IN: Indiana University Press, 2007: pp. 327–39.
14. Laan E, Both S. Sexual desire and arousal disorders in women. *Adv Psychosom Med* 2011; 31: 16–34.

15. Petersen JL, Hyde JS. A meta-analytic review of research on gender differences in sexuality, 1993–2007. *Psychol Bull* 2010; 136: 21–38.

16. Meuleman E, van Lankveld J. Hypoactive sexual desire disorder: an underestimated condition in men. *BJU Int* 2005; 95, 291–6.

17. Bancroft J, Graham CA. The varied nature of women's sexuality: unresolved issues and a theoretical approach. *Horm Behav* 2011; 59: 717–29.

18. Bachmann G, Bancroft J, Braunstein G, *et al.* Female androgen insufficiency: the Princeton consensus statement on definition, classification, and assessment. *Fertil Steril* 2002; 77: 660–5.

19. Wierman ME, Basson R, Davis SR, *et al.* Androgen therapy in women: an Endocrine Society clinical practice guideline. *J Clin Endocrinol Metab* 2006; 91: 3697–710.

20. Traish A, Guay AT, Spark RF and the Testosterone Therapy in Women Study Group. Are the Endocrine Society's clinical practice guidelines on androgen therapy in women misguided? *J Sex Med* 2007; 4: 1223–35.

21. Burrows LJ, Basha M, Goldstein AT. The effects of hormonal contraceptives on female sexuality: a review. *J Sex Med* 2012; 9: 2213–23.

22. Lottes IL. Sexual health policies in other industrialized countries: are there lessons for the United States? *J Sex Res* 2002; 39: 79–83.

23. van Lunsen RHW, Laan ETM, Brauer M. Sex, pleasure and dyspareunia in liberal Northern Europe. In Hall K, Graham C. (eds) *The Cultural Context of Sexual Pleasure and Problems: psychotherapy with diverse clients*. New York, NY: Routledge, 2012: pp. 356–70.

24. Diamond M, Jozifkova E, Weiss P. Pornography and sex crimes in the Czech Republic. *Arch Sex Behav* 2011; 40: 1037–43.

25. van Moorst BR, van Lunsen RHW, van Dijken DKE, Salvatore CM. Backgrounds of women applying for hymen reconstruction, the effects of counselling on myths and misunderstandings about virginity, and the results of hymen reconstruction. *Eur J Contracept Reprod Health Care* 2012; 17: 93–105.

26. van Lunsen RHW, Laan ETM, van Dalen L. Contraception and sexuality. In Milsom I. (ed.) *Contraception and Family Planning*. Philadelphia, PA: Elsevier, 2006: pp. 5–19.

27. Harrison AT, Gavin L, Hastings PA. Prepregnancy contraceptive use among teens with unintended pregnancies resulting in live births – pregnancy risk assessment monitoring system (PRAMS), 2004–2008. *MMWR Morb Mortal Wkly Rep* 2012; 61: 25–9.

28. American College of Obstetricians and Gynecologists. Over-the-counter access to oral contraceptives. Committee Opinion No. 544. *Obstet Gynecol* 2012; 120; 1527–31.

29. Amphis. Clitoris anatomy. Drawing free for public domain. http://commons.wikimedia.org/wiki/File:Clitoris_anatomy_unlabeled.jpg (accessed 18 March 2013).

30. O'Connell HE, Eizenberg N, Rahman M, Cleeve J. The anatomy of the distal vagina: towards unity. *J Sex Med* 2008; 5: 1883–91.

31. Foldes P, Buisson O. The clitoral complex: a dynamic sonographic study. *J Sex Med* 2009; 6: 1223–31.

32. De Graaf H, Meijer S, Poelman J, Vanwesenbeeck I. Seks onder je 25ᵉ. *Seksuele gezondheid van jongeren in Nederland anno 2005*. Delft, the Netherlands: Uitgeverij Eburon, p. 63.

33. Elmerstig E, Wijma B, Sandell K, Berterö C. 'Sexual pleasure on equal terms': young women's ideal sexual situations. *J Psychosom Obstet Gynecol* 2012; 33: 129–34.

34. Elmerstig E, Wijma B, Swahnberg K. Young Swedish women's experience of pain and discomfort during sexual intercourse. *Acta Obstet Gynecol* 2009; 88: 98–103.

Chapter 3

The history of contraception

Lesley Smith

Deep in the Egyptian Museum in Cairo, sits a glass display case. Within the case are a number of exhibits, amongst them number 745, which is a small, plain finger-shaped piece of linen with strings attached to be worn around the waist to hold the linen in place. It is not a glamorous item and considering it was found in the tomb of Tutankhamun, the boy pharaoh, it may to the casual observer be considered of hardly any interest at all, compared to the other finds in the tomb. Surrounded by golden figures, precious oils and a dynastic royal bed, such a small crinkled piece of cloth might easily have been lost in the rush of the excavation that stunned the world. Fortunately, it was saved and is arguably one of the most interesting finds and, certainly from a medical point of view, a treasure.

That simple piece of linen is believed to be a condom, and is displayed as such by the Egyptian Museum. Not only that, but if correctly identified it is the earliest condom known of today, either as a surviving object or in written evidence. However, a note of caution should be applied here as the condom may have been used as a prophylactic against disease rather than a form of contraceptive. The other consideration in linking the condom to Tutankhamun himself is that the existence of such an item does not necessarily mean it was meant to be used by the pharaoh in the afterlife, as funerary goods were also left for the use of servants accompanying the pharaoh on his post-death travels [1]. It has also been suggested by some that this may be a form of ritual dress rather than a condom, and certainly there is no other evidence of condoms at such an early date.

Tutankhamun ruled Eygpt between 1332 and 1323 BC, but there is evidence of even earlier contraception from the land of the pharaohs. In 1889, an English archaeologist, Flinders Petrie, working near the modern Eygptian town of Lehun, excavated some papyri. These are in fact the oldest known collection of medical texts of any kind, one of which is dated around 1825 BC and therefore written around 500 years before Tutankhamun lived. We can be sure of the age because someone, probably a physician, helpfully recorded the 29th year of the reign of Amenemhat on the back of a papyrus. Some of the other texts in the collection may be older. Amongst the largest of the texts is one related entirely to women's medicine, which is now known as 'The Kahun Gynaecological Papyrus' (now housed at University College London, ref. UC 32057). Although this cannot be precisely dated, it can be attributed to the period of the late Middle Kingdom (1850–1700 BC) [2].

The document apparently included several receipts for 'preventing' (contraception) but unfortunately fragments are missing, and none of these receipts is complete. One of these reads, 'For preventing […] crocodile dung chopped over HsA and awyt-liquid, sprinkle […]

Contraception, eds Paula Briggs, Gabor Kovacs and John Guillebaud. Published by Cambridge University Press. © Cambridge University Press 2013.

lasts […]'. The 'awyt liquid' is sour milk, and although the exact meaning of 'HsA' is uncertain, it is thought to be a reference to *HsA-n-Sbb* (a dough-like vegetal substance) [2].

This is a recipe for a preparation that is to be burned as a fumigant, probably for the woman to stand over. Fumigation has been used in many periods and places, including North Africa, as an aid both to contraception and conception, dependent upon the content of the recipe. Descriptions of conditions contained within the papyri give an insight into how people perceived anatomy such as, 'it is discharges of womb in her eyes', 'terror of the womb' and 'wandering womb'. This may explain why the ancient Eygptians thought foul smelling *materia medica* when burned might cause the womb to flee, and therefore act as contraception, whilst sweet smelling incense might be used to attract the womb to the neck of the cervix, ready to receive the male seed during intercourse.

Another form of contraception which has been attributed to ancient Egypt is the presence of gold coins in the uterine region of two female mummies, supposedly discovered at the British Museum in London. If this story is correct, these could perhaps be seen as a symbolic contraceptive or perhaps a payment to the gods for a child already born or for another conception in the afterlife. However, this story provides a warning against simply accepting traditions: this 'discovery' has been mentioned to me independently by a number of different individuals, but enquiries at the British Museum provided no evidence of coins ever having been found in mummies (most of which pre-date the introduction of coinage to Egypt), and the origin of the tale is likely to be a garbled account of gold amulets found in the wrappings of mummies, a tradition which is well known in the archaeological record.

Another account of ancient contraception which is equally difficult to verify, but which does certainly date back to antiquity, at least as a story, can be found in the Bible, in Genesis 38:9. This is the story of Onan. According to the scriptures, Onan does not wish to have children by his dead brother's wife, although he has a duty under levirate marriage to ensure the continuation of a family line, with the firstborn of such a marriage being seen as the son of the deceased brother. To avoid fathering a child who will not be his own, Onan deliberately 'spills his seed', when 'going into' his wife. This has traditionally been interpreted by the Church as a reference to masturbation, but might equally be seen as a reference to *coitus interruptus*. In either case, it demonstrates awareness that the male seed was necessary to engender a child, and that by spilling that seed outside the female body a male reduced the chances of conception. This reference from the Old Testament not only proves ancient knowledge of how conception may be avoided, but also formed part of the basis for later canon law when addressing contraception and other sexual issues in the Catholic Church.

There is also a great deal of evidence relating to birth control practices in Ancient India going back as far as 2000 BC, particularly in relation to spiritual beliefs. Writings such as the *Atharvaveda* and many other texts leading into and beyond the epic period in Indian antiquity frequently show reference to contraception and other fertility issues. The early works suggest prayers as well as some brutal surgical measures such as crushing the testicles and, for women, hysterectomies.

Medieval Indian writings give an extraordinarily wide range of anti-fertility options, some of which may be found in other continents, such as the observance of celibacy, religious restrictions and the use of talismans tied to the man or woman. The content of some of the talismans is fascinating. For example, one recipe states that some hair from the man's right hand should be tied up with the hair from the trunk of an elephant and the tail of a horse. These collected hairs plus the tooth of a boar are to be tied to the right hand of the man to provide a talisman designed to avoid conception. It is not clear whether this should be worn only during intercourse [3].

Mantras were also believed to produce sterility in both men and women, just like prayers of intercession in the Christian Church in Europe. In a writing known as *Yoga Ratnakara* there appears to be reference to an intrauterine device. The device is described as made up of a root collected on the 14th day of a 'black fortnight', which is then inserted into the *yoni*, believed to mean the uterus by some scholars despite the word in Sanskrit meaning vagina. It would be interesting to research further to see if this method was recommended to be carried out immediately after birthing which would mean the word *yoni* could indeed mean uterus in this context [3].

The range of *materia medica* in ancient Indian texts is very broad, with roots, flowers, leaves and seeds prepared in various ways to make oral contraceptives for women. There is even an oral contraceptive for men made in part of goat's urine which is described as highly efficacious because once taken the man would supposedly be instantly sterile. Pessaries to act either as a physical barrier or spermicide appear in many cultures across the globe. In India, writings suggest using a mix of rock salt and oil pushed high into the vagina before or after intercourse. It is a method of contraception that continued to be used right until modern times. The range of fertility controls in ancient and medieval Indian writings is striking, proving that this was culturally a very important issue, and whilst there was a moral and religious obligation for people to have children, particularly male children of honourable character, contraception was still desirable [3].

The next period of antiquity to consider is the lives of the Greeks and Romans, who produced the great medical philosophers who would shape the thoughts and practices in Europe for over 1500 years. During this period it is important to consider the role that abortion played as a form of contraception. Hippocrates, who lived on the Greek island of Kos in the fifth century BC, is viewed as the Father of Medicine in Western culture and his work helped form the ethics of professional medical practitioners up until relatively modern times. The translation of the Hippocratic Oath is the subject of much debate, as some scholars claim that the translations over the years through the medieval period and beyond have been general rather than specific. Some historians state that the line on abortion in the original Hippocratic Oath translates that the physician must not 'give a suppository to cause an abortion', which in a broader sense has been interpreted (particularly through the medieval ecclesiastical courts) as a prohibition on abortion caused by any means [4]. What is undeniable in this debate is that abortion was discussed in the fifth century BC and considered a moral and medical matter that should have boundaries and ethics applied to it.

Both Greek and Roman texts discuss late-term abortions by the use of medicines or violent forms of manipulation that were also recognized as potentially dangerous to the mother. Whilst surgical procedures for abortion are referred to in early works, most academics agree this was only resorted to in the most desperate of medical emergencies.

An early example of suggested violent physical exercise to bring on an abortion was known as the *Lacedaemonian leap* in which a woman was advised to jump high in the air and have her heels strike at her buttocks. This record is found in a medical treatise believed to have been written by Hippocrates, *On the Nature of the Child*. The hard blow from the heels and the angle the woman attained at the moment of the strike was believed to open the cervix and force the embryo out. The principle of this type of vigorous exercise is reflected as late as the twentieth century when anxious young women following unprotected sex would lift weights, jump up and down or run up and down stairs in an attempt to 'bring on a period'.

Soranus was a highly influential Greek physician who was also the leading writer in the classical world on obstetrics and gynaecology. He points out in his texts that abortions undertaken in the first 30 days following conception were relatively easy and certainly less dangerous than late-term abortions. The writings of Soranus are rather confusing as he specifically states he would not give an abortion, whilst also giving the recipe for abortifacients. One explanation may be that the ancients did not believe an abortion could be so termed until the fetus was 'quick', e.g., living. Aristotle tells us that life in the sense of animation happened in a fetus 40 days after conception for a male and 90 days after conception for a female. More importantly, is the drug given purely to start menstruation or to force termination of pregnancy? That moral difference in terms of intent was vitally important when it was considered by the ecclesiastical courts in later centuries [5].

Receipts for abortifacients can be found in medical texts from the ancients to recent times. The content of these recipes does have some *materia medica* that can be found repeatedly such as rue, wormwood and penny royal. Silphium is also mentioned by Soranus, who suggests the juice of Silphium 'the size of a chick pea' should be taken in water once a month to avoid conception and cleanse away any existing conception. Abortifacients were not always necessarily taken orally, and were sometimes administered topically on the lower abdomen in the form of a poultice, whilst laxatives taken in large doses were also thought to cause termination of a pregnancy. Pessaries were also certainly used for the same purpose. Unsurprisingly, it was also suggested that soaking for a long time in a warm bath after drinking alcohol could cause the womb to open, causing termination. This range of options from manipulation to potions and poultices proves that even in ancient times women needed medical termination services. In terms of contraceptives, Roman women are known to have used sponges dipped in vinegar before introducing into the vagina prior to intercourse. There is also evidence that a sea sponge wrapped in silk was used by the Ancient Jewish people and acted as what was considered a most effective form of birth control [4].

Natural sea sponges would be easy to obtain and therefore an inexpensive choice with the added bonus of neither the man nor the woman being made uncomfortable by the presence of a small sponge. Waxy pessaries inserted into the body containing what was thought to be herbal spermicides also appear in classical texts.

In the medieval period medical schools started to spring up across Europe in places such as Paris, Montpellier, Bologna and the earliest of all, Salerno, which was already a thriving medical school in the eleventh century. In early 1076 a local writer, Alfanus, describes Salerno in his youth: 'Salerno then flourished to such an extent in the art of medicine that no illness was able to settle there'. The concentration of medical knowledge at Salerno resulted in the writing or compilation of a number of medical textbooks there. One of the most important of these is a collected treatise on women's medicine dating from the twelfth century, known as the *Trotula*. This not only includes a number of recipes for contraception, but also some discussion of why contraception might be appropriate, despite the fact that, as mentioned, the general attitude of the medieval Church was broadly opposed to contraception. Amongst other authorities, the *Trotula* quotes an African Benedictine monk, Constantine, who states that some women had such anatomical limitations that childbirth could cost them their lives. Constantine also states that as sexual activity was vital for a woman to enjoy good health, they should be given contraceptives [6].

The recommendations for contraceptives are fascinating to say the least: 'In another fashion, take a male weasel and let its testicles be removed and let it be released alive. Let the woman carry these testicles with her in her bosom and let her tie them in goose skin or in another skin, and she will not conceive'. Another alternative was that she could carry the womb of a barren goat against her naked flesh, which is likely to have had a significant smell after a few days. Finally, a woman who had been badly torn during childbirth could put the number of grains of barley and or caper spurge into the afterbirth for as many years ahead as she wished to remain barren [6].

What makes the study of contraception and sexual health generally so interesting is that the medieval medical schools were run by specialists who promoted their own disciplines and beliefs rather than in a spirit of shared knowledge or for the good of all. This means there are often contradictions from one university to another at the same time in history. There was also great caution about moral issues and the worth of physicians as seen by the people and the Church. Many physicians and other medical professionals such as midwives were licensed directly by Bishops.

The year 1446 proved to be a significant date in terms of society's view of sex and marriage as The Council of Florence, after 15 years of debate, declared that marriage, according to the Catholic Church, was a sacrament. The deeply held suspicion that sex was a smear on human lives carrying with it the title Original Sin was now in question, as sex within the married state was desirous of God and man. Despite this declaration, the Medieval Catholic Church still gave strict guidelines on sexual behaviour even in the matrimonial bed. Fridays were forbidden as a day on which intercourse might take place, as were Sundays. Both were viewed as holy days, with the tradition of the Crucifixion taking place on a Friday. The whole of Lent and the whole of Advent were also periods of sexual restraint, both being periods of four to six weeks. If one had consumed alcohol excessively, intercourse was not to take place, and, finally, in times of menstruation. The fact that menstruation was a time when a woman may not conceive was known and therefore if intercourse took place knowing the woman could not conceive and therefore just for the sinful purposes of pleasure and not for procreation as intended by God, then the those involved might be called up in front of the courts. Records prove that some people ignored these restraints whilst the Church continued to condemn some sexual practices that would be considered perfectly usual now. Intercourse standing up, from behind or with the woman astride the man were all viewed as attempts to avoid conception as the semen was seen to fall out of the woman's body. Fellatio and cunnilingus fell under the banned practices as this would cause wastage of seed for the man and woman whilst anal intercourse was particularly frowned upon. It is important to appreciate that medieval medicine believed in the concept of dual ejaculation at the moment of orgasm and therefore the deliberate wasting of a woman's seed was considered as much of a sin as the 'pollution' of men. Despite the canon laws of restrictive behaviour there is evidence in a wide range of matter of all three activities. Pornography in terms of illustrations, sculpture and bawdy songs provide vital information in understanding the behaviour of our ancestors [7].

A major change in approaches to contraception came about as an accidental result of venereal disease. In 1493, a disease was recorded in the British Isles which had also recently been seen in other parts of Europe. It was first thought to be a skin disorder and treated with the ancient Arabic treatment of painting the skin with mercury also known as 'quicksilver'. The vacillating blisters proved to be what was termed a 'pox', a particular pox that was known as 'The French Disease', syphilis. Condoms started to be used in an attempt to control the spread of disease and in some countries the brothels were closed. In England they were closed by order of King Henry VIII in 1546. The link between the brothels and the spread of syphilis was being recognized, whilst mercury continued to be used in a desperate attempt to heal victims for hundreds of years. There is some, if scanty, evidence of the use of leather or gut condoms kept in jars of oil and used repeatedly [8]. Soon, it would be noticed that the use of such condoms meant that the woman did not conceive, although no doubt this method sometimes failed, and that would be of great interest. Prostitutes were very valuable commodities to the brothel owners as well as to the church or state as the brothels, also known as 'stews', were taxed. An experienced woman at the top of her profession would generate considerable income and as it was known that abortion, mechanically or by abortifacients could mean death or disability, a contraceptive that was safe and effective would certainly be welcomed.

The really strong evidence of the use of condoms as a protection against venereal diseases comes from Gabriele Falloppio, also known as Gabriel Fallopius, who was an outstanding Italian anatomist of the sixteenth century. He, like many other physicians, trained initially as a priest as well as in the Classics. Falloppio carried out what we would now call a medical trial on the effectiveness of using a condom as a prophylactic against syphilis. The condoms in the trial were made of linen and wrapped around the penis: 'I tried the experiment on 1,100 men, and I call immortal God to witness that not one of them was infected'. Animal gut condoms were also available and some were found, wrapped inside each other, down a privy within Dudley Castle in England. They date from the mid-sixteenth century [9].

The advent of printing in the late fifteenth century meant that books began to be published for general audiences. These included many popular books aimed at the housewife, which gave advice across a range of subjects from cookery to home surgery and also recipes for how to 'bring on flowers' (encourage menstruation). Some authors make an effort to advise the reader to ensure she is not pregnant prior to trying a recipe, but this may be as much to protect the writer against criticism or even litigation [10]. There are also references to the top of lemons or limes being used as a contraceptive cap, inserted high into the vagina. Experiments have been able to prove that the juice from highly acid fruits can kill sperm, candida and some forms of venereal disease [11]. Evidence exists of such fruits being used for the same purpose in parts of Africa and also in countries such as Malaysia where the lime juice was squeezed over a piece of kapok and then introduced into the body.

Moving forwards into more modern time, the use of a douche immediately following intercourse was widely considered an effective system of birth control in the nineteenth century. In 1920 'Lysol' was marketed as an intimate vaginal douching product able to prevent infection, and this promotion of prevention of infection enabled advertising such a product without mentioning birth control, which would have been considered an outrage to public decency if widely seen. What is known is that douches were used in many societies as a form of contraception.

From the mid-nineteenth century, the arrival of rubber meant the first condoms were produced of the new material. Some of the early condoms are described as being rather thick and uncomfortable to wear. A sponge left in a jar of oil with a thread for removal was in use in the early twentieth century, but there is little evidence of this method being used widely.

Family planning pioneer Marie Stopes and other medical professionals across the world were also attempting to come to grips with family planning. Large families with high birth and child mortality rates and the despair combined with abject poverty this could cause meant there was a real drive by some medical professionals to address fertility and contraception. Education, including that of sexual health started to become available to married couples. Some sexual health pioneer nurses say they were ostracized at times by other nurses who thought their work indecent or not real nursing as it did not address illness or injury.

Gradually great benefits could be seen in helping the poorest families reduce the number of conceptions.

North American studies in the 1920s and 1930s in New York and New Jersey found that the most common form of birth control was coitus interruptus. This method was popular despite the concerns voiced by doctors believing it could cause a nervous disposition in their patients, particularly the men. The reality is that people have used withdrawal as a form of birth control not only in America but also in Africa, Australasia, Europe, India and the Middle East.

The Catholic Church allowed the use of what became known as the 'rhythm method' of contraception, by advising a married couple to calculate from menstruation dates when a woman is most likely to ovulate. This process then involved abstention for approximately a week each month. Jewish women are said to have had their own methods of attempting abortion by sitting over a pot of steam or hot stewed onions. By the mid-twentieth century, rubber condoms were widely if discreetly available, and given out free to many armed service personnel in the First and Second World Wars in an attempt to not only ensure troops did not leave a trail of unwanted children in their wake but also as a protection against venereal diseases. Cervical barriers of material such as grass or cloth can be found in many cultures including Africa. Tissue made of bamboo was rolled into balls and pushed into the vagina by Japanese prostitutes. Such basic barrier systems would not only be readily available and cheap, but would also be discreet.

In the 1960s came a new wonder drug, the contraceptive pill. This medical breakthrough would have such a massive impact on societies across the world it became known simply as 'The Pill'. Despite the fact that some doctors initially insisted on receiving signed permission from a woman's husband before prescribing the contraceptive pill, the sense of freedom both sexually and culturally for women was immense. Decisions could be made about education, careers and financial restraints in a way that was unimaginable just half a century before.

There was some resistance. In 1961 a birth control clinic opened by a medical practitioner in New Haven, Connecticut was quickly closed and the owners arrested and fined. A battle then ensued in the US Supreme Court, which ended when it was agreed that the 1879 birth control law was unconstitutional, and so birth control became legal in Connecticut at least. More than one battle was fought in many places to enable society to be educated openly and have the right to make choices about birth control.

Sexual health became an important part of consideration for companies producing contraceptives and suddenly condoms could be bought in most places in the world from open shelves in chemists and supermarkets, sold in brightly coloured packets. This was a tremendous move forward from discreet packets hidden away in men-only environments, like barber shops, and sold in plain brown paper bags.

Public toilets for men and women had dispensing machines, ensuring that buying contraceptives that also acted as prophylactics against sexual diseases did not have to be shameful, but open, and that the purchaser was making a choice that was desirable and sensible. Condoms themselves became a fashionable commodity as they were no longer thick and uncomfortable but made of the finest, yet strongest materials that could be bought in a range of colours, including luminous for a dark room, and flavours. Some had patterned surfaces such as ribbed for extra stimulation during intercourse. All had the added benefit of spermicides. The invention of a female condom has also enabled a woman to make yet another form of choice if she wished to prevent both pregnancy and disease.

Vasectomy and sterilization operations are available and accessible across the globe.

Intrauterine devices have become more sophisticated in design from the new wave in the mid-twentieth century, and medical trials have started to show signs that a whole new generation of contraceptives, although inserted into the womb, would be highly effective and remain in place for some years. Later, some would have the benefit of slow release hormones. Implants in the arm and regular injections have become the birth control choice of many and still science moves on to find the best possible forms of contraception with the least possible negative impact on the human body for the man or woman in today's modern society.

Despite all these extraordinary scientific breakthroughs, many societies are still terribly overcrowded and wracked with poverty, as yet another overcrowded household receives yet another child to feed and nurture. In Western societies in particular, contraceptives are given out, often free to all who ask either at a medical practice, hospital or family planning clinic close to their home or a short bus ride away. There is carefully considered sex education in schools such as might have caused moral outrage 40 years ago. People are well informed from an early age.

Still the teenage pregnancy rate is at very high levels, much higher in ratio than in the sixteenth century in England. Some young people would rather use a plastic film that goes around their sandwiches as a contraceptive around the penis prior to intercourse than simply ask for free condoms. Terminations of pregnancy are also at a high level.

For most societies it is no longer seen as immoral to educate people about contraception and give people a choice about the life they lead within the family unit. There are still many pressures that test the birth control and education systems we have in place. The pressures are on moral, religious or cultural grounds.

There is still a great deal of work to be done.

References

1. News Roundup. Condom from Cromwell's time goes on display in Austria. *BMJ* 2006; 333: 10.3.

2. The Kahun Gynaecological Papyrus. http://www.reshafim.org.il/ad/egypt/timelines/topics/kahunpapyrus.htm (accessed February 2013).

3. Rgveda, 1:164:32, referenced in Dash B, Basu RN. Methods for sterilization and contraception in Ancient and Medieval India. *IJHS* 1968; 3.1: 9–24.

4. Riddle JM. *Contraception and Abortion from the Ancient World to the Renaissance.* Cambridge MA: Harvard University Press, 1994.

5. Muller WP. *The Criminalization of Abortion in the West.* New York, NY: Cornell University Press, 2012.

6. Green MH. (ed.) *The Trotula.* Philadelphia, PA: University of Pennsylvania Press, 2001.

7. Haynes A. *Sex in Elizabethan England.* Stroud, UK: Sutton Publishing, 1999.

8. Brown, K. *The Pox.* Stroud, UK: Sutton Publishing, 2006.

9. Gaimster D, Boland P, Linnane S, Cartwright C. The archaeology of private life: the Dudley Castle condoms. *Post-Medieval Archaelogy* 30: 129–42.

10. Markham G. (ed by M. R. Best) *The English Housewife.* Montreal, Canada: McGill-Queen's University Press, 1994.

11. Smith L. Contraception in the sixteenth century. *J Fam Plann Reprod Health Care* 2006; 32: 59–60.

Chapter 4

Physiology of the menstrual cycle and natural family planning

Gabor Kovacs and Paula Briggs

Understanding menstrual physiology is the basis of understanding the whole concept of fertility, including the mechanism of action of contraceptives. It is also the basis for understanding natural family planning methods.

Hormonal control of ovulation

The menstrual cycle is controlled by the hypothalamo–pituitary axis. The pituitary is a small gland, the size of a cherry, which sits at the base of the brain, anteriorly, behind the bridge of the nose. It is just under the hypothalamus where gonadotrophin-releasing hormone (GnRH), a deca-peptide (a hormone made up of 10 amino acids), is secreted passing into the pituitary via venous channels in a pulsatile manner. It is the frequency and the amplitude of these pulses that determines the response from the pituitary gland, which then secretes follicle stimulating hormone (FSH), the hormone responsible for stimulating the developing Graafian follicles. Follicle stimulating hormone levels are higher in the early phase of the cycle (when it initiates follicular development) than in the later phase. There is a small rise in the level of FSH, which accompanies the very important luteinizing hormone (LH) peak, just prior to ovulation. The anterior pituitary also secretes LH, which remains at basal levels throughout the cycle, with the exception of the LH peak. The rise in the level of LH commences about 36 hours prior to ovulation, and it lasts for 24 hours, with the peak occurring about 24 hours prior to ovulation. This pattern of LH secretion became well understood during the development of the in vitro fertilization programme where women were monitored three hourly in order to detect ovulation, so the oocyte could be collected in a natural cycle and just prior to spontaneous ovulation.

Development of the Graafian follicle

As the follicles start to develop from day 1 of the cycle, the granulosa cells of the follicles start to secrete the steroid hormone, oestrogen. The oestrogen as well as affecting many parts of the body also has the effect of regulating the pituitary, so that FSH secretion is reduced, similar to the thermostat of a central heating system. This is called negative feedback, meaning that as the follicle is maturing, secreting more and more oestrogen, FSH secretion is turned off. This interaction between the secreted oestrogen and the pituitary gland ensures that usually only one oocyte matures and is released most of the time. Various follicles have different sensitivity to FSH, and it is the most sensitive follicle which becomes dominant, the one destined to

Contraception, eds Paula Briggs, Gabor Kovacs and John Guillebaud. Published by Cambridge University Press. © Cambridge University Press 2013.

ovulate, the other developing follicles undergoing atresia. The hormone Inhibin (type A and B) is also secreted from the ovary and also has an inhibitory effect on the pituitary with respect to FSH secretion.

The effect of oestrogen and progesterone on the endometrium

The most overt function of the circulating oestrogen is to cause the endometrium to prolif-erate, and both the glands and the supporting tissue (stroma) thicken, so that after ovulation with the secretion of progesterone it can become secretory, containing tortuous glands with lots of glycogen and thus be able to provide a welcoming nutritional environment should an embryo arrive.

Ovulation of the follicle

When the follicle is ready to ovulate, the oestrogen also primes the pituitary gland to secrete LH (positive feedback). Luteinizing hormone levels rise acutely (LH peak) for 24 hours like a flash of lightning. This is responsible for the release of the ovum from the follicle about 36 hours after the start of the rise, and 24 hours after the LH peak (Figure 4.1). The hormone would more accurately be called 'ovulating hormone' and that is what luteinizing hormone means (as it induces the corpus luteum 'yellow body' after ovulation). The Graafian follicle, as well as providing the gamete to form a new embryo, is also responsible for the secretion of the steroid hormones, oestrogen and progesterone. At the start of each menstrual cycle, several follicles commence to develop, but usually only one matures, with the other follicles degenerating (atresia). Only the 'leading follicle' which is destined to ovulate matures and that is why humans usually only produce single babies. If two ova are released, twins may result. This concept of the 'dominant follicle' is what differentiates humans from animals who have litters rather than single offspring.

As the leading follicle matures, it reaches a diameter of nearly 20 mm, and bulges out from the surface of the ovary. It is similar to a hen's egg where the yoke corresponds to the ovum and the egg white, the granulosa cells. The 'egg shell' in the Graafian follicle is represented by the outer covering of theca interna and theca externa.

At ovulation, when the follicle is 16–18 mm in diameter, in response to the LH peak, the shell of the egg is cracked and the yoke (the ovum) is released to find its way into the Fallopian tube looking for spunky sperm.

During the development of the Graafian follicle, the female germ cell also has to mature and to reduce its chromosome complement from 46 (diploid) to 23 (haploid).

When the mature oocyte is released from the ovary at ovulation, it is about 135 micron (0.135 mm) in diameter and is surrounded by cells called the cumulus oophorus.

The tissue forming the theca interna and externa (the human equivalent to the egg shell) remain as the corpus luteum – the yellow colour comes from the deposition of carotene in the cytoplasm of the thecal cells – and is responsible for secreting hormones essential for a pregnancy to be established (oestrogen and progesterone) which stimulate the uterine lining (endometrium) to thicken, in anticipation of an embryo arriving in a few days time, if a sperm has fertilized the ovum.

It is the combined secretion of oestrogen and progesterone that induces the secretory changes in the endometrium.

Menstrual cycle regulation

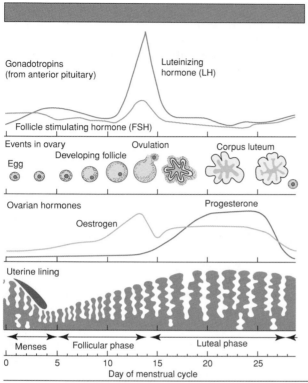

1. Hypothalamus releases GnRH, stimulating the pituitary

2. FSH secreted from pituitary stimulates follicle

3. Follicles produce oestrogen- negative feedback turning off FSH release

4. Critical level of E_2 stimulates- LH peak-positive feedback- ovulation

5. Corpus luteum secretes E_2 and P_4 life span 12–14 days

Figure 4.1 Hormonal changes during the menstrual cycle. (GnRH, gonadotrophin-releasing hormone.)

The corpus luteum and pregnancy

The corpus luteum has an inherent life span of about 14 days, and as it succumbs, in the absence of a pregnancy, the levels of oestrogen and progesterone decline, resulting in an influx of inflammatory white blood cells (leucocytes) and the release of chemicals called prostaglandins and cytokines. This results in the endometrium sloughing off, and the commencement of the next period, the first day of bleeding being defined as 'Day 1' of the next cycle. However if fertilization occurs, the early embryo secretes beta human chorionic gonadotrophin (β-hCG), which has a stimulatory effect on the corpus luteum, rescues it and maintains its hormonal function, so that the levels of oestrogen and progesterone do not decline but rather continue to increase. This maintains the endometrium, and prevents the onset of the next menstrual period. It is the role of the corpus luteum to secrete adequate oestrogen and progesterone during the first three months of the pregnancy, a role which is then taken over by the placenta at about three months.

As oestrogen and progesterone circulate throughout the body they affect many tissues and organs. As we stated above, the most overt is the effect on endometrium and menstruation.

Basal body temperature

Progesterone is thermogenic – it elevates the body's temperature. Therefore measuring a woman's basal body temperature on awakening on a daily basis will show an elevation of about 0.5°C once ovulation has taken place and progesterone is secreted. Whilst the pattern is not always clear, in many women it is a useful method of determining if and when ovulation has occurred. This phenomenon of luteal temperature rise is the basis of the 'temperature method' of natural family planning (NFP), and can also be used for assessing whether, when and how well ovulation is taking place, in the assessment of a subfertile couple, and in the management of ovulation stimulation with clomiphene citrate (see Chapter 22).

Cervical mucus changes and the basis of the Billings method of NFP

Another very important effect of oestrogen and progesterone is on the secretions of the cervical glands – the cervical mucus. Following the observations of the Billings [1] we can use the changes in cervical mucus as a bioassay of the menstrual cycle, thus pinpointing fertile and infertile days.

The quantity and quality of cervical mucus varies depending on the relative circulating levels of oestrogen and progesterone.

The effect of oestrogen is to stimulate the production of copious amounts of mucus from the cervical glands. The physical composition of cervical mucus depends on its water and salt concentration – oestrogen encourages slippery/watery mucus often described as 'egg whitey', referred to in the Billings method of NFP as 'basic fertile pattern' (BFP). As soon as progesterone is secreted and reaches the cervical glands, it changes the salt concentration to result in a 'gluey' or 'snotty' consistency, referred to as 'basic infertile pattern' (BIP). It is this defined change from BFP to BIP that defines the time of ovulation, and enables couples to use it for NFP.

A woman commences her menstrual cycle with menstruation for a few days. Following the end of her menses she experiences only small amounts of mucus, but the quantity of the mucus gradually increases as the developing follicle commences to secrete more and more oestrogen. This also results in the oestrogenic BFP mucus, which is maximal just prior to ovulation. As soon as ovulation occurs, the mucus changes to BIP, and this persists until menstruation, when the cycle recommences. These changes can be used to suggest whether a woman is ovulating or not, when assessing her cycle.

These physiological changes are logical, as at the time just prior to ovulation it is important that the mucus facilitates the passage of the sperm through the cervix, uterus and Fallopian tubes. After ovulation the thickened BIP mucus is protective from allowing sperm (which no longer have any physiological function), and maybe micro-organisms from entering the uterus.

Fertilization

The human ovum is released from the surface of the ovary at ovulation and needs to find its way into the Fallopian tube with the help of the finger-like projections on the tubes called fimbriae. The ovum then progresses along the Fallopian tube with fertilization taking place in the lateral one third (called the ampulla). It is believed that the human ovum can only be

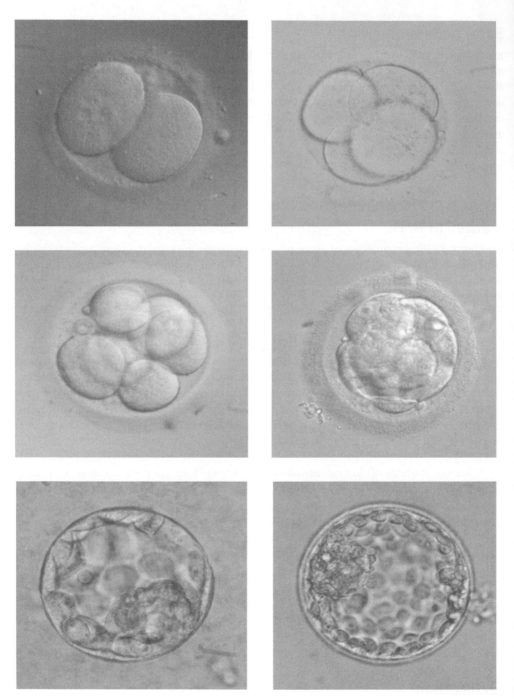

Figure 4.2 Division into 2 cells usually occurs by 24 hours after fertilization, with the embryo reaching 4–8 cells by 48 hours.

fertilized during a few hours. It is therefore important that the oocyte is exposed to live, fertile sperm during its first few hours in the Fallopian tube. Consequently, sperm deposited in the vagina enter the cervical canal where they are protected by the mucus from the acidic environment of the vagina. To maximize the chance of fertilization, sperm need to be deposited into the vagina prior to ovulation. It is believed that sperm will survive for two to three days in the mucus environment, so couples who want to conceive are advised to undertake intercourse at least every second day from when menstruation finishes until ovulation is thought have occurred.

Conversely, couples using NFP must abstain around the ovulatory period. The problem is that it is uncertain how long a sperm may survive, and pregnancy has been documented even when intercourse did not occur for several days prior to ovulation.

This will be discussed in more detail under NFP below.

Fertilization commences with contact between the oocyte and sperm, and climaxes with the fusion of their two haploid pronuclei (each containing 23 chromosomes) resulting in a diploid embryo (with 23 pairs of chromosomes (46)). After the attachment of the sperm to the ovum, the acrosomal cap of the sperm releases enzymes (known as hyaluronidase) which help to break through the zona pellucida membrane surrounding the oocyte. As the successful sperm enters the oocyte, it stimulates the zona pellucida to undergo what is called the acrosome reaction which prevents any further sperm from entering the oocyte.

Early embryonic development and implantation

After fertilization, the embryo undergoes repeated cell division known as cleavage and segmentation, which transforms it into a solid clump of cells. At the 16 cell stage it is called the 'morula'. Our understanding of this stage of human embryo formation is now much improved due to in vitro fertilization and the ability to observe embryos in the laboratory. Division into 2 cells usually occurs by 24 hours after fertilization, with the embryo reaching 4–8 cells by 48 hours (Figure 4.2).

As the embryo keeps dividing it is also travelling along the Fallopian tube towards the uterine cavity. This movement is accomplished by both the movement of the fine hairs (cilia) lining the tube as well as contractions of the muscles within the tubal walls. The clump of embryonic cells on about the fifth day undergoes cavitation, and accumulates fluid to become a *blastocyst*. It is about this time when it reaches the uterine cavity. The cells then differentiate into the *inner cell mass* which will form the embryo, and the *trophoblast* which forms the placenta and membranes. Nutrition during this journey is provided by the tubal and uterine secretions. The trophoblast then burrows into the superficial layer of the endometrium, and begins to establish the placenta, which will become the route of nutrition to the embryo, as well as the source of oestrogen and progesterone during the pregnancy.

Natural family planning

For couples in whom artificial methods of contraception are unacceptable for religious or other reasons, the only option is NFP. Cynically, an old joke amongst family planners is: 'What do you call couples who use NFP?' – 'Parents'. This is unfair, as NFP is based on the physiological principles described above. There are a couple of problems with NFP. First, it limits sexual intercourse to times in the cycle that are 'safe' and these days may not correspond to the time when a couple feel loving or feel the need to have sex. So the couple need very strong willpower. Secondly, as stated above, there is no guarantee that sperm may not survive longer than the expected two to three days, so despite abstinence during the peri-ovulatory period, fertilization and pregnancy may still occur.

There have been a number of modifications of NFP as our understanding of reproductive physiology has improved. Another complication of NFP is that not all women have the perfect pattern of temperature and mucus changes every month. It is particularly difficult when women have irregular cycles with irregular ovulation.

The rhythm method

This is the oldest and least efficient form of NFP, also referred to as 'Vatican roulette'. The rhythm method is based on the fact that the corpus luteum usually survives about 14 days, and therefore the luteal phase is approximately 14 days long. Thus, to calculate the fertile days, a number of cycles are studied, and 14 days are then subtracted from the longest and from the shortest cycles, thus estimating a range for the expected days of ovulation for that woman. Again, we have to allow for sperm survival, so the couple need to abstain from sexual intercourse a few days earlier. The problem with the rhythm method is that we are trying to predict what is happening in this cycle from what happened in previous cycles, and whilst that is probably reasonable in many situations, it is by no means certain.

Temperature method

A refinement of the rhythm method is to record a basal temperature chart, which will give additional information in the current cycle about when ovulation is occurring. As described above, the progesterone secreted after ovulation is thermogenic, so if a woman records her basal body temperature (Figure 4.3) she will see an elevation after ovulation, and combined with her 'menstrual rhythm' can be reasonably confident that she has ovulated, and that intercourse should not result in conception.

There is still the problem that there is no warning of imminent ovulation, so there are relatively few days in a cycle when intercourse is 'safe'.

The Billings (mucus) method

What the Billings method offers in addition to the rhythm and temperature methods is that it actually studies the current cycle, and also gives some warning about ovulation approaching.

First, couples are advised that they can have sexual intercourse after menstruation, but only on alternate days so that the semen does not interfere with the cervical mucus inspection. As the oestrogen rises, the quantity and quality of cervical mucus changes resulting in the BFP, thus warning that ovulation is approaching. The couples then abstain from intercourse, until the distinct change from BFP to BIP, which suggests ovulation. After the estimated day of ovulation, they abstain for a couple more days, and then hopefully they are 'safe' until the next period.

Clinical trials of the Billings method in the 1980s have shown remarkable effectiveness, as long as couples who broke the rules were excluded from the analysis. This of course is no surprise, as the physiology that the concept is based on is sound. The problems are that human beings are human and emotion often over-rules logic; that sperm are sometimes surprisingly virile and can survive several days; and of course not every cycle in every woman shows the typical signs described. Nevertheless, using NFP compared to no contraception will decrease the number of conceptions.

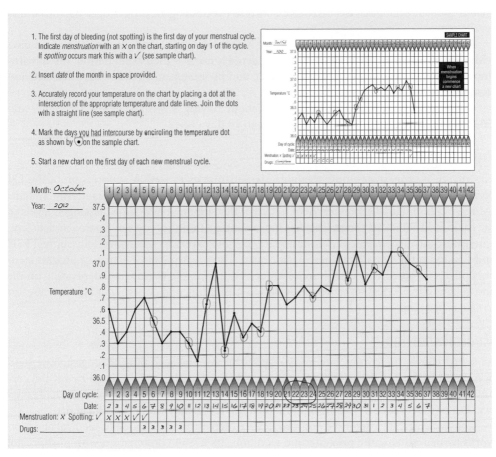

Figure 4.3 Basal body temperature chart. Clomiphene citrate 150 mg (3 tablets) were taken from day 5 to day 9. Ovulation appears to have occurred on day 18. Intercourse occurred on days 10, 12, 14, 16, 18 and 19. Temperature elevated for 19 more days – patient conceived in this cycle. On day 44 (26 days post ovulation) her beta human chorionic gonadotrophin (β-hCG) was 8400 and progesterone 139.

Practical messages from this chapter

The mechanism of action of the combined hormonal contraceptives

The principal mechanism of action of combined hormonal contraceptives (CHC) is inhibition of ovulation. This is due to the oestrogen supressing FSH release (negative feedback), whereas the progestogen inhibits LH release. Although ethinyl oestradiol (EE) is a potent synthetic oestrogen, with lower doses, follicular development can occur. As a backup, the progestogen should inhibit LH release and prevent ovulation.

We also explained that sequential secretion of oestrogen and progesterone is essential for endometrial development, the steady combined administration of oestrogen and progestogen in a pharamacological dose throughout the cycle induces an inactive endometrium with few glands developing, thus making implantation unlikely even if an oocyte is fertilized and an embryo arrives in the uterine cavity. It is also said that the progestogen in CHC has an anti-mucus effect, but it is hard to calculate how the oestrogen : progestogen balance works on the mucus.

The other important point to remember is that when women have hormone-free days with CHC they are not having what is considered a normal menstrual period, but a 'withdrawal bleed'. When the exogenous oestrogen and progestogen is ceased, the endometrium sloughs, thus causing a bleed.

Consequently there is nothing natural about having 4 weekly bleeds on CHC, and extended regimes are no less physiological than 28 day cycles.

Progestogen-only methods

The effects of progestogen-only methods are anti-mucus as well as suppression of the LH peak. Consequently progestogen-only implants (Nexplanon®) and intrauterine systems (Mirena®) both allow some degree of follicular development and allow oestrogen levels in the early–mid-follicular range. This has the advantage that they are not oestrogen deficient, whereas depot-medroxyprogesterone acetate (Depo-Provera®) seems to totally supress FSH and LH and results in a hypo-oestrogenic state. The mechanism of action of progestogen-only pills is less predictable, with some women continuing to ovulate and depending on the anti-mucus effect, whilst others have ovulation inhibition, and consequent amenorrhoea or irregular bleeding.

Medical abortion

As stated above, the corpus luteum is responsible for the secretion of progesterone (and oestrogen) in the first few weeks of pregnancy. It has long been recognized that if the corpus luteum was surgically removed during an early pregnancy, before the placenta had taken over the production of steroid hormones, then the pregnancy would fail and abort.

Consequently, the use of the anti-progestin mifepristone as a mode of medical abortion works by neutralizing the progesterone secretion. Its use in combination with misoprostol then induces uterine contractions.

Reference

1. Billings EL, Brown JB, Billings JJ, Burger HG. Symptoms and hormonal changes accompanying ovulation. *Lancet* 1972; 1: 282–4.

Chapter 5

The oestrogen component of currently used steroidal contraceptives

David Crook

Background

The issues relating to the clinical applications of oestrogens have traditionally been easier to review (and are certainly far less controversial) than those relating to progestogens. In the area of contraception, especially combined oral contraceptives (COCs), ethinyl oestradiol (EE) has been the clear market leader for many decades. Attempts to substitute alternative oestrogens, such as drugs structurally identical to a woman's own natural oestradiol, have resulted in COCs with poor cycle control, unsuitable for the majority of women and so rarely receiving marketing approval. Although perhaps desirable from a theoretical basis, exogenous oestradiol is rapidly inactivated by the liver, resulting in unpredictable plasma levels of the active steroid and hence these problems with cycle control.

Only within the last few years have oestradiol-based COCs emerged as true competitors to those containing EE. Progress has been made through strategies such as careful matching with innovative progestogens and manipulation of the dosing cycle. These developments have resulted in currently licensed COCs containing either oestradiol valerate (E_2V) or the natural hormone 17β-oestradiol (E_2, hereafter referred to as oestradiol) (Figure 5.1). As E_2V is a prodrug (being rapidly converted to E_2), both of these new formulations rely on E_2 for their therapeutic efficacy.

The primary driver for the development of the oestrogen component has been a widespread concern that EE-containing COCs may in some women – especially those who are genetically predisposed – increase their risk of venous thromboembolism (VTE) and other rare adverse events. The ethinylation of the oestradiol protects the steroid from hepatic degradation and so improves efficacy when administered orally, but also leads to widespread metabolic changes, for instance in aspects of coagulation and fibrinolysis, that in theory might increase the risk of VTE [1]. The simplest approach to reducing these metabolic disturbances has been to reduce the oestrogen *dose*, but attention is now focused on the potential benefits of changing the oestrogen *type*.

The purpose of this brief review is to set out the rather peculiar background to the inclusion of oestrogens in contraception as well as to review some simple pharmacology. The more clinical aspects of oestrogens in contraception are covered elsewhere in this book.

Contraception, eds Paula Briggs, Gabor Kovacs and John Guillebaud. Published by Cambridge University Press. © Cambridge University Press 2013.

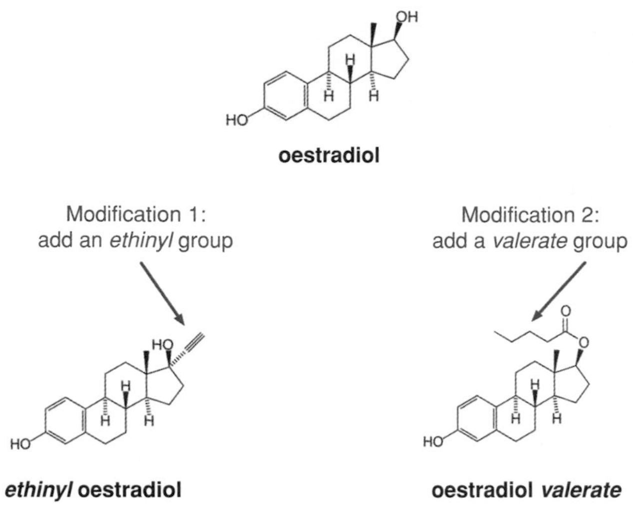

Figure 5.1 The three oestrogens currently used in oral contraception.

oestradiol

Modification 1:
add an *ethinyl* group

Modification 2:
add a *valerate* group

***ethinyl* oestradiol**

oestradiol *valerate*

What are oestrogens?

Oestrogens are steroid hormones that act primarily on ovulation regulation and other aspects of female reproduction and sexual development, as well as on a wide range of organs including bone, brain and blood vessels. The classic mechanism of action for all steroid hormones is to bind to specific intracellular receptors and induce change in their shape, encouraging dimerization (two pairs of hormone/receptor complexes forming a single unit) and leading to recruitment of co-regulators. The complexes formed through this route are able to influence gene transcription and hence the production of proteins with biological activities. Other, more direct, mechanisms may be involved in which the steroid binds at the level of the cell membrane and so induces cytoplasmic signalling pathways.

The predominant oestrogen (and the one with the highest biological activity) in the premenopausal woman is E_2, synthesized predominantly in the ovaries using the enzyme aromatase to modify raw material such as testosterone. Other oestrogens used in clinical practice, including those that have been chemically modified, are shown in Table 5.1.

The development of oestrogen as a contraceptive component

The first piece of evidence that chemical contraception may be possible – that ovarian extracts might inhibit ovulation – followed on from Haberland's demonstration in 1919 that rabbits implanted with the ovaries of pregnant rabbits became temporarily infertile [2]. He clearly recognized the potential of this discovery in terms of human fertility control and by 1930 had persuaded a Hungarian pharmaceutical company to develop an ovarian extract ('Infecundin'). Nothing much came of this development – the very idea of chemical contraception became immensely unpopular with the public, leading to his suicide – but presumably this extract would have contained oestrogens and progesterone, albeit with weak activities.

At about the same time as Haberland's death, the American Margaret Sanger was just starting her crusade for birth control, although there would be a 30-year interval before she became interested in the concept of hormonal contraception [3]. When Sanger and the

Table 5.1 Classification of oestrogens. Those currently used in contraception in **bold**.

Natural and human
- oestrone (E$_1$)
- **oestradiol** (E$_2$)
- oestriol (E$_3$)
- oestetrol* (E$_4$)

Natural but non-human
- e.g., equilin and equilenin (from horses)
- e.g., phytoestrogens (from plants)

Synthetic steroidal**
- e.g., **ethinyl oestradiol (EE)**
- e.g., **oestradiol valerate (E$_2$V)**

Synthetic non-steroidal
- e.g., diethylstilbestrol

* Only produced during pregnancy.
**Structure is modified to increase therapeutic potency.

equally redoubtable Katherine McCormack approached the reproductive biologist Gregory Pincus about hormonal contraception he was quite sure that effective oral contraception could be achieved using progestogen alone and had no interest in using any form of oestrogen. Once Pincus had accepted the commission to develop an oral contraceptive he looked at various candidate molecules. Carl Djerassi's brilliant team at Syntex had recently published their synthesis of norethindrone, the first orally active progestogen, but for commercial reasons Pincus decided to work with a rather more mundane steroid, norethynodrel, marketed by G. D. Searle (now part of Monsanto).

Preliminary testing showed that oral norethynodrel administration did indeed inhibit ovulation, leading to large field trials in Puerto Rico and elsewhere. During these trials there was a sudden increase in menstrual cycle abnormalities, subsequently traced to a new batch of the drug that had been produced by a more refined synthesis that reduced the levels of a synthetic intermediate, *mestranol*. Guessing that this 'contaminant' had been critical to the efficacy of the earlier batches, Pincus's team deliberately reintroduced mestranol into subsequent batches in order to achieve the original levels of 'contamination' and showed that subsequent batches restored cycle control. We now know that the oestrogen component not only benefits cycle control, but also can contribute to the overall effectiveness of COCs, for instance through effects on the hypothalamus and pituitary [4].

In 1959, G. D. Searle obtained a license in the USA for a version of Pincus's contraceptive (Enovid®: 9.85 mg norethynodrel plus 150 µg mestranol). The license was for various gynaecological applications, including contraception, but the company chose not to openly promote this combination as a contraceptive. Instead, in 1960 they released a lower dose compound Enovid 5 mg® (5 mg norethynodrel plus 75 µg mestranol) and this is now regarded as the first COC. Schering in Germany (now part of Bayer HealthCare) were quick to follow Searle's lead and by 1961 had launched Anovlar® (50 µg ethinyl oestradiol – not mestranol – plus 4 mg norethisterone) in West Germany.

Mestranol is now only rarely used; although clearly effective in terms of cycle control it is a prodrug, being converted to the active steroid EE. There is simply no merit in using mestranol rather than EE, and indeed the conversion of mestranol to EE is vulnerable to inhibition by a long list of CYP2C9 inhibitors, such as anti-fungal azoles.

Currently used contraceptive oestrogens

Ethinyl oestradiol (EE)

Schering's Berlin laboratories were the crucible of steroid synthesis for many decades. In 1938, Inhoffen and Hohlweg (and others [2]) developed the first synthetic oestrogen by substituting an ethinyl group at carbon 17 of oestradiol (Figure 5.1). EE is well-absorbed when orally administered and once in the blood is highly resistant to degradation by the liver and so has exceptionally high biological activity. EE was approved by German regulators for various gynaecological applications in 1949, marketed as Progynon C®. Clearly this was the 'off-the-shelf' option for Schering when it came to developing their own COC, quickly picked up by other manufacturers as the logical choice for a COC oestrogen given the potential concerns with mestranol as a prodrug.

Over the next few decades EE doses of $\geq$ 50 µg fell out of fashion and there was a downwards shift towards EE doses of 30–35 µg. Subsequently 20 µg EE doses became popular, initially targeted at the older woman with reduced fertility; they turned out to be remarkably well-tolerated and effective. Even lower doses of EE are available. The primary driver for this strategy of dose reduction has been a continued concern that an apparent increased risk of VTE reported in COC users was related to the oestrogen (rather than the progestogen) component (reviewed in [1]). A dose-effect response had been detected in earlier observational studies involving very high ($\geq$ 50 µg EE) doses and the evidence to justify the move to low doses tends not to be evidence based. Indeed, in observational studies the 20 µg EE COC formulations appear to be associated with higher, not lower, VTE risk. There may be a biological basis for this anomaly or it may indicate that observational epidemiological studies are always, despite the best efforts of statisticians, susceptible to residual prescribing bias. This situation is further confused by terminology, with yesterday's 'low-dose' formulations becoming the 'medium-dose' formulations in future comparative studies.

Most COCs are packaged as a 21 day sequence of active ingredients with either placebo pills to be used for the rest of the arbitrary 28 day cycle in order to induce a withdrawal bleed or a 7 day pill-free interval. Some women dislike these bleeds and various approaches, such as 3 and even 12 monthly formulations, are now available (see Chapter 12). Phasic formulations (in which the dose of EE and/or progestogen varies throughout the cycle) can also be used.

EE can also be delivered as part of non-oral contraception. Following the high acceptability of transdermal ('patch') administration of steroid hormones for many post-menopausal women, in 2002 Ortho-McNeil released Ortho Evra®, a contraceptive patch delivering EE at a target rate of 20 µg/day in combination with the progestogen norelgestromin (a prodrug of norgestimate) at an intended delivery rate of 150 µg/day. These patches, to be applied to buttocks, abdomen, upper arm or upper torso (other than the breasts), were to be changed every week for three weeks, with a patch-free week to complete the arbitrary four week cycle. These patches are acceptable to women, but it was subsequently found that plasma EE levels were higher than with oral administration of EE. An increased risk of VTE (compared to COCs), detected in some non-randomized studies, led to demands from European Union and US regulators for labelling updates, as well as extensive litigation. These higher plasma levels of EE levels are a disappointment as, at least in theory, non-oral administration of EE might lead to more subtle metabolic changes and perhaps a reduced VTE risk.

In 2002, Organon (now part of Merck Sharp and Dohme) marketed NuvaRing®, a flexible vaginal ring releasing EE at an intended delivery rate of 15 µg/day in combination with the

Table 5.2 Oestrogens currently used in contraception, with examples.

OC oestrogen	Typical OC dose (mg/day)	Example
Ethinyl oestradiol (EE)	0.020–0.035	**Microgynon® (Bayer)** Days 1–21: EE 0.03 mg/day + levonorgestrel 0.15 mg/day Days 22–28: no tablets or placebo (Microgynon® ED)
Oestradiol valerate (E_2V)	2.0	**Qlaira®/Klaira®/Natazia® (Bayer)** Days 1–2: E_2V 3.0 mg/day Days 3–7: E_2V 2.0 mg/day + dienogest 2.0 mg/day Days 8–24: E_2V 2.0 mg/day + dienogest 3.0 mg/day Days 25–26: E_2V 1.0 mg/day Days 27–28: placebo
Oestradiol (E_2)	1.5	**Zoely® (Merck Sharp and Dohme)** Days 1–24: E_2 1.5 mg/day + nomegestrol acetate 2.5 mg/day Days 25–28: placebo

OC, oral contraceptive.

progestogen etonorgestrel (an active metabolite of desogestrel) at an intended delivery rate 120 µg/day. Such devices are designed to be used continuously for three weeks and then removed by the user for a ring-free week to complete the cycle. Plasma EE levels are notably low with NuvaRing®, especially when compared to the transdermal contraceptives, but the studies needed to show whether such a difference has clinical significance have yet to be performed. To date neither E_2V nor E_2 have been shown to be suitable for any form of non-oral contraception: this remains the territory of EE.

Oestradiol valerate (E_2V)

One trick that pharmacologists use in order to ensure reliable blood levels of an orally administered drug is to add a carboxylic acid to form an ester. After the modified drug enters the body the ester is rapidly cleaved away to reveal the native molecule. There is an assumption that 'cloaking' the molecule in this way delays drug degradation at the level of gut and liver. In the case of E_2, valeric acid can be added to carbon 17 to form oestradiol valerate (Figure 5.1). This compound has been widely used both orally and as an injection (primarily in the treatment of menopausal symptoms) but until recently had not proven reliable as a COC oestrogen.

In 2009 a multiphasic COC containing oestradiol valerate (1.0–3.0 mg) together with the progestogen dienogest (2.0–3.0 mg) (Table 5.2) was shown to result in acceptable cycle control and contraceptive efficacy [5]. This major development presumably derives from (a) the use of the valerate ester, (b) the choice of partner progestogen, and (c) the results of experimentation with new multiphasic dosing schedules. Marketed by Bayer HealthCare as Qlaira®/Klaira® in the European Union and as Natazia® in the USA, this formulation is claimed to result in better cycle control than an EE comparator formulation (despite the rather complex dosing schedule and 'missed pill' concerns) and indeed may prove useful in the treatment of heavy menstrual bleeding [6].

In terms of VTE risk there is evidence that the impact on coagulation and fibrinoloysis is 'similar or less pronounced' than with EE formulations [7], but whether these surrogate studies will translate into a difference in clinical endpoints is not known.

Oestradiol (E$_2$)

The dienogest/oestradiol valerate formulation described above showed that it was indeed possible to develop a clinically effective alternative to EE, albeit one requiring a complex dosing sequence and an oestradiol ester. The molecule was developed initially by Teva, and then Merck (Organon initially) collaborated on the clinical trial development. The global intellectual property (IP) is owned by Teva and marketing approval in the European Union was gained by them, but there is an agreement between the two companies on which countries Zoely® is marketed within. The UK is a Merck (Merck Sharp and Dohme) territory for Zoely®.

Zoely®, a monophasic oral contraceptive containing E$_2$ at a dose of 1.5 mg, combined with the progestogen nomegestrol acetate (NOMAC) at 2.5 mg for days 1–24, with 4 placebo tablets being taken on days 25–28 of the arbitrary 4 week cycle (Table 5.2). Compared to a drospirenone/EE formulation the combination appeared to be acceptable, with some suggestion of a benefit in terms of cycle control [8, 9] as well as less effect on various putative markers of haemostasis [10].

Conclusions

Until the last few years a prescriber discussing contraceptive options with a woman could bring in issues such as the route of administration of contraceptive steroids, their doses and dosing schedules and the type of progestogen. The one thing that was never on the table was the nature of the oestrogen: it more or less had to be EE. More recently, new formulations containing the natural hormone oestradiol have become available. Preliminary evidence from comparative trials indicates that many women find these oestradiol-based COCs to be effective alternatives to those containing EE.

Any evidence-based extension of choice in contraceptive prescribing has to be welcome. The very large unanswered (unanswerable?) question is whether there are advantages to these new formulations in terms of VTE and other conditions thought to be linked to EE.

References

1. Godsland IF, Winkler U, Lidegaard Ø, Crook D. Occlusive vascular diseases in oral contraceptive users: epidemiology, pathology and mechanisms. *Drugs* 2000; 60: 21–869.

2. Frobenius W. 'The rabbits are prepared ...' The development of ethinylestradiol and ethinyltestosterone. *J Reproduktionsmed Endokrinol* 2011; 8: 32–57.

3. Marks LV. *Sexual Chemistry: a history of the contraceptive pill.* London: Yale University Press, 2010.

4. Hahn DW, McGuire JL, Kuhnke, J. Contraception. *Ullmann's Encyclopedia of Industrial Chemistry.* Wiley Online Library: Published online, 15 October 2011.

5. Fruzzetti F, Trémollieres T, Bitzer J. An overview of the development of combined oral contraceptives containing estradiol: focus on estradiol valerate/dienogest. *Gynecol Endocrinol* 2012; 28: 400–8.

6. Borgelt LM, Martell CW. Estradiol valerate/dienogest: a novel combined oral contraceptive. *Clin Ther* 2012; 34: 37–55.

7. Klipping C, Duijkers I, Parke S, *et al.* Hemostatic effects of a novel estradiol-based oral contraceptive: an open-label, randomized, crossover study of estradiol valerate/dienogest versus ethinylestradiol/levonorgestrel. *Drugs R D* 2011; 11: 159–70.

8. Westhoff C, Kaunitz AM, Korver T, *et al.* Efficacy, safety, and tolerability of a monophasic oral contraceptive containing nomegestrol acetate and 17β-estradiol: a randomized controlled trial. *Obstet Gynecol* 2012; 119: 989–9.

9. Mansour D, Verhoeven C, Sommer W, *et al.* Efficacy and tolerability of a monophasic combined oral contraceptive containing nomegestrol acetate and 17β-oestradiol in a 24/4 regimen, in comparison to an oral contraceptive containing ethinylestradiol and drospirenone in a 21/7 regimen. *Eur J Contracept Reprod Health Care* 2011; 16: 430–43.

10. Ågren UM, Anttila M, Mäenpää-Liukko K. Effects of a monophasic combined oral contraceptive containing nomegestrol acetate and 17β-oestradiol compared with one containing levonorgestrel and ethinylestradiol on haemostasis, lipids and carbohydrate metabolism. *Eur J Contracept Reprod Health Care* 2011; 16: 444–57.

Chapter 6

The risk of oestrogens in contraceptives

Sven O. Skouby

Introduction

It is estimated that more than 100 million women worldwide use an oral contraceptive [1]. Modern oral contraceptives (OCs) afford not only excellent birth control but also a variety of non-contraceptive benefits, ranging from regulation and reduction of both menstrual bleeding and dysmenorrhoea to treatment of premenstrual syndrome, menstrual migraines, acne and hirsutism. Long-term benefits include reduced rates of endometrial, ovarian and colorectal cancer. However the cardiovasular safety is still under debate because thombotic events, even with rare occurrence, can have an impact on a clinically significant number of women. This chapter will review the estimated thrombotic risks associated with the oestrogen content of combined hormonal contraception.

Until recently, most combined hormonal contraception used ethinyl oestradiol (EE) as the oestrogen component, which yields satisfactory results in terms of ovulation inhibition and effects on the endometrium. The earliest pills contained doses of 100–150 μg of mestranol or EE. Over the past 50 years, considerable attention has been directed to dose reduction of EE, first to 50 μg, then to low dose 30–35 μg, and then to very low dose 20 μg pills with the lowest dose of 10 μg introduced most recently, but at the same time this is associated with some compliance problems due to more frequent episodes of unscheduled bleeding.

The oestrogen content in combined hormonal contraception is linked to the reported increased risk of thrombotic events. The first report of an increased risk of venous thrombosis appeared in 1961 [2] with a report of pulmonary embolism in a nurse, who had just begun taking an OC. In 1963, the first case of myocardial infarction in an OC user was reported and a connection with ischaemic stroke was noted in 1968 [3]. Subsequently, numerous reports have been published on the increase in thrombotic risk, indicating a 2 to 6-fold increased risk of deep vein thrombosis associated with current OC use [4]. Concern about the venous thromboembolism (VTE) risk of hormonal contraceptive options has triggered a number of 'pill scares', each of which resulted in panic stopping and a spike in unplanned pregnancies. Cardiovascular disease has a multifactorial aetiology with a number of potentially modifiable risk factors. The preferred method of creating evidence would be prospective randomized controlled trials (RCTs). However, given the infrequency of thrombosis in women on hormonal contraception, this is neither feasible nor ethical. Instead, data from alternative studies using a variety of epidemiological techniques, i.e., review of large prescription databases, centralized national and hospital registries and cohort studies, together with clinical studies

Contraception, eds Paula Briggs, Gabor Kovacs and John Guillebaud. Published by Cambridge University Press. © Cambridge University Press 2013.

using biomarkers such as changes in the haemostatic system, have to be considered to determine the possible rate of thrombosis and other complications When results are consistent and in agreement this leads to acceptable evidence on risk, but when results are unexpected or inconsistent the level of evidence is obviously questionable. Current guidelines indicate that, as with all medication, contraceptive hormones should be selected and initiated by weighing risks and benefits for the individual patient.

Thrombotic diseases

Arterial thrombosis

The risk of arterial thrombosis, including stroke and myocardial infarction, is reported to be increased in users of combined hormonal contraception. Such events may be fatal, or lead to disabling sequelae. The level of risk was the highest in the early years of pill use when the oestrogen dose was very high, and large numbers of women using them were heavy smokers or had existing vascular risk factors such as uncontrolled hypertension. A multicentre study by the World Health Organization (WHO) showed a 5-fold increased risk of myocardial infarction with currently used OCs as well as a 3-fold increased risk of ischaemic stroke and a 1.5- to 2-fold increased risk of haemorrhagic stroke [5]. In more recent studies, this risk has decreased, with reduced oestrogen dosing and exclusion of women with cardiovascular risk factors from pill use as the most important factors. As OCs are increasingly used in the later reproductive years, further research is needed to define the risks in older women for whom the prevalence of risk factors and the incidence of cardiovascular disease are higher.

In fact, the most striking point about the risk of arterial thrombosis is the marked increased in risk in women with established risk factors:

- Smoking: 14-fold increase
- Hypertension: 6-fold increase
- Adverse lipid profile: 25-fold increase
- Diabetes: 17-fold increase

Strokes in young women are rare with an absolute incidence rate of 3 per 100 000 person years. The risk is also increased in combined hormonal contraception users with the already established risk factors of smoking (24-fold), hypertension (78-fold), and adverse lipids profile (1011-fold) [6].

One particular risk factor for stroke is migraine with aura.

Women with migraine *without aura* who take OC have a low risk of stroke, similar to women without migraine. The risk of stroke is increased 11-fold for women who have migraine *with aura* and who do not use OC, and increases to 23-fold for women with migraine *with aura* using OC [7].

Peripheral arterial disease (PAD) is rare in young women. However, co-morbidity in patients with premature onset of PAD is high, and carries a poor prognosis, because of a high incidence of vascular occlusion. In one study devoted to PAD, risk was also increased in combined hormonal contraceptive users with a further 3.8 overall increase in risk and with an additional increase seen with concomitant smoking or diabetes [7].

In summary, while oestrogen may play a role in arterial thrombosis, the effect is primarily related to an interaction with traditional, and to some extent modifiable, risk factors for arterial disease. The overall risk of arterial disease in young healthy women is low and seems

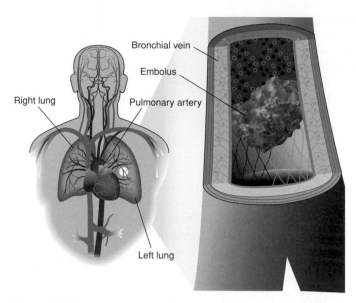

Figure 6.1 Pulmonary embolism.

not to be significantly impacted by low oestrogen containing hormonal contraceptives. In women with an established risk profile, detection of the risk factors at the time of considering a prescription for combined hormonal contraception is essential. This is important not only to assess oestrogen-related risk, but also to consider alternative methods on an individual basis. If no other method seems applicable, it is a professional duty to establish timely intervention to modify these risk factors early and to provide extensive information to the patient about treatment options and their effects and/or side effects.

Venous thrombosis

Venous thrombosis has an annual incidence of 1–3 per 10 000 individuals per year (background rate). It is uncommon in young individuals and becomes more frequent with advancing age. It mostly manifests in the deep veins of the leg, but may occur in other sites, such as the upper extremities, cerebral sinus, liver and portal veins or retinal veins. Venous thrombi are composed predominately of red blood cells, but also platelets and leucocytes bound together by fibrin. Embolization occurs when parts of the clot dislodge and are transported by the blood flow, usually through the heart to the vasculature of the lungs (Figure 6.1). There are a number of risk factors for VTE. They fit into an extended version of Virchow's triad (stasis, hypercoagulability, endothelial damage) and they change the haemostatic balance toward clot formation. This can be achieved by decreasing blood flow and lowering oxygen tension, by activating the endothelium, by activating innate or acquired immune responses, by activating blood platelets, or by increasing the number of platelets and red blood cells or modifying the concentrations of pro- and anticoagulant proteins in the blood. Numerous risk factors are known, which can be divided into genetic and acquired (Table 6.1).

A contemporary multiple-hit hypothesis implies that more than one risk factor is present at any one time. One of the most well-known acquired risk factors is the use of combined hormonal contraception, with most research conducted on oral administration. For reference,

Table 6.1 Venous thrombosis: genetic and acquired risk factors.

Genetic			Acquired		
Risk factor	Prevalence (%)	RR	Risk factor	Prevalence (%)	RR
Leiden factor V heterozygous	6.0	8	Age > 30 vs 30 years	50	2.5
Leiden factor V homozygous	0.2	64	Adiposity (BMI > 25)	30	2
Protein C insufficiency	0.2	15	COCs	30	2–6
Protein S insufficiency	0.1	10	Varicose veins	8	2
Antithrombin III insufficiency	0.02	50	Pregnancy	4	8
Prothrombin 2021A	2.0	3	Medical diseases	5?	2–5
Hyperhomo-cysteinaemia	3.0	3	Immobilization/trauma	?	2–10

BMI, body mass index; COCs, combined oral contraceptives; RR, relative risk.

the baseline absolute risk of thrombosis in non-users is in the range of 1–6 per 10 000 user-years. If no valid observations on the absolute risk are available, the reported relative risk increase caused by the use of hormonal contraceptives should be multiplied by this baseline risk. This gives an overall risk of venous thrombosis with combined hormonal contraception use in the range of 4–20 per 10 000 user-years with estimates of increased risk ranging from 3-fold to 8-fold [8].

Population studies have demonstrated a reduction in the risk of venous thrombosis with oestrogen dose reduction. Going from an oestrogen dose of 50 μg to 35–30 μg reduced the risk by 30% and reducing to 20 μg the risk is further reduced by 18%, but still remains elevated compared to non-users [9]. The most prominent pharmacological development has been the recent introduction of natural oestrogens (17β oestradiol and 15α hydroxyestriol, oestetrol) in OCs. The former, 17β oestradiol is the major oestrogen endogenously produced in the ovaries during the fertile period, whereas oestetrol is only produced during pregnancy. While there seems to be evidence of a lower impact on thrombotic risk markers, these changes are small, albeit pursuing the accepted consensus idea of least changed compared to pre-treatment values as being the gold standard for new hormonal products [9]. Given the rarity of thrombosis, the performed studies are thus promising and have led to marketing approval, but are still insufficient to demonstrate whether these new products are safer than existing EE pills.

Risk factors

Length of use

It is now generally accepted that the risk of VTE in users of OCs decreases with length of use. There is a marked increased risk in thrombosis during the first year of use with the odds ratio as high as 12 reported for the first 3 months of use ('the starter effect'). Comparisons of the thrombosis risks between different hormonal contraceptives must therefore account for length of use and ensure that new users of one agent are truly being compared to new users of another agent. With time, the risk of thrombosis decreases, but always remains higher than non-users. This risk disappears during the first months after stopping the pill.

Age

The risk of VTE is strongly associated with age, with thrombosis rates doubling between the ages of 20 and 40. Most recent studies have clearly demonstrated age as an additional thrombotic risk factor with pill use [9]. In women under 30 years of age the increase in thrombosis rate with pill use is 2–4 per 10 000 user-years (absolute increase of 1.5 per 10 000 user-years), but in the 30–40 age group the risk rises from 2 to 6 per 10 000 user-years (absolute increase of 8 per 10 000 user-years). It is notable that most studies look at women 20–35 years of age and the risk of thrombosis tends to be higher in women older than 35 years. Thus, due to an increase in baseline risk of thrombosis in older women and an increasing number of women in the elder group of reproductive age using combined hormonal contraceptives, the number of thromboses attributed to oestrogen increases. It needs to be remembered that age is also a risk factor for pregnancy-induced thrombosis and other complications. Mortality among women 40 years of age or older is five times that of women between 25 and 29 years of age.

Obesity

The world is experiencing an obesity pandemic, with rates of obesity (body mass index (BMI) > 25 kg/m^2) rising for more than two decades. Although obesity has been suggested to be a risk factor for fatal pulmonary embolism, its role as an independent risk factor has only recently been established in a systematic review [10]. Investigations that reported an increased risk because of obesity have been criticized because they failed to control for hospital confinement or other risk factors, and although high proportions of patients with VTE disease have been found to be obese the importance of the association is diminished because of the high proportion of obesity in the general population. To date, however, there is notable and consistent evidence of an association of obesity with venous thrombosis, more so in women compared to men. The risk appears to be at least double that for normal weight subjects (BMI 20–24.9 kg/m^2) [11]. Obviously this is of importance for users of combined hormonal contraception. Obese women are at similar risk of unintended pregnancy as normal weight women, but unfortunately there is little data establishing a link between contraceptive use, its attendant risks of complications and obesity because most studies, in particular on hormonal contraception, have excluded overweight women. The risk of VTE may be additive when using a combined hormonal method, and with the continuous and global rise in obesity this interaction with combined hormonal contraception will become a more prevalent risk issue.

Thrombophilia

Thrombophilia is a term used to describe a group of conditions in which there is an increased tendency, often repeated and over an extended period of time, for excessive clotting. These include inherited conditions, based on a demonstrated genetic mutation such as factor V Leiden, protein C and S deficiencies, antithrombin deficiency and prothrombin 20210A mutations (which may be suspected on family history). There are also acquired conditions such as lupus anticoagulant or antiphospholipid antibody syndrome, which can occur alone as a manifestation of an autoimmune disorder or as part of a syndrome such as systemic lupus erythematosus. The presence of an inherited thrombophilia is a major modifier of thrombosis risk in users of combined hormonal contraception. Therefore, WHO recommendations state that OC use in women with thrombophilic mutations is associated with an unacceptable health risk. These recommendations are mainly based on case-control studies reporting increased relative risks of venous thrombosis during OC use in women with hereditary thrombophilic defects [12]. However, to qualify all hereditary thrombophilic defects as similarly strong risk factors might be questioned. The absolute risk of venous thrombosis in factor V Leiden heterozygous carriers is estimated at being 0.15 per 100 person-years, whereas in antithrombin, protein C or protein S-deficient persons these estimates range from 0.7 to 1.7 per 100 person-years, indicating a considerably higher degree of risk. One study showed yearly thrombosis rates of 2, 7 and 5% per year respectively in patients with protein S, protein C and antithrombin deficiency [13]. This risk increase has led to questions regarding the need to screen young women for thrombophilia prior to OC use. However, in the absence of a clear family history of venous thrombosis, i.e., in the general population, the number needed to be tested to withhold OCs in carriers and to prevent a single death from pulmonary embolism would exceed half a million. Consequently the number women who will be denied effective contraception is of concern. Screening should therefore be considered only in women with a family history of venous thrombosis (at least one first-degree relative).

Women with a personal history of venous thrombosis

There is consensus that combined OCs should not be prescribed to women with a history of venous thrombosis. Whilst no randomized trials of this issue have been conducted in contraceptive users, women with a history of previous thrombosis were randomized to hormone replacement therapy (HRT) versus placebo; this trial was stopped due to a rate of thrombosis of 8.5% per year in the oestrogen arm versus only 1% in the placebo arm [14]. Also indirect evidence for an adverse effect exists: venous thrombosis that occurred during combined OC use is less likely to recur when the OCs were stopped. In a prospective study of 272 women after a first episode of venous thrombosis, the recurrence rate was 1.3% per person-year in women who did not use OCs, as compared with approximately 3% per year in those who used OCs at some point during follow-up. There was no apparent difference between women who used OCs at the time of their first venous thrombosis event and those who did not [15]. It is noteworthy that there is no indication to immediately discontinue OCs in women who are diagnosed with venous thrombosis. Anticoagulants effectively prevent the extension and recurrence of venous thrombosis, whereas effective contraception is crucial while women are using vitamin K antagonists, because these agents may lead to warfarin embryopathy. Thus, OCs may be continued until shortly before discontinuation of anticoagulant therapy.

Biological mechanism of oestrogen-induced thrombosis risk

Oestrogens have many different effects on haemostasis, lipids and inflammatory risk markers. The changes in the coagulation system include increases in the levels of procoagulant factors VII, X, XII and XIII and reductions in the anticoagulant factors protein S and antithrombin. These changes predict a change toward a more procoagulant state which is confirmed in studies examining global tests, such as activated protein C (APC) resistance or global coagulation capacity measured with the thrombin generation test (TGT). With increased levels of coagulation factors VII, IX, X, XII and XIII and reduced levels of the natural anticoagulants protein S and antithrombin, the overall effect is a prothrombotic shift in the haemostatic

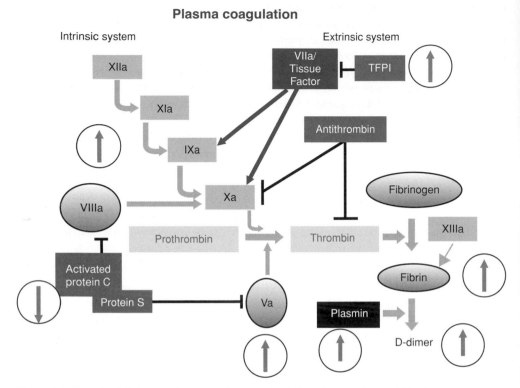

Figure 6.2 Thrombophilic impact of oestrogen hormone. (TFPI, tissue factor pathway inhibitor.)

balance [16] (Figure 6.2). Epidemiological studies have shown that high levels of many of these factors are thrombotic risk factors. It is currently unclear how these effects are brought about at the molecular level of the oestrogen receptor. It is likely that these effects at the cellular level are also under genetic control which translates to the described thrombophilia conditions above, and therefore some women appear to be more sensitive to the effect of oestrogens than other women. The oestrogen-induced changes in fibrinolysis are less straightforward. Oestrogen use enhances the fibrinolytic activity in plasma. The main enzyme in fibrinolysis, plasmin, dissolves the fibrin clot, producing fibrin degradation products such as D-dimers (Figure 6.2). Levels of plasminogen-activator inhibitor 1 (PAI-1) are decreased while tissue plasminogen activator tPA increases. The decreased concentration and activity of PAI-1 and the increased plasma levels of tPA and plasminogen during the use are, however, at least partially counteracted by elevated thrombin-activatable fibrinolysis inhibitor (TAFI). It is, however, not clear whether the effects of OC on fibrinolysis parameters have clinical implications, since there is no firm evidence that changes in the fibrinolytic system affect the risk of venous thrombosis. The haemostatic effects are due to oestrogen effects on liver synthesis of these proteins. For EE this is due to direct chemical action on the liver rather than a first-pass effect, which is seen for oestradiol. Several tests have been proposed as surrogate markers of thrombotic risk. As mentioned, a correlation has been demonstrated between the risk of venous thrombosis and APC resistance determined with the thrombin generation-based assay. Prothrombin, protein S and tissue factor pathway inhibitor (TFPI) are considered to be the major determinants of the thrombin generation-based APC resistance test. The plasma levels of these proteins are affected by hormonal contraceptive use, which might account for increased APC resistance. The changes in the APC resistance during hormonal contraceptive use correlate remarkably well with the changes in the levels of sex hormone-binding globulin (SHBG), suggesting that contraceptives with higher 'total oestrogenicity' cause more pronounced changes in the APC resistance, which may explain their higher risk of venous thrombosis. Moreover, changes in the SHBG levels have been shown to be positively associated with the hormone-induced increase of the venous thrombosis risk [17]. Therefore, although not directly related to the haemostatic system, plasma SHBG levels were proposed as a surrogate marker for the venous thrombosis risk in users of hormonal contraceptives although some discrepancy exists [18]. Apart from these tests we have also looked at factor VII-activating protease (FSAP), which is a plasma serine protease with potential roles in the regulation of coagulation and fibrinolysis, and therefore with an association to both venous and arterial thrombosis formation. A similar impact on FSAP activity and antigen levels was detected with combined OCs containing from 20 to 50 μg EE [19]. However, like any surrogate endpoints, it is not clear how these laboratory markers correlate absolute thrombotic risk with clinical use of oestrogen, and to date these markers have not been prospectively verified.

Conclusion

The oestrogen content in combined hormonal contraception is linked to increased risk of thrombotic events. Prospective observational studies have shown that all currently marketed combined OCs increase the risk of venous thrombosis 2 to 6-fold, and that this risk is highest in the first year of use with a regression thereafter. Oestrogen is therefore the most common risk factor for venous thrombosis in young women, but nowhere is the concept of absolute versus relative risk as important as in advising patients about the risk of thrombosis with oestrogen use. Whilst for an 18 year old a 3-fold risk may appear concerning, the additional risk of thrombosis is 1 per 2000 users per year. The currently marketed preparations seem to carry no increased risk of arterial thrombosis in healthy women. Another important point is that pregnancy is a far more profound thrombophilia risk. In the absence of reliable contraception, women of reproductive age face risks of VTE associated with pregnancy of up to 29 per 10 000 woman-years and in the immediate postpartum period this risk is as high as 300–400 per 10 000 woman-years and the death rate from thrombosis in the 1–4 per 100 000 women-years. Overall, combined hormonal contraception includes some of the most tested and safe preparations available. In women with a history of thrombosis, oestrogen should not be used unless the woman is to remain on anticoagulation. In anticoagulated women, the anticoagulant blunts any prothrombotic effect of the combined hormonal contraception, and the oestrogen offers the advantages of a reduction in menstrual blood loss and protection from a high risk pregnancy. Future research should strive to reduce the venous thrombosis rate further. Clinical prediction models for incident thrombosis should be developed on the basis of clinical variables (age, BMI, smoking, family history, etc.) or clinical variables plus screening for genetic thrombophilia defects in women with a positive family history. Each of the thrombophilia tests should be subjected to a cost-effectiveness analysis. In addition, the value of the proposed biochemical markers of VTE in OC users (APC resistance, SHBG, etc.) must be assessed in large clinical studies, and the assays need to be standardized by international consensus.

References

1. World Health Organization. Cardiovascular disease and steroid hormone contraception. Report of a WHO Scientific Group. *World Health Organ Tech Rep Ser* 1998; 877: 1–89.
2. Jordan WM. Pulmonary embolism. *Lancet* 1961; 2: 1146–7.
3. Boyce EJ, Fawcett JW, Noall EW. Coronary thrombosis and Conovide. *Lancet* 1963; 1: 111.
4. ESHRE Capri Workshop Group. Hormones and cardiovascular health in women. *Hum Reprod Update* 2006; 12: 483–97.
5. WHO Collaborative Study of Cardiovascular Disease and Steroid Hormone Contraception. Acute myocardial infarction and combined oral contraceptives: results of an international multicentre case-control study. *Lancet* 1997; 349: 1202–9.
6. Rosendaal FR, Van Hylckama Vlieg A, Tanis BC, Helmerhorst FM. Estrogens, progestogens and thrombosis. *J Thromb Haemost* 2003; 1: 1371–80.
7. van den Bosch MA, Kemmeren JM, Tanis BC, et al. The RATIO study: oral contraceptives and the risk of peripheral arterial disease in young women. *J Thromb Haemost* 2003; 1(3): 439–44.
8. Lidegaard Ø, Nielsen LH, Skovlund CW, Skjeldestad FE, Løkkegaard E. Risk of venous thromboembolism from use of oral contraceptives containing different progestogens and oestrogen doses: Danish cohort study, 2001–9. *BMJ* 2011; 343: d6423.
9. Sex steroids and changes in the cardiovascular system. In Oral contraceptives and cardiovascular diseases. From Myths to Realities, *Gynecol Endocrinol* 1996; 10 (Suppl 2): 71–2.
10. Ageno W, Becattini, C, Brighton T, Selby S, Kamphuisen PW. Cardiovascular risk factors and venous thromboembolism: a meta-analysis. *Circulation* 2008; 117: 93–102.
11. Alman-Farinelli MA. Obesity and venous thrombosis: a review. *Semin Thromb Hemost* 2011; 8: 903–7.
12. Department of Reproductive Health, World Health Organization. *Medical Eligibility Criteria for Contraceptive Use*, 4th edn. Geneva, Switzerland: World Health Organization, 2009. http://whqlibdoc. who.int/publications/2010/ 9789241563888_eng.pdf (accessed 27 February 2013).
13. de Groot AN, van Dongen PW, Vree TB, Eskes TK. Oral administration of methylergometrine shows a late and unpredictable effect on the non-pregnant human menstruating uterus. *Eur J Obstet Gynecol Reprod Biol* 1995; 60: 101–7.
14. Hoibraaten E, Qvigstad E, Arnesen H, et al. Increased risk of recurrent venous thromboembolism during hormone replacement therapy. Results of the randomized, double-blind, placebo-controlled estrogen in venous thromboembolism trial (EVTET). *Thromb Haemost* 2000; 84: 961–7.
15. Christiansen SC, Cannegieter SC, Koster T, Vandenbroucke JP, Rosendaal FR. Thrombophilia, clinical factors, and recurrent venous thrombotic events. *JAMA* 2005; 19: 2352–61.
16. Reitsma PH, Versteeg HH, Middeldorp S. Mechanistic view of risk factors for venous thromboembolism. *Arterioscler Thromb Vasc Biol* 2012; 32: 563–68.
17. Odlind V, Milsom I, Persson I, et al. Can changes in sex hormone binding globulin predict the risk of venous thromboembolism with combined oral contraceptive pills? *Acta Obstet Gynecol Scand* 2002; 81: 482–90.
18. Kluft C, Skouby SO, Jespersen J, Burggraaf J. Sex hormone-binding globulin as a marker for the thrombotic risk of hormonal contraceptives: a rebuttal. *J Thromb Haemost* 2013; 11: 394–5.
19. Sidelmann JJ, Skouby SO, Kluft C, et al. Plasma factor VII-activating protease is increased by oral contraceptives and induces factor VII activation in-vivo. *Thromb Res* 2011; 128: e67–72.

Progestogens used in contraceptives

Susanna Hall and Ailsa E. Gebbie

Progestogens in contraceptive usage

Progestogens are a class of steroid hormones, which like all major steroid hormones, originate from the cholesterol molecule and are characterized biochemically by a C-21 carbon skeleton (Figure 7.1). They are derivatives of progesterone, the hormone that maintains pregnancy and regulates the normal menstrual cycle. Synthetic derivatives of progesterone are variously known as progestogens, progestagens or progestins and have a key role in hormonal contraception, either alone or in combination with oestrogen.

The knowledge that progesterone inhibited ovulation led to pioneering biochemical work in the 1940s and 1950s to manufacture potent orally acting progestogens to help menstrual problems. The natural extension and breakthrough with this work was the development of hormonal contraception, and the first oral contraceptive pill containing the progestogen norethynodrel in combination with an oestrogen was approved for use in the USA in 1960.

Types of progestogen

Progestogens are usually rather loosely described in terms of groups or 'generations' related to their biochemical characteristics and the natural history of their development (Table 7.1). Not all progestogens fit neatly into this classification. Progestogens will have different generic and trade names in different countries.

Third-generation progestogens

The newer third-generation progestogens were developed in the 1980s in an attempt to reduce cardiovascular risk with combined oral contraception. These progestogens have less affinity for the androgen receptor and therefore a more favourable effect on lipid profile. It has been difficult to establish an evidence base that combined oral contraception containing third-generation progestogens is safer in respect of cardiovascular disease because the overall risk of arterial disease in young women is so low. It was a major surprise in 1995 when four well-designed studies showed a doubling of risk of venous thromboembolism (VTE) in users of combined pills containing third-generation progestogens, compared to those containing second generation. There has been extensive debate on the significance of this finding, but there is general agreement that any difference in VTE risk is probably very small and all combined pills can be prescribed as first line.

Contraception, eds Paula Briggs, Gabor Kovacs and John Guillebaud. Published by Cambridge University Press. © Cambridge University Press 2013.

Table 7.1 Classification of progestogens.

	Progestogens
First generation	Norethindrone Norethynodrel Ethynodiol diacetate
Second generation	Levonorgestrel Norgestrel Norethisterone
Third generation	Gestodene Desogestrel Norgestimate
Fourth generation	Dienogest Drospirenone Nesterone Nomegestrol Trimegestone

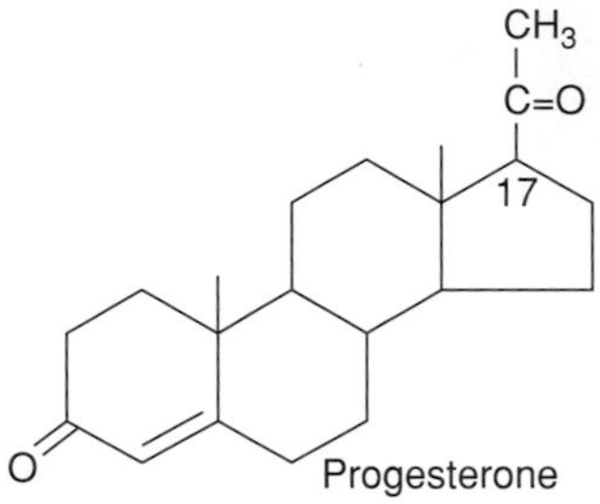

Figure 7.1 Progesterone molecule.

Fourth-generation progestogens

Recently, other novel progestogens are being used in contraception (fourth generation) and, although they may appear to have biochemical advantages, it is difficult to translate that into a definite clinical benefit for women. Anecdotally, women may feel that a particular preparation suits them well and if this prescription is continued then good compliance is likely. In general, third or fourth-generation progestogens are less androgenic and can be helpful for women with acne, greasy skin and mood symptoms.

Cyproterone acetate

Cyproterone is classified as an anti-androgen, but has weak progestogenic activity. It is combined in low dose with oestrogen in a preparation, which is both a contraceptive and effective for the treatment of symptoms of hyperandrogenism, e.g., polycystic ovarian syndrome and severe acne. The regulatory authorities in some countries suggest use of preparations containing cyproterone is limited in duration because of a potentially higher risk of VTE; once the symptoms of hyperandrogenism have resolved, the woman may consider changing to a more conventional combined hormonal contraceptive preparation.

Anti-progestogens

Drugs have been developed which antagonize or suppress the actions of progesterone. Currently anti-progestogens are licensed for use in emergency contraception, abortion and gynaecology. There are also exciting prospects for using anti-progestogens as hormonal contraception.

Progestogen-only contraceptive methods

Progestogen-only methods of contraception include pills, subdermal implants, injectables and the intrauterine system. They vary in dosage and potency but share many common features in terms of safety profile and side effects. Table 7.2 gives the relative failure rates of the progestogen-only methods [1, 2].

Table 7.2 Efficacy of progestogen-only contraception [1, 2].

Type of progestogen-only method	Efficacy
Progestogen-only pill	Variable depending on compliance 0.3–8.0 per 100 women-years Lower failure rate in women > 40 years
Progestogen-only subdermal implant (Nexplanon®)	Not user dependent Fewer than 1 per 1000 pregnancies over 3 years use (none in clinical trials)
Progestogen-only injectable	If administered at the correct time interval, fewer than 4 per 1000 pregnancies over 2 years
Progestogen-releasing intrauterine system	Not user dependent Failure rate 1–2 per 1000 users per year of use

In general progestogen-only methods are extremely safe. However, all women wishing to start a progestogen-only method should have their medical history taken in order to identify any conditions that would contraindicate or caution their use. The World Health Organization Medical Eligibility Criteria for Contraceptive Use (WHOMEC) are evidence-based recommendations on the appropriateness of contraceptive prescription, without imposing unnecessary restrictions [3]. There are relatively very few WHOMEC 3 and 4 conditions (which represent situations where there is unacceptable risk from the contraceptive method) for progestogen-only methods and these are summarized in Table 7.3. Individual countries often adapt WHOMEC for their own particular requirements and evidence base.

The non-oral methods of progestogen-only contraception, along with copper intrauterine devices, are classified as long-acting reversible contraception (LARC). These are methods of contraception that require administration less than once per cycle or month, and have very low failure rates as they are not user dependent. In view of this and their cost effectiveness compared to oral methods at one year, it is suggested that women should be offered a choice that includes all LARC methods when starting contraception [1].

Progestogen-only pills

There are two main groups of progestogen-only pills (POPs). Pills containing 'traditional' progestogens include levonorgestrel and norethisterone preparations, and pills containing the 'newer generation' of progestogen, desogestrel (Cerazette®). Traditional POPs exert their main effect on cervical mucus, making it more viscous and therefore impenetrable to sperm. This effect is quick to be initiated, and quick to dissipate, necessitating very regular pill taking. To a lesser extent, POPs exert their effects on the endometrium, which prevents implantation. The main mechanism of action of the desogestrel POP is to disrupt the luteinizing hormone (LH) surge and prevent ovulation in addition to similar effects on cervical mucus and the endometrium.

Benefits

1. Everyday preparations are easier for some women to remember than preparations with a pill-free interval (combined oral contraception). There is a shorter time interval to re-initiate contraceptive cover should there be a missed pill (two versus seven days for combined hormonal preparations).

Table 7.3 Conditions that attract a WHOMEC category 3 or 4 classification [3].

Condition	WHOMEC category			
	POP	Progestogen-only subdermal implant	Progestogen-only injectable	Progestogen-releasing IUS
Pregnancy				4
Breastfeeding < 6 weeks postpartum	3	3	3	
Postpartum: < 48 hours including insertion immediately after delivery of the placenta and breast feeding				3
> 48 hours–< 4 weeks				3
Puerperal sepsis				4
Immediately post-septic abortion				4
Multiple risk factors for cardiovascular disease including older age, smoking, diabetes, hypertension and obesity			3	
Hypertension Systolic > 160 mmHg or diastolic > 100 mmHg or			3	
Vascular disease			3	
Acute DVT/PE	3	3	3	
Current history of IHD	3 (continuation only)	3 (continuation only)	3	3 (continuation only)
Stroke including history of cerebrovascular accidents and TIA	3 (continuation only)	3 (continuation only)	3	
SLE with positive or unknown antiphospholipid antibodies	3	3	3 (plus with severe thrombocytopenia)	3
Migraine with aura at any age	3 (continuation only)	3 (continuation only)	3 (continuation only)	3 (continuation only)
Unexplained vaginal bleeding		3	3	4 (initiation only)
Gestational trophoblastic disease with decreasing or undetectable β-hCG; persistently raised β–hCG or malignant disease				3 4
Current breast cancer	4	4	4	4
Breast cancer in the past where there has been no evidence of current disease for 5 years	3	3	3	3
Diabetes with nephropathy, neuropathy or retinopathy; or other vascular disease or diabetes of > 20 years duration	2	2	3	

Table 7.3 (cont.)

Condition	POP	WHOMEC category		
		Progestogen-only subdermal implant	Progestogen-only injectable	Progestogen-releasing IUS
Cirrhosis (severe decompensated disease)	3	3	3	3
Liver tumours: hepatocellular adenoma (benign) or hepatoma (malignant)	3	3	3	3
Cervical cancer (awaiting treatment)				4 (initiation only)
Endometrial cancer				4 (initiation only)
Ovarian cancer				3 (initiation only)
Uterine fibroids with distortion of the uterine cavity				4
Anatomical abnormalities that distort the uterine cavity in a manner that is incompatible with IUD insertion				4
Current PID				4 (initiation only)
Current purulent cervicitis or chlamydial infection or gonorrhoea				4 (initiation only)
Known pelvic tuberculosis				4 (initiation) 3 (continuation)

β-hCG, beta human chorionic gonadotrophin; DVT, deep vein thrombosis; IHD, ischaemic heart disease; IUD, intrauterine device; IUS, intrauterine system; PE, pulmonary embolism; PID, pelvic inflammatory disease; POP, progestogen-only pill; SLE; systemic lupus erythematosus; TIA, transient ischaemic attack; WHOMEC, World Health Organization Medical Eligibility Criteria for Contraceptive Use.
Note: Initiation = starting a method of contraception by a woman with a specific medical condition.
Note: Continuation = Continuation of a method already being used by a woman who develops a new medical condition.

2. Oestrogen free and therefore avoids oestrogen-associated risks, including VTE, cardiovascular and cerebrovascular risks. There are very few women who are not eligible for POP.
3. Suitable for immediate start regimes ('Quick Starting') or using as a 'bridging' method of contraception.
4. Twenty per cent of women have amenorrhoea, which is perceived by many as a benefit [2].
5. The desogestrel POP inhibits ovulation so may be useful in the management of other gynaecological conditions including endometriosis and premenstrual symptoms.
6. Progestogen-only pills can be used during breastfeeding, and there is no effect on the quality or quantity of breast milk and no effect on infant growth [2].

Safety concerns and medical eligibility for prescribing

See Table 7.3 for WHOMEC 3 and 4 contraindications for progestogen-only pills. Although evidence is limited, it appears that there is little or no increased risk of VTE, stroke or myocardial infarction from taking POPs, and there does not appear to be a causal relationship with breast cancer (see Chapter 15).

Drug interactions

Enzyme-inducing drugs interact with POPs reducing their contraceptive efficacy. This includes ritonavir-boosted protease inhibitors for human immunodeficiency virus (HIV) treatment, enzyme-inducing anticonvulsants and enzyme-inducing antibiotics including rifampicin and rifabutin. An alternative method should be advised if the drug is likely to be used long term. Women on a short course of enzyme-inducing drugs should be advised to use condoms in addition to the pill while taking treatment and to continue for 28 days after stopping the enzyme inducer.

How is the method used?

Progestogen-only pills are taken every day and women should be advised to take the pill at the same time, i.e., every 24 hours. Pill taking instructions should be backed up with appropriate written information [4]. Traditional POPs have a narrow 'window' in which the pill should be taken and should this be extended longer than 27 hours from the previous pill, (i.e., > 3 hours late), missed pill rules apply (Box 7.1). The desogestrel POP maintains its ability to inhibit ovulation if taken up to 36 hours from the previous pill (i.e., no longer than 12 hours late), and missed pill rules apply if the pill is taken at a greater interval than this.

Some countries used to recommend double dose POP if the woman weighed greater than 70 kg. This practice was not evidence-based and is no longer recommended.

Box 7.1 Missed pill rules for POPs

If you are more than 3 hours late (12 hours if you are taking the POP, Cerazette®):

- Take a pill as soon as you remember. If you have missed more than one, only take one
- Take your next pill at the usual time. This may mean taking two pills in one day. This is not harmful
- You are not protected against pregnancy. Continue to take your pills as usual, but use an additional method of contraception, such as condoms, for the next two days
- You may need to consider emergency contraception

Initiation of contraception

The POP can be initiated up to and including day 5 of the menstrual cycle without the need for additional contraceptive precautions.

The POP may also be started at any other time during the menstrual cycle if the clinician is 'reasonably certain' that the woman is not pregnant (known as 'Quick Starting') [5]. In this situation, 48 hours are required for the pill to become effective for contraception. If there has been a potential risk of conception, an assessment should be made for the need for emergency contraception, and if the woman is likely to continue to be at risk of pregnancy or has expressed a preference to initiate contraception without delay then the POP can be started immediately. 'Quick Starting' is outside the product licence of individual preparations.

The POP can also be useful to consider as a 'bridging' method of contraception; that is, providing contraception immediately when the desired method is either unavailable or would not be suitable until pregnancy can be reliably excluded.

Common side effects

Potential hormonal side effects of the POP include weight changes, headaches and mood changes. Women can be informed that there is no causal relationship between weight changes or headaches and the POP. Mood changes can occur with the POP, but there is no causal relationship with depression [2].

Altered bleeding patterns are the most common reason for discontinuation of the POP, with 10–25% of women discontinuing within 1 year. Approximately 40% of women will bleed regularly, 40% will have erratic bleeding and 20% will be amenorrhoeic [2].

Progestogen-only implants

There are several different types of subdermal implant licensed for contraceptive use across the world. The old six-rod system Norplant® has largely been superseded. The Nexplanon® implant contains etonogestrel (replacing the Implanon® device) and is the most widely available subdermal contraceptive implant. Other progestogen-only contraceptive implants are licensed or being developed and include Jadelle®, a two-rod implant containing levonorgestrel, and Capronor™, a biodegradable single-rod implant also containing levonorgestrel.

Nexplanon® is a single radio-opaque rod measuring 40 mm × 2 mm, made of an ethylene vinylacetate copolymer which allows for controlled release of 68 mg of etonogestrel (bio-equivalent to Implanon®). It is licensed for use for three years and its main mode of action is inhibition of ovulation. It also has an effect on cervical mucus, preventing sperm penetration, which helps maintain its very high efficacy levels. Efficacy does not appear to be affected by weight [6]. Nexplanon® has radio-opaque properties that allow for easy identification of the deep or non-palpable implant on X-ray in contrast to its predecessor, Implanon® which was not radio-opaque. Following removal of the implant, etonogestrel concentrations are usually undetectable by 10 days (mean 6 days), with ovulation returning to 94% of women within 3 weeks [6].

Jadelle® consists of two silicone rods containing a total of 150 mg of levonorgestrel and is licensed for contraceptive use for 5 years. It replaced Norplant®, which was withdrawn around 2002. Jadelle® primarily works by thickening the cervical mucus, preventing sperm penetration as well as causing endometrial changes preventing implantation. There is an effect on ovulation, though this changes with time (90% of cycles are anovulatory in year 1 changing to only 50% by year 5) [1]. The cumulative pregnancy rate at 3 years is 0.3% and 1.1% at 5 years for Jadelle®. Jadelle® is not available in the UK.

Benefits

1. Highly effective (more effective than female sterilization)
2. Does not have a user failure rate
3. Nexplanon® lasts for three years; Jadelle® lasts for five years

4. As this is an oestrogen-free method, there are no significant concerns about the risk of VTE, stroke or myocardial infarction.
5. Around 20% of women have amenorrhoea, which is perceived by many as a benefit.
6. In common with other methods of contraception whose mechanism of action is inhibition of ovulation, the implant may be used to treat some gynaecological conditions.

Safety concerns and medical eligibility for prescribing

See Table 7.3 for WHOMEC 3 and 4 conditions for progestogen-only implants. Although there is very little specific evidence, it seems reasonable to extrapolate from data on other low dose progestogen-only methods, that there is likely to be no significant increased risk of VTE, stroke or myocardial infarction from using progestogen-only implants. There do not appear to be concerns about bone mineral density associated with use of implants [6].

Drug interactions

The contraceptive efficacy of the etonorgestrel-releasing implant is reduced by liver enzyme-inducing drugs, including ritonavir-boosted protease inhibitors for HIV treatment, enzyme-inducing anticonvulsants and enzyme-inducing antibiotics including rifampicin and rifabutin. Women using enzyme-inducing drugs for short-term treatment who wish to continue to use the implant should be advised to use additional contraceptive precautions (e.g., condoms) during treatment and for 28 days after stopping treatment. If the woman needs to remain on enzyme-inducing drugs long term, an alternative method of contraception should be used.

How is the method used?

Nexplanon® can be inserted up to day 5 of the menstrual cycle and is immediately effective (no additional contraception needed). The implant may also be inserted at any other time in the menstrual cycle providing the clinician can be 'reasonably certain' that the woman is not pregnant or if there is a risk of pregnancy, i.e., 'Quick Starting'. In this situation, additional contraception is required for 7 days until the implant provides reliable contraception (e.g., condom use). This should always be considered for women with and without an existing pregnancy risk who will often continue to be at risk of pregnancy [5]. 'Quick Starting' guidance suggests that if a pregnancy is subsequently diagnosed and the woman wishes to continue with the pregnancy, the implant should be removed. The implant may be retained for future contraception if the woman chooses to terminate the pregnancy. Women changing from another hormonal method of contraception can ensure ongoing contraceptive cover by continuing with their previous method for a further 7 days or more.

Health professionals who insert and remove progestogen-only subdermal implants should have training in the correct technique, maintain their competence and regularly update their skills [6].

Insertion and removal of Nexplanon®

Nexplanon® should be inserted subdermally using local anaesthesia in the non-dominant arm. The manufacturer suggests that the implant should be inserted 8–10 cm from the medial epicondyle of the humerus (Figure 7.2). The implant is inserted subdermally using a specially designed applicator (Figure 7.3). After placement of the implant it is recommended that both

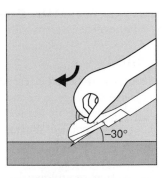

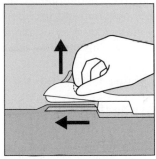

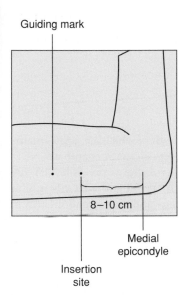

Figure 7.2 Position of subdermal implant in arm.

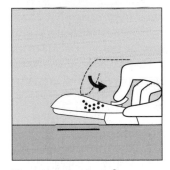

Figure 7.3 Nexplanon® insertion.

the woman and the health professional palpate the implant under the skin to confirm its placement as non-insertions have been described. Bleeding and bruising can be minimized after the procedure by applying a pressure bandage.

Removal of the implant is done with a small amount of local anaesthetic placed under the distal end of the palpable implant. A small incision is then made and the implant may be 'popped-out', or grasped with mosquito forceps. The implant may need to be freed from a fibrous scar capsule prior to removal. Following removal, the incision should be closed and covered. A pressure bandage may help reduce bleeding and bruising. A further implant can be inserted into the same site where an implant has been removed.

Problems associated with removal

Deep and impalpable implants should only be removed by experienced operators. Most experts use high frequency ultrasound imaging to locate the non-palpable implant. The implant is removed using careful blunt dissection [7] or a special technique described where a needle is inserted under the implant with the assistance of real time ultrasound scanning.

Common side effects

Hormonal side effects may be experienced by women using progestogen-only implants. These may include weight change, acne and headache. Women can be informed that there is no evidence of a causal relationship between weight gain or headache and the implant. Acne may improve, occur or worsen with the implant [6].

Changes in bleeding pattern are universal among women who use any progestogen-only implant, with approximately 20% experiencing amenorrhoea and approximately 50% experiencing infrequent, frequent or prolonged bleeding. Around one third of women discontinue using progestogen-only implants because of unscheduled bleeding [6]. As this contributes to the high discontinuation rates of implants (43% at 1 year), women should be provided with information about this potential side effect at the time of initiation of the method and encouraged to return to their healthcare provider if they experience problems. Discontinuation from non-bleeding side effects is less common.

Injectable progestogens

Types and mode of action

The two types of progestogen-only injectable contraception, both of which are LARC methods, are depot-medroxyprogesterone acetate (DMPA) and norethisterone oenanthate (NET-EN). The former, DMPA is much more commonly prescribed across the world while NET-EN only has a licence for short-term use in some countries. Both DMPA and NET-EN inhibit ovulation. They also have secondary effects on cervical mucus and on the endometrium, impairing sperm penetration and preventing implantation.

Benefits

1. Effective and safe method that is not user dependent.
2. Discreet and easy to administer.
3. Most women experience a change in bleeding pattern, with 70% being amenorrhoeic at 1 year of use, which many perceive as a benefit.
4. Progestogen-only injectables inhibit ovulation and suppress ovarian activity, so can be very useful to help gynaecological conditions such as menstrual dysfunction, endometriosis and premenstrual syndrome.
5. Free from oestrogen and avoid oestrogen-related health risks.

Safety concerns

See Table 7.3 for WHOMEC 3 and 4 contraindications for progestogen-only injectables.

Cardiovascular disease

WHOMEC suggests caution with use of progestogen-only injectables where there are several existing risk factors for vascular disease. Use of progestogen-only injectable contraception is not associated with changes in blood pressure or an increased risk of cardiovascular disease, stroke or myocardial infarction [1]. Most evidence suggests that progestogen-only injectables are not associated with an increased risk of VTE [8].

Bone mineral density

Bone mineral density is slightly reduced at all ages in women who use DMPA [1]. This effect is of most concern in adolescents as they have not yet attained their peak bone mass.

Reduction in bone mineral density, however, does not equate to fracture risk or osteoporosis and there is little evidence that use of DMPA translates to an increased fracture risk [1]. Evidence also suggests that bone mineral density recovers when women stop using DMPA.

In many countries, the regulatory authorities have issued guidance on this issue, and in the UK the following advice was issued to healthcare professionals [9].

- In women aged under 18 years, DMPA may be used as first line contraception only after other options have been discussed and considered unsuitable or unacceptable.
- A re-evaluation of the risk and benefits of treatment for all women should be carried out every two years in those who wish to continue use.
- For women with significant lifestyle and/or medical risk factors for osteoporosis other methods of contraception should be considered.

Drug interactions

DMPA is not affected by drug interactions and the dose and delivery intervals do not need to be changed in women taking enzyme-inducing drugs.

How is the method used?

DMPA is given as a dose of 150 mg administered every 12 weeks. NET-EN is given as a dose of 200 mg every 8 weeks. DMPA and NET-EN should both be administered by deep intramuscular injection in the gluteal muscle. Ideally both should be administered in the first five days of the menstrual cycle, when immediate contraceptive effect is achieved. 'Quick Starting' is also acceptable at any time in the menstrual cycle, providing the clinician is reasonably certain that the woman is not pregnant. When initiated outside days 1–5, 7 days of additional precautions should be advised.

Late injection

Repeat injections for DMPA and NET-EN should be planned for 12 and 8 weeks respectively. The evidence suggests that repeat injections can be administered up to 2 weeks late (i.e., up to 14 weeks for DMPA and 10 weeks for NET-EN) whilst maintaining their contraceptive effect [8]. If more than two weeks has passed since the injection is due, the woman should be assessed for her risk of pregnancy and need for emergency contraception. If there is no risk of conception, the injection can be administered and the woman should be advised to use additional contraceptive precautions (e.g., condoms) or abstain for seven days while the contraceptive effect is re-established.

Return of fertility

There is a delay in return to fertility following discontinuation of the progestogen-only injectables, but no evidence of impaired fertility after 18 months when compared to other methods of hormonal contraception.

Common side effects

Changes to bleeding pattern

The majority of women experience a change in their bleeding pattern while using progestogen-only injectables. Bleeding patterns that may be experienced include amenorrhoea, infrequent bleeding and prolonged bleeding. Amenorrhoea is often very acceptable to women and is more common with prolonged use. Seventy per cent of women are amenorrhoeic at 12 months. Unscheduled bleeding is extremely common, particularly after the first injection and practitioners sometimes give the next injection early in this circumstance, though there is no evidence to support this practice.

The most common reasons for discontinuation of the progestogen-only injectables are changes in bleeding pattern and weight gain, with up to 50% discontinuing the method at 1 year in some studies.

Weight gain

There is an association between the use of progestogen-only injectables and weight gain, with evidence suggesting an average gain of 3 kg over 2 years [8]. Evidence also suggests that women with a body mass index (BMI) greater than 30 at initiation of the injection had significantly greater weight gains than those with a BMI less than 25 [8].

Other hormonal side effects

Women may experience other hormonal side effects such as mood changes, changes to libido and headaches. There have been no causal relationships found between these effects and progestogen-only injectables [8].

Progestogen-releasing intrauterine system

Types and mode of action

The most commonly used progestogen-releasing intrauterine system in most countries is the levonorgestrel-releasing intrauterine system (LNG-IUS) known as Mirena® (Figure 7.4). This T-shaped device releases 20 μg of levonorgestrel daily from its medicated stem and is licensed for use for 5 years for contraception [10]. It primarily exerts its contraceptive effect by causing marked endometrial atrophy, resulting in an unfavourable environment for implantation. The levonorgestrel effect on cervical mucus also inhibits sperm transport and contributes to its contraceptive efficacy. There is no reliable effect on ovulation inhibition.

New intrauterine systems are currently in development with smaller frames and lower doses of progestogen. Other progestogen-releasing intrauterine devices have been available; for example, Progestasert®, now withdrawn, and FibroPlant®, a frameless device implanted into the myometrium.

Benefits

1. Safe and highly effective contraception (and a lower rate of ectopic pregnancy than copper-bearing intrauterine devices).
2. Not user dependent
3. Licensed for the treatment of heavy menstrual bleeding and recommended as first line by the National Institute for Health and Clinical Excellence (NICE), with an average 90% reduction in menstrual blood loss.

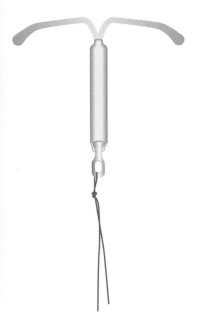

Figure 7.4 Mirena® intrauterine system.

4. Useful for other gynaecological conditions such as endometriosis or premenstrual symptoms.
5. May be used for endometrial protection as the progestogenic arm of hormone replacement therapy (HRT), enabling women to choose the type and dose of oestrogen preparation and often resulting in bleed-free HRT in the peri-menopause (see Chapter 14).

Safety concerns

See Table 7.3 for WHOMEC 3 and 4 contraindications for the IUS. Although there is very little specific evidence, it seems reasonable to extrapolate from data on other low dose progestogen-only methods, that there is likely to be no significant increased risk of VTE, stroke or myocardial infarction from using the IUS [10]. The IUS has limited data on its association with breast cancer, but what exists is reassuring (see Chapter 22).

Other risks are associated with the insertion procedure, and include infection (increased risk in the first 20 days after insertion), expulsion (risk of 1 : 20 insertions, most common in the first few months after insertion) and perforation (a rare risk of 1 : 1000 insertions) [10].

Drug interactions

The contraceptive efficacy of the IUS is not affected by drugs and it does not affect the efficacy or safety of any concomitant medication.

How is the method used?

If an IUS is inserted within the first five days of the menstrual cycle, the contraceptive effect is immediate. Insertion can also take place at other times in the menstrual cycle, providing the healthcare professional is reasonably certain that there is no risk of pregnancy. In this circumstance, women should be advised to use additional contraceptive precautions (e.g., condoms) for seven days. The IUS should not be inserted when there is a risk of pregnancy because it does not have a proven emergency contraceptive effect and the safety of a potent progestogen in close proximity to a developing fetus is uncertain. This contraindicates 'Quick Starting' after emergency contraception.

Women should be advised that there may be a period, on average, of three to six months of irregular bleeding following insertion of an IUS.

It is generally accepted that in women over the age of 45 years an IUS can remain in situ for seven years.

Insertion principles are in common with insertion of all other intrauterine devices and practitioners should have training in the correct technique, maintain their competence and regularly update their skills.

The newest IUS device (Mirena® EvoInserter™) is 4.4 mm diameter wide. This is narrower than the previous applicator. There are no specific contraindications for the use of the IUS in nulliparous women.

Common side effects and reasons for discontinuation

Hormonal side effects may be experienced by IUS users, particularly in the early months after insertion. Breast tenderness is often described and usually decreases with time. Women may experience changes in their skin and acne may develop or worsen.

Altered bleeding patterns and pain are the commonest reasons for discontinuation of the IUS. Persistent irregular bleeding is common, but usually settles with time. Amenorrhoea with an IUS, although welcomed by many women, may not be perceived as a benefit by all, as some may be concerned regarding possible pregnancy. It is extremely important to warn women what to expect and the likely timescale for problems to settle. There are no evidence-based recommended treatments for irregular bleeding.

Tips for clinical practice with progestogen-only contraception

1. Promote progestogen-only LARC methods.
2. Counsel women carefully about potential bleeding patterns before initiating progestogen-only methods. Women who are forewarned are more likely to be accepting of a change in menstrual bleeding pattern.
3. If there is troublesome bleeding in the short term, women can be advised to take a non-steroidal anti-inflammatory drug (NSAID) or use an additional hormonal method unless contraindicated.
4. Consider the possibility of sexually transmitted infections or underlying gynaecological pathology with persistent, new onset or heavy bleeding.

References

1. National Institute for Health and Clinical Excellence. *Long Acting Reversible Contraception*, Clinical Guideline 30, October 2005. http://www.nice.org.uk/nicemedia/live/10974/29909/29909.pdf (accessed 15 October 2012).
2. Faculty of Sexual and Reproductive Healthcare. *Clinical Guidance. Progestogen-only Pills*, November 2008 (updated June 2009). http://www.fsrh.org/pdfs/CEUGuidanceProgestogenOnlyPill09.pdf (accessed 15 October 2012).
3. Department of Reproductive Health, World Health Organization. *Medical Eligibility Criteria for Contraceptive Use*, 4th edn. Geneva, Switzerland: World Health Organization, 2009. http://whqlibdoc.who.〈?PMU?〉int/publications/2010/

9789241563888_eng.pdf (accessed 5 November 2012).

4. FPA. *Your Guide to the Progestogen-only Pill*. Patient information leaflet, 2011. http://www.fpa.org.uk/media/uploads/ helpandadvice/contraception-booklets/ progestogen-only-pill-your-guide.pdf (accessed 20 October 2012).

5. Faculty of Sexual and Reproductive Healthcare. *Clinical Guidance. Quick Starting Contraception*, September 2010. http://www.fsrh.org/pdfs/ CEUGuidanceQuickStartingContraception. pdf (accessed 20 October 2012).

6. Faculty of Sexual and Reproductive Healthcare. *Clinical Guidance Progestogen-only Implants*, April 2008 (updated January 2009). http://www.fsrh. org/pdfs/CEUGuidanceProgestogen OnlyImplantsApril08.pdf (accessed 20 October 2012).

7. Mansour D, Walling M, Glenn D, *et al*. Removal of non-palpable etonorgestrel implants. *J Fam Plann Reprod Health Care* 2008: 34(2); 89–91.

8. Faculty of Sexual and Reproductive Healthcare. *Clinical Guidance. Progestogen-only Injectable Contraception*, November 2008. http://www.fsrh.org/pdfs/CEU GuidanceProgestogenOnlyInjectables09.pdf (accessed 22 October 2012).

9. MHRA. *Updated Guidance on the Use of Depo-Provera Contraception*, 18 November 2004. http://www.mhra.gov.uk/ Safetyinformation/ Safetywarningsalertsandrecalls/ Safetywarningsandmessagesformedicines/ CON1004262 (accessed 4 November 2012).

10. Faculty of Sexual and Reproductive Healthcare. *Clinical Guidance Intrauterine Contraception*, November 2007. http://www. fsrh.org/pdfs/CEUGuidanceIntrauterine ContraceptionNov07.pdf (accessed 22 October 2012).

Chapter

8

The contraceptive consultation

Caroline Harvey, Kathleen McNamee and
Deborah J. Bateson

Introduction

The contraceptive consultation differs across international healthcare systems in relation to the setting, scope of practice, provider-responsibility and the available time frame. The service may range from a straightforward repeat contraceptive pill script for a medically well long-term user to more complex situations which require consideration of multiple factors. These include personal circumstances and preferences, the medical history, access to ongoing services and cost considerations. Contraceptive advice may be provided opportunistically or be part of a planned consultation and the patient may be well informed about her or his options or conversely have minimal or even no prior knowledge.

Despite this variability, the basic principles which should be embedded in any consultation include an evidence-based approach to assessment, advice and service provision and a patient-centred approach to contraceptive choice, regardless of life stage.

Role of the healthcare practitioner

The role of the healthcare practitioner is to take a relevant medical and social history from the patient (Box 8.1). The history underpins the provision of balanced and easily understood contraceptive information to assist the patient in making an individually tailored and safe choice. Providing evidence-based information about the wide range of options at the same time as responding to the patient's individual needs can present a challenge to practitioners. The key to a successful consultation is to ensure that the patient leaves with their contraceptive needs met, either with the immediate provision of a contraceptive method or a plan for initiation at a specified future date. This chapter provides guidance on how to fulfil this outcome.

The patient

In many instances the patient will be an individual woman but couples may present together, or on occasions, men may present alone. Young people may attend the consultation alone, with parents or other significant adults or friends. It is a generally accepted best practice for the young person to be seen alone for at least part of the consultation. This facilitates the practitioner in obtaining an accurate history, ensures that sensitive information is kept private and allows a full assessment of the young person's decision-making competency, psychosocial situation and safety. While couples may prefer to be seen together, the healthcare

Contraception, eds Paula Briggs, Gabor Kovacs and John Guillebaud. Published by Cambridge University Press. © Cambridge University Press 2013.

Box 8.1 A contraceptive consultation framework

- Development of rapport and empathy
- Systematic history-taking in order to set the scene for discussion of medically appropriate contraceptive options (based on application of a MEC framework)
- A flexible approach to either 'narrow down' the range of contraceptive options or 'broaden out' the discussion to include methods that the patient hasn't considered
- Explanation of the evidence-based advantages and disadvantages of selected methods (including LARC methods)
- Explanation of method-related relative risks and side effects in a way that is easily understandable (and which dispels common myths and misunderstandings)
- A flexible approach to method initiation (determining the advantages and disadvantages of an immediate contraceptive start against allowing time for patient to absorb and consider options)
- Information about available emergency contraceptive options
- Advice on 'doubling up' with condoms for those at risk of STIs or those requiring dual contraceptive cover
- Clear directions for follow-up and instructions for 'when things don't go according to plan' such as missed pills or late insertion of a vaginal ring
- Directions to written or web-based information

---

practitioner must be sensitive to issues of coercion or intimate partner violence and consider strategies to see an individual alone if this is suspected. Women with an intellectual disability may be accompanied by family members or carers, unpaid or paid, who may be very important in relation to assisting with communication and facilitating decision making. However, it is important to be aware of the possibility that the family member or carer may have an alternative agenda to the patient, such as the control of menstruation or a desire for sterilization.

The setting

In a generalist setting, posters inviting patients to discuss sexual health issues, brochures on contraception and information on confidentiality may be of assistance in setting the scene for the consultation. Availability of drop in appointments and a same day service for long-acting reversible contraceptive (LARC) methods may assist with timely initiation of methods.

General principles of a consultation

The development of rapport and empathy are crucial to a successful consultation outcome since they allow the practitioner to gain insight into the patient's individual circumstances. The consultation can then be shaped according to the individual's needs. It may include, for example, a discussion about the different LARC methods, directions about how to access emergency contraception or the additional use of condoms to prevent sexually transmitted infections (STIs). The contraceptive consultation can also be an opportune time for health promotion messaging and health screening interventions.

Box 8.2 Important points in history taking

1. Previous pregnancies and outcomes
   - unintended pregnancies and if a contraceptive method was used at the time
2. Previous difficulty with maintaining a regular pill-taking schedule, e.g., shift working
3. Menstrual history
4. Previous gynaecological procedures
5. Risk of STIs
6. Current relationship status
7. Frequency of sex
8. Medical history including
   - factors that increase the risk of coronary artery disease or cerebrovascular disease: migraine with aura, past or family history of stroke, transient ischaemic attack or coronary artery disease, smoking, hypertension, diabetes, lipids
   - factors that increase the risk of deep venous thrombosis (DVT): past or family history of venous thromboembolism, known thrombogenic mutation, immobilization
   - hepatobilary disease
   - hormone-dependent cancer
   - concurrent use of medications
   - lactation
   - smoking
   - conditions that might benefit from the use of hormonal contraception
   - heavy menstrual bleeding
   - dysmenorrhoea
   - acne
9. Plans for future pregnancies
10. Value placed on method efficacy/preventing pregnancy
11. Ability to pay for contraception and attend for repeat visits
12. Need to conceal use of contraception
13. Need to conceal irregular or persistent bleeding
14. Ability to cope with non-scheduled bleeding or amenorrhoea

Consideration of medical contraindications and drug interactions

Given the wide range of contraceptive options, narrowing down the options by consideration of medical contraindications and drug interactions is an important first step. Except for the lactational amenorrhoea method, withdrawal and fertility awareness based methods, which need to be carefully considered due to their high typical use failure rates, all methods of contraception have absolute or relative medical contraindications. Taking a succinct but thorough personal and family medical history is central to an effective consultation (Box 8.2). For example, eliciting information about risk factors for venous and arterial vascular disease is essential during a consultation for an oestrogen-containing method while asking about a latex allergy is important when discussing condom use. It is important to obtain information on the use of liver enzyme-inducing drugs (many of the anti-epileptics) as concurrent use decreases the efficacy of many hormonal methods.

Table 8.1 Definition of MEC categories.*

MEC category	Definition
1	A condition for which there is no restriction for the use of the contraceptive method
2	A condition where the advantages of using the method generally outweigh the theoretical or proven risks
3	A condition where the theoretical or proven risks generally outweigh the advantages of using the method. The provision of a method requires expert clinical judgement and/or referral to a specialist contraceptive provider, since use of the method is not usually recommended unless other more appropriate methods are not available or acceptable
4	A condition which represents an unacceptable risk if the contraceptive method is used

MEC, Medical Eligibility Criteria.
*Adapted from [1].

Medical Eligibility Criteria system

The Medical Eligibility Criteria (MEC) system is a useful internationally recognized tool that allows health professionals to safely match a woman's medical and personal history with her preferred methods of contraception. It was initially developed by the World Health Organization [1] and has been adapted for local use in the UK [2], USA [3] and Australia [4]. Table 8.1 gives a summary of the definition of each MEC category [2].

The risk of pregnancy needs to be balanced against the known or potential risks of the method of contraception. It is important to ensure that women are not denied suitable methods of contraception on the basis of misplaced non-evidence-based concerns. Unnecessary restriction of methods of contraception due to perceived health risks may lead to even greater pregnancy-related risks. The MEC system is a useful way to direct choice for women with either pre-existing or new onset medical conditions. The decision can of course be particularly difficult where the medical risk of both the contraceptive method and pregnancy are high.

A woman's continued medical eligibility to use a method should be considered at each review consultation.

Examination

Most methods of contraception require minimal if any physical examination or investigation [5].

Important information to include in contraceptive consultations

Benefits of LARC methods

The superior efficacy of the LARC methods, including injectables, intrauterine methods and contraceptive implants, is well established [6]. LARC methods are highly effective as a result of their 'fit and forget' technology with minimal user input. They are relatively cost effective compared to shorter acting methods.

Emergency contraception

Information should be given about emergency contraceptive options, including mechanism of action, efficacy and where to access all options if relevant. Emergency contraceptive options include insertion of a copper intrauterine device (IUD), a stat 30 mg oral dose of ulipristal acetate or a stat dose of 1.5 mg levonorgestrel. This is covered in more detail in Chapter 18. Availability, accessibility and cost are highly variable between countries. Advance provision can be appropriate in some circumstances.

Dual protection with condoms

Patients at risk of STIs should be provided with information about 'doubling up' with condoms (either male or female) at the same time as an effective method of contraception to prevent both STIs and unintended pregnancy.

Screening for other conditions

The contraceptive consultation can be a good opportunity for health promotion messaging and opportunistic health screening. Depending on the life-stage and individual context this may include cervical and STI screening, a cardiovascular risk assessment and screening for abuse and intimate partner violence. Whilst it is acknowledged there may be benefit to this additional screening, it is important to weigh this against the risk of diluting the contraceptive message and the risk of the patient perceiving this as intrusive and unwelcome, which may act as a deterrent to ongoing contraceptive care.

Available time: shaping the consultation

Where time is limited, an effective contraception consultation lies in its shaping. The practitioner needs to determine in the first few minutes whether the consultation needs to begin broadly and narrow down or conversely whether it could be broadened out to provide more information than the patient initially requests (Box 8.1). Available time, medical eligibility considerations and whether this is a first or subsequent consultation for a particular method will influence this structure. While there is no strong evidence for the superiority of any one template for a structured consultation over another, following some sort of a framework is important. This needs to give comparative information about available contraceptive methods and should include:

- Method advantages and disadvantages
- Efficacy of the chosen method
- Method-related costs
- Other method specific considerations including when to initiate the method, follow-up required, information for 'when things don't go according to plan' such as when pills are missed or late insertion of a vaginal ring.

Use of additional tools

There are a variety of tools ranging from websites to models that can be useful to support a contraceptive consultation (Box 8.3).

The following cases illustrate approaches and principles in a sample of contraceptive consultations across the reproductive lifespan. While the consultation focus differs, the basic principles remain the same for patients of all ages.

Box 8.3 Contraceptive consultations: additional tools

- Computer prompts
- Checklists
- Assessment tools, e.g., HEADSS
- Demonstration devices, models and pill swatches
- Written information with appropriate literacy and language
- Websites
- 'Motivational' interviewing skills
- Self-assessment online resources

Case scenario 1: Mandy

Mandy is 15 years old and presents requesting the contraceptive pill. She has been having sex for 3 months with her boyfriend, also aged 15, and they use condoms 'mostly'. Her last menstrual period started about two weeks ago and her last unprotected sex was yesterday. Her menstrual cycles vary in length from four to five weeks. She has no medical conditions or family history of venous thromboembolism (VTE) and is not taking any medications.

You determine that all sexual activity has been consensual and assess her as being a 'mature minor'. She does not want her parents to know of her visit to the clinic. Discussion is broadened to include the benefits of LARC methods; however, Mandy decides to try the combined pill initially while taking home further written information on implants and injectables. The additional use of condoms is reinforced to prevent STIs. Mandy is advised to take the emergency contraceptive pill to reduce the risk of pregnancy. The combined pill is started immediately using the 'Quick Start' method and condoms are supplied.

Issues raised by the consultation

Consent, parental involvement and confidentiality

Most countries allow young women to consent to their own medical treatment and to confidentiality if they are assessed as a 'mature minor'. Using a structured psychosocial assessment tool allows the practitioner to gain insight into the family situation, cognitive development and potential risks in the young person's life. These include the use of alcohol and drugs, a significant age difference compared with the sexual partner and being a child in care [7]. Although it is important to discuss parental involvement with the young woman, she is in the best position to judge whether this is appropriate and generally this should not be a barrier to provision of contraception. Confidentiality is an issue identified as extremely important to young people in their use of health services and requires explicit discussion [8]. In rare situations confidentiality may need to be breached; for example, where child sexual abuse is suspected and therefore one should also discuss the limitations to confidentiality.

Efficacy, access, costs, LARC methods and emergency contraception

Each contraceptive method has a perfect and typical use efficacy rate. The perfect use efficacy reflects the method being used in perfect research type conditions while the typical rate reflects what happens in real life. Mandy's chosen method, the combined pill, is estimated to have a failure rate of 0.3% with perfect use, meaning the pill is taken correctly every day and there is no vomiting, drug interactions or severe diarrhoea to consider. Unfortunately in typical use its failure rate is estimated at 9% in the first year of use [9]. Missed pills, without use of back up contraception, are a common occurrence. In addition there is a need to obtain, and in many countries pay for, ongoing prescriptions.

As a young person, Mandy is likely to be highly fertile. It is important to discuss LARC options. Although their use is encouraged, ultimately it is Mandy's decision as to her preferred method of contraception. Whilst availability of the combined pill is high in most countries, timely access to intrauterine methods and implants might be limited by practitioner availability and costs. Condoms are readily accessible, but young people may fail to access them for a variety of reasons including embarrassment.

It is important to inform Mandy of guidance in the case of missed pills and of the availability of emergency contraceptive options. The levonorgestrel emergency contraception pill is available from pharmacists without a prescription in many, but not all, countries. Barriers vary by country, but include the pharmacist's interpretation of local regulations regarding supply to young people, embarrassment and cost. Ulipristal acetate is becoming increasingly available in many countries and clinical trials suggested that it has a higher efficacy for women who have unprotected sex around the time of ovulation. The copper IUD is the most effective method of emergency contraception, can be inserted up to five days after unprotected sexual intercourse and continued as a long-term method. All women presenting for emergency contraception should have the option of a copper IUD.

Immediate start

Since Mandy had intercourse yesterday, a negative test will not exclude recent conception. However, waiting for her next menstruation could put her at risk of pregnancy in the interim. In addition by the time she next menstruates she may have forgotten the instructions about correct pill start and use. Numerous studies have shown that there are fewer unplanned pregnancies in women using the 'Quick Start' method on the day of the consultation. There is no known risk of teratogenesis if the low dose combined oral contraceptive (COC) pill is taken during early pregnancy. Mandy is given the emergency contraceptive pill (levonorgestrel 1500 μg) and is shown which active pill to start in the pack. She is informed she will not be protected against pregnancy for seven days. A pregnancy test is advised in four weeks time regardless of bleeding [10].

By virtue of her age, Mandy is at high risk of chlamydia infection. You advise her to have a test and recommend using condoms, which will provide the best available protection from STIs.

Case scenario 2: Saidie

Saidie is a 23-year-old student requesting a repeat prescription of her COC pill. She is not currently in a relationship and has had three male partners in the last year. On further questioning she tells you she is quite busy with her studies and ran out of pills three weeks ago. She has not had sex during the last five days. She sometimes forgets to restart her active pills after her placebo break. She likes the pill as it helps her acne and she enjoys the ability to skip periods. She has not developed any new medical conditions and is on no other medication. She remains a non-smoker.

Saidie is at risk of unplanned pregnancy and STIs. You encourage consistent condom use and alternative combined hormonal methods are discussed as an option, but Saidie acknowledges that getting to the pharmacist for an ongoing supply may be difficult. You also discuss the LARC methods including the contraceptive implant, injection, copper IUD and intrauterine system (IUS) using a pictorial chart that compares the typical use efficacy of each method. She decides to try the implant, and is prepared to accept the chance of unscheduled bleeding as the method is rapidly reversible. You inform her that she may not experience the same beneficial effect on her skin with a progestogen-only implant as she did with the COC pill.

Issues raised by the consultation

LARC methods, missed pills and maintaining an ongoing supply

Although Saidie is happily established on COCs, a review is a good opportunity to discuss the more effective LARC methods and alternative delivery routes including the patch and ring. A review needs to include a discussion on missed pills, late patch application, ring insertion or injection and information on how to deal with this. For continuing users who have difficulty maintaining a regular schedule, use of phone apps or reminders may be of assistance. Maintaining a contraceptive supply may be affected by cost, time constraints or other access issues in some countries.

Review of continued medical eligibility for the method

Checking for new risk factors affecting continued medical eligibility or new medications is particularly important for women using combined hormonal methods.

Access

In many countries contraceptive implants and intrauterine devices are inserted in primary care settings and are generally accessible. Even though Saidie is potentially at risk of STIs, the benefits of an IUD or IUS would outweigh the disadvantages. However in some situations access to a skilled inserter can be an issue and may necessitate a referral to another agency, clearly an issue for busy women, like Saidie.

Side effects and reversibility

For Saidie concern about side effects is quite an issue. The ease of insertion of the implant compared to the IUD or IUS, combined with its rapid reversibility compared to depot-medroxyprogesterone acetate (DMPA) makes it an acceptable choice. Although Saidie is not considering a pregnancy in the near future, use of DMPA can be associated with a delay in the return to fertility.

With any hormonal method of contraception, side effects can be problematic and may be difficult to predict. If she changes from the COC to a progestogen-only method, she must understand that she will experience loss of cycle control.

Opportunistic health promotion

The contraceptive consultation can be an opportune time to consider other health issues. You have taken the opportunity to screen for chlamydia. It is important to encourage and motivate Saidie with positive suggestions about the benefits of condom use rather than pointing out her past failings in this regard. Fear of criticism from staff has been identified as a deterrent to young people's attendance at sexual health services [8].

Case scenario 3: Polly

Polly is 37 years old and had her third child 4 months ago. She is fully breastfeeding and remains amenorrhoeic. She is desperate for a 'very effective' method as she could not cope with another child. She has previously used a contraceptive implant which caused unacceptable vaginal bleeding and spotting. As a teenager she used several contraceptive pills, but says that they caused irritability and low libido.

Polly seems anxious during the consultation and reveals that her husband would like another child, but she doesn't. Intrauterine and injectable methods are discussed and after consideration Polly chooses to use DMPA and is given the first injection during the consultation. A cervical smear test is performed as she is overdue for screening.

Issues raised by the consultation

Postnatal assessment and screening for other conditions

The contraceptive consultation is an ideal time to consider postnatal depression. Polly does seem quite stressed, but on screening does not fulfil the criteria for a diagnosis of depression. She reveals she is a little frightened of telling her husband she doesn't want any more children and would like to conceal her use of contraception at least in the short term. Careful questioning reveals he has on occasions hit her, but never their children. She doesn't feel at risk at the moment; however, you give her information on services for victims of partner violence and make it clear you are happy to discuss it with her at any time. In the UK, the recommendation is to refer all cases of domestic violence to social care, but Polly can be reassured that her children will not be taken away from her.

Postnatal contraception

There are some restrictions on the use of hormonal contraception in the postpartum period for women who are breastfeeding, particularly in the first six weeks after childbirth. Polly still fulfils the criteria for using the lactational amenorrhoea method (LAM) as she has not yet had a period, is fully breastfeeding and less than six months post partum. However, her strong desire to avoid a further pregnancy has prompted her to seek out an additional highly effective method. As Polly is fully breastfeeding, combined methods are relatively contraindicated (MEC 3) until six months post partum, so progestogen-only and intrauterine methods are offered.

Side effects and past contraceptive experience

Polly is concerned about use of DMPA because of her previous personal experience of side effects with hormonal contraception. She is particularly concerned about low libido and irritability. You inform her that although these are side effects commonly attributed to the contraceptive pill there is no strong evidence of a causal effect. She is pleased to hear that she has a high chance of amenorrhoea while using DMPA, but is prepared to accept unscheduled bleeding as a possible side effect.

Reversibility

The potential delay in return to fertility with use of DMPA is seen by Polly as a benefit.

Contraceptive effectiveness and concealment

The two key factors influencing Polly's choice of contraception are high efficacy and method privacy/concealment. While COC pills can potentially be hidden and partners may not always be aware of an IUD thread or a subdermal implant, concealment is not guaranteed. Injectable methods provide the greatest degree of privacy for those wishing to conceal contraceptive use.

Case scenario 4: Anya

Anya is 47 years old and presents for a prescription for her regular antihypertensive. In passing she tells you she has recently met a new partner after being single for five years following the break-up of her marriage. Anya has three children, now teenagers. She has a body mass index (BMI) of 32, stopped smoking 6 months ago and has a family history of heart disease. Anya has a history of regular menses and has no peri-menopausal symptoms. She says she and her partner are using condoms some of the time and that her partner is considering having a vasectomy.

Anya previously used a COC pill without any problems and wonders if she should go back on the pill again. You explain that the benefits of using an oestrogen-containing method are outweighed by the risks now that she is in her 40s and has additional risk factors for arterial vascular disease. After a broad discussion about suitable options, Anya remains undecided but takes some written information about emergency contraception, intrauterine methods, implants and vasectomy.

Issues raised by the consultation

Need for contraception

Although Anya's chance of pregnancy after the age of 40 is reduced compared to when she was in her 20s and 30s, you need to advise her that some women continue to be fertile even into their early 50s. Contraception is advised until there is no longer a chance of ovulation, and since Anya continues to menstruate she is at risk of pregnancy. Women aged 50 years no longer require contraception after 12 months of amenorrhoea, while those below the age of 50 are advised to wait for 2 years of amenorrhoea. The natural loss of fertility can be assumed for most women at the age of 55 years.

Method eligibility

The principles of contraceptive choice are the same regardless of age. The woman's medical history as well as her social, cultural and economic factors all need to be considered when choosing her method of contraception. It is important to ask about previous contraceptive experiences including any side effects. Since increasing age itself is an independent risk factor for conditions such as venous and arterial vascular disease, osteoporosis and gynaecological problems, it is essential to take a thorough history for women aged over 40.

Anya has an elevated risk of arterial and venous disease as a result of her family history, elevated BMI, recent smoking and hypertension as well as her age. An oestrogen-containing method is contraindicated and the DMPA injection would generally not be a first choice due to its adverse effect on lipids as well as bone mineral density. Other progestogen-only or non-hormonal methods would all be potentially suitable.

Additional benefits of hormonal contraception at the peri-menopause

Women may experience heightened premenstrual symptoms as well as heavy menstrual bleeding in the peri-menopause. This can be effectively treated with hormonal contraception. All combined hormonal contraceptive options can be used to control heavy menstrual bleeding as well as relieving menopausal symptoms and maintaining bone mineral density. However, methods containing oestrogen are contraindicated for Anya. Oestrogen-containing methods are generally not advised for any woman beyond the age of 50, when the risks outweigh the benefits and switching to a non-hormonal or progestogen-only method should be advised.

Since the risk of serious pathology, including endometrial cancer, is increased in women in their 40s and 50s it is essential to carry out appropriate investigations in order to rule out serious causes in those with heavy menstrual bleeding before initiating treatment. The IUS is a useful first line option for controlling heavy menstrual bleeding during the peri-menopause, while simultaneously providing effective contraception. This is discussed in detail in Chapter 14.

Anya's periods are not heavy and therefore insertion of either a copper IUD or IUS can be considered.

Opportunistic contraception consultations and broadening the options

Anya presented for other reasons and mentioned contraception only in passing. She was not fully aware of her risk of pregnancy and using condoms inconsistently as she believed that she was unlikely to become pregnant in her 40s. She had considered starting the combined pill, but had very little knowledge of intrauterine methods, implants and of the availability and place of emergency contraception. Available time in the consultation was used to consider her medical eligibility and provide information on a broader range of options. While interested in intrauterine methods, Anya indicated that she wanted to do further reading before making a decision. She will talk with her partner about vasectomy again and they will use condoms more consistently. A further appointment is made in two weeks.

Conclusion

While there is no single formula for an effective contraceptive consultation, this chapter illustrates the basic elements that underpin every interaction for the effective provision of contraception. The approach to the consultation, whether it is a brief encounter or a complicated interaction, requires the application of a systematic yet flexible framework. This framework allows the practitioner to combine the arts of listening and empathy with a knowledge-driven evidence-based approach to increase the chance of a successful patient outcome, regardless of life stage.

References

1. Department of Reproductive Health, World Health Organization. *Medical Eligibility Criteria for Contraceptive Use*, 4th edn. Geneva, Switzerland: World Health Organization, 2009. http://whqlibdoc.who.int/publications/2010/9789241563888_eng.pdf (accessed 4 November 2011).
2. Faculty of Sexual and Reproductive Healthcare. *UK Medical Eligibility Criteria for Contraceptive Use*, 2009. http://www.fsrh.org/pdfs/UKMEC2009.pdf (accessed 4 November 2012).
3. Farr S, Folger SG, Paulen M, *et al.* US medical eligibility criteria for contraceptive use, 2010: adapted from the World Health Organization Medical Eligibility Criteria for Contraceptive Use, 4th edition. *MMWR Recomm Rep* 2010; 59(RR-4): 1–86.
4. Bateson D, Harvey C, McNamee K. *Contraception: an Australian clinical practice handbook*, 3rd edn. Brisbane: Family Planning Queensland, 2012.
5. Tepper NK, Curtis KM, Steenland MW, Marchbanks PA. Physical examination prior to initiating hormonal contraception: a systematic review. *Contraception* 2012.08.010 (Epub ahead of print).
6. Winner B, Peipert JF, Zhao Q, *et al.* Effectiveness of long-acting reversible contraception. *N Engl J Med* 2012; 366(21): 1998–2007.
7. Goldenring J, Rosen D. Getting into adolescent heads: an essential update. *Contemp Pediatr* 2004; 21: 64.
8. Baxter S, Blank L, Guillaume L, Squires H, Payne N. Views of contraceptive service

delivery to young people in the UK: a systematic review and thematic synthesis. *J Fam Plann Reprod Health Care* 2011; 37(2): 71–84.

9. Trussell J. Contraceptive failure in the United States. *Contraception* 2011; 83(5): 397–404.

10. Faculty of Sexual and Reproductive Healthcare. *Clinical Guidance. Quick Starting Contraception*, September 2010. http://www.fsrh.org/pdfs/CEUGuidance QuickStartingContraception.pdf (accessed 28 February 2013).

Menarche and associated problems

Mary Hernon and Victoria Sephton

Case scenario: Alex

Alex is referred to the adolescent gynaecology clinic. She is 13 years old and has a history of infrequent but extremely heavy periods. Her menarche was age 9. She is tall for her age and overweight with a body mass index (BMI) of 42. She has acne.

Her mum is also overweight with polycystic ovarian syndrome (PCOS). She had difficulty conceiving and had clomiphene citrate treatment in order to conceive.

Alex is having frequent absences from school when she is bleeding. She is refusing to participate in physical education (PE). This is not helping her to reduce her weight.

Her general practitioner (GP) has tried her with the desogestrel-containing progestogen-only pill (POP) Cerazette®. This has resulted in continuous bleeding.

Alex is now having trouble relating to her peer group and is suffering from low mood. This is having a further detrimental effect on her school attendance.

Introduction

Menarche is the name given to the first menstrual bleed of a young woman. The word comes from the Greek '*men*' meaning moon and '*arkhe*' meaning beginning. This recognizes that subsequent bleeds are cyclical like the four weekly phases of the moon.

Menarche is a milestone in a young woman's life and in many cultures it is marked by special celebration. In other cultures, however, it marks the possibility of fertility. This can result in girls being taken out of school by their parents and entered into child or adolescent marriage, which is associated with higher maternal mortality rates, lower socioeconomic standing and a greater chance of domestic violence.

A review of the qualitative literature on young women's experiences of menarche revealed that menarche had a major impact on lives physically, psychologically, socially and culturally [1]. It showed that preparation for menarche by a knowledgeable person such as a school nurse was beneficial.

Timing of menarche

The stages of puberty were described by Tanner in the 1960s. There are five Tanner stages from pre-pubertal appearance of breasts and pubic hair (stage 1) to adult appearance (stage 5) [2].

Contraception, eds Paula Briggs, Gabor Kovacs and John Guillebaud. Published by Cambridge University Press. © Cambridge University Press 2013.

Subareolar breast bud development is usually the first sign of puberty with a normal age range of 8.8–12.8 years. This is followed around six months later by early pubic hair growth, although one third of girls will get the pubic hair first. Increased growth velocity is usually the next step, but in some girls can precede the early secondary sex characteristics.

Menarche is usually one of the last events of puberty occurring about 6 months after the maximum growth velocity and when breast development is at Tanner stage 3–4 and pubic hair growth is at Tanner stage 4. It is closely related to bone age with 80% of girls reaching menarche at bone age 13–14.

Growth of the uterus takes place at Tanner stage 4 to more than four times its pre-pubertal volume. The length of a pre-pubertal uterus is 2.6–3.0 cm and it is tubular in shape. After puberty the uterus will be 5–8 cm long and it becomes pear shaped [3]. Prior to puberty it is normal to see occasional ovarian follicular cysts of up to 10 mm in diameter. The ovaries start to increase in size at age five with a further increase under hormonal stimulus. There is also an increase in follicular growth at the onset of hormonal stimulus so that the ovary develops a multicystic appearance, which can be confused with the appearances of a polycystic ovary by sonographers not experienced in scanning younger girls. There are no set criteria, but less than 12 follicles with an ovarian volume of up to 10 ml are considered normal [3].

Pubertal development before the age of eight and menarche before the age of nine should be investigated by an endocrinologist [2]. The initial investigations are an X-ray of the wrist for bone age and a pelvic ultrasound scan. It is helpful to order these prior to the appointment. Blood tests for follicle stimulating hormone (FSH), luteinizing hormone (LH), oestradiol, testosterone and androgen profile are required, but may be deferred until the luteinizing hormone-releasing hormone (LHRH) test to avoid multiple venesections. Further scans of the head and adrenal glands may be left to the endocrinologist's discretion.

It is preferable to refer these girls early, as early puberty can be caused by intracranial, adrenal or ovarian tumours and their eventual adult height may be affected if they are not treated. It is noted that it is sometimes difficult to differentiate breast budding from adiposity in obese children.

Premature isolated menarche in the absence of any pubertal development has been reported very rarely [2]. This is a diagnosis of exclusion, which requires a full endocrinological work up. If the work up is normal, an examination under anaesthetic is required to exclude a foreign body and vaginal or cervical tumours. Foreign body, such as a piece of toilet tissue, is the most common cause of vaginal bleeding in this group. Tumours such as the rhabdomyosarcoma, sarcoma botryoides are extremely rare, but should be excluded in this circumstance. It is not possible to obtain a thorough examination in clinic due to discomfort and this should be done in theatre under a general anaesthetic with a cystoscope or hysteroscope.

On the other hand, failure to menstruate in girls by the age of 14 where there is **no** secondary sexual development and in girls by the age of 16 where there **is** secondary sexual development can be considered abnormal and should be investigated [2]. This is known as primary amenorrhoea and requires investigation.

As a general rule, girls with primary amenorrhoea **without** secondary sexual development will have a hormonal problem. These can be associated with constitutional delay, chronic systemic disease or absence of ovarian or hypothalamic pituitary function. Girls with amenorrhoea **with** secondary sexual development will often have an anatomical problem. These include imperforate hymen or transverse vaginal septum or, in cases of Mayer–Rokitansky–Küster–Hauser (MRKH) syndrome or complete androgen insensitivity syndrome (CAIS), absent uterus and upper vagina.

Polycystic ovarian syndrome is a rare cause of primary amenorrhoea and in this case patients will have secondary sexual development with a hormonal problem. It is more commonly a cause of secondary amenorrhoea or oligomenorrhoea. It can be diagnosed using the Rotterdam Criteria which states that the patient must have two out of three of the following symptoms or signs: hyperandrogenism (acne and/or hirsuitism), oligomenorrhoea, the appearance of polycystic ovaries on pelvic ultrasound scanning (USS) [4]. Hormone levels are no longer required to make the diagnosis, however they may be necessary if PCOS is only one of the differential diagnoses. Anti-Müllerian hormone (AMH) is significantly raised in PCOS due to the increase in number of antral follicles in the condition and can be used to help make the diagnosis. This is the blood test used in older women as a predictor of ovarian reserve to see if it is possible for them to delay child bearing or to inform fertility treatment regimes.

In primary amenorrhoea, pregnancy should be considered and excluded and blood tests taken for FSH, LH, oestradiol, prolactin, thyroid function, urea and electrolytes, sex hormone binding globulin (SHBG), androstenedione and testosterone. A USS of the pelvis should be organized. The authors advocate a chromosomal analysis in the initial set of blood tests to avoid extreme prolonged patient anxiety if performed at a later stage, but some practitioners would perform this only in the presence of a raised FSH or the absence of a uterus on ultrasound.

Primary amenorrhoea with secondary sexual development and **cyclical pain** plus or minus a pelvic mass should raise the suspicion of a blockage in the genital tract with accumulation of non-draining menses (cryptomenorrhoea). Imperforate hymen is relatively common with an incidence of 1 in 1000 girls and is simply dealt with in theatre by excising the hymen and draining the collected old blood. A transverse vaginal septum is less common (1 in 80 000) and requires more expert surgery depending on the location and thickness of the septum.

There is thought to be a genetic component to the age of menarche and studies have shown a correlation to the age of the girl's mother at menarche [5]. The KISS1 gene and its receptor G protein coupled receptor 54 (GPR54) are considered to have a key role. A single nucleotide polymorphism of LIN28B on chromosome 6 has been associated with early puberty. Most of the genetic studies have been performed in Caucasian populations, however, and need to be confirmed in other populations.

The age of onset of menarche has decreased over the last 150 years by 3–4 months per decade [5]. In 1840 the average age of menarche was 16.5 years. It is now 12.8 years. This is thought to be due to better nutrition and general health and socioeconomic factors, although there are differences in racial and ethnic groups and by geographic location. For example, in the USA, African-American girls menstruate on average three months earlier than Mexican-American girls who menstruate earlier than Caucasian-American girls. These differences exist even when the data were adjusted for BMI and several social and economic variables. In Europe, girls in the Southern Mediterranean areas start to menstruate earlier than girls in Northern Europe. Asian girls attain menarche at a similar time to Southern European girls [5].

This decrease in age at menarche has reversed in the last 20 years however. The reasons for this are not clear but may be linked to the current cultural trend for young girls to be very thin and to exercise more.

Both BMI and height strongly correlate with age at menarche. A raised BMI at age five to nine years is associated with earlier menarche. Blood leptin levels are associated with increased gluteofemoral fat. Leptin may give information regarding fat distribution to the hypothalamus around and during puberty.

Intense exercise has been shown to have a negative effect on the hypothalamus. Athletes and ballerinas achieve menarche later than controls but swimmers do not, suggesting a link to fat distribution as these girls have different physiques.

Environmental factors are also known to have an effect, with high socioeconomic status, high parental education and urban environment being associated with earlier menarche. In addition, girls adopted from developing countries and brought up in Western Europe will have an earlier menarche. Later puberty is associated with chronic illness, living in a war zone and a rural environment.

Endocrine disruptor chemicals are industrial solvents, plastics and pesticides, which are structurally similar to oestrogen and work through oestrogen receptors or directly on the central nervous system. Exposure to these can delay or accelerate puberty and cause disorders of sexual differentiation (DSD) or cancers.

There are health risks associated with achieving early menarche. These are increased risk of raised BMI, increased cardiovascular risk and increased risk of breast cancer. This is due to abdominal type obesity with increased insulin, testosterone and insulin-like growth factor 1, which are growth factors for mammary tissue proliferation and promote carcinogenesis.

Early menarche is also associated with an increase in all cancer mortality [5]. It is linked to earlier first intercourse and more negative experiences with male partners. It is a risk factor for adolescent depression, anxiety and violent behaviour. There may be a small increased risk of having endometriosis.

Late menarche is associated with increased risk of osteoporosis and fractures.

It would be useful to study which girls in particular are at risk of adverse events due to abnormal timing of menarche and if medical manipulation of pubertal events would be beneficial.

Peri-menarchal dysfunctional uterine bleeding

Although the age at menarche has decreased, there appears to be an increase in the time taken to achieve regular ovulatory cycles. In the first year after menarche, 80% of cycles are anovulatory, 50% in the 3rd year and 10% are still anovulatory 6 years after menarche [2]. This is due to the failure of the feedback mechanism causing the LH surge in the imma-ture hypothalamic–pituitary–gonadal axis. Simply put to patients, without being patroniz-ing – the hormones are not in a grown-up pattern yet. This means the endometrium is often under unopposed oestrogen stimulation causing it to become thick and unstable. It breaks down in an irregular manner resulting in extremely heavy menstrual loss. Histology of the endometrium shows a hyperproliferation or simple hyperplasia.

Obtaining a history from any woman regarding the volume of blood loss during men-struation can be difficult. This is said with no disrespect to women, but in the knowledge that women do not normally physically compare menstrual loss. The average blood loss is 40 ml with a normal range of 25–70 ml. Over 80 ml blood loss is abnormal and may result in anaemia. A super plus tampon can absorb 12–15 ml of blood so calculations can be made on this basis but most women will not be able to supply objective information on the volume of blood loss. Younger women often do not use tampons and the loss absorbed on pads is more difficult to measure. Therefore, discussions around the presence and size of blood clots in the menstrual loss and the presence of flooding, where the loss escapes the tampons and pads and goes onto clothes or bedding, are useful. Frequency of pad change can be helpful – more frequently than two-hourly is significant, but only if the pads are soaked. Reports of having to miss school or daily activity are significant.

Often the patient's mother will frequently inform you of her own dreadful periods that resulted in a hysterectomy at a young age. We would try to reassure her and her daughter that the patient only has half of Mum's genes and may escape a similar fate.

There is no role for pelvic or rectal examination in these girls and they tolerate it poorly. It is unlikely that there will be any pelvic pathology and a USS can be used to detect anomalies of the genital tract. It is important not to put young girls off visiting a GP or gynaecologist in the future. Abdominal palpation can be useful to exclude a pelvic mass such as a haematocolpos.

Investigations can include full blood count (FBC), iron levels, clotting factors, if there is a family history of bleeding disorders or the girl has failed to respond to hormonal treatments, and USS of the pelvis. Testing for AMH may be included if PCOS is suspected. Hormone levels such as FSH, LH, oestradiol, testosterone and SHBG are not essential. Thyroid function is usually done only if there are other signs suspicious of thyroid disease.

There is no role for hysteroscopy or dilation and curettage (D&C).

Reassurance may be all that the patient and parents need in managing this condition, but treatment can be considered if there is a decrease in quality of life.

Research in this area may result in better treatments for women. It must also be noted that very few studies have been conducted in the adolescent population and that treatment options are frequently extrapolated from adult data.

Girls with regular periods are likely to be ovulating and the mechanism for menorrhagia in them is less well understood but is thought to be due to increased endometrial fibrinolysis and an alteration in prostaglandin balance. This explains the rationale for treating with tranexamic acid (an anti-fibrinolytic agent) and mefenamic acid (a non-steroidal anti-inflammatory drug with anti-prostaglandin effects on the uterus to reduce swelling and contractility). This is a standard first line non-hormonal treatment for menorrhagia and dysmenorrhoea. Tranexamic acid 1 g 6–8 hourly has been shown to reduce menstrual flow by 54% and mefenamic acid 500 mg 8 hourly by 20%. Both drugs can cause nausea, headache and gastrointestinal disturbance. Tranexamic acid does not increase the risk of thrombosis, but the tablet is quite large. This can be a problem for some girls as is the frequency of administration of these tablets. We usually suggest taking the tablets before and after school and before bed.

If non-hormonal treatments are not effective or not desired we usually move on to hormonal tablets. These would include progestogen-only (POP) or the combined oral contraceptive (COC) pill. Treatment with hormones will impose an artificial cycle, but will not correct the underlying disorder, so stopping therapy may result in recurrence of irregular periods. Rather, treatment can be viewed as a way of 'getting through' the first few years of heavy and/or irregular periods until a grown up pattern of hormones is established. We recommend treatment is given for at least a year. The patient can decide at that point if she wishes for a trial without treatment to see if her symptoms have improved. If a girl is happy on her treatment she can continue it. The years of disruptive menstruation coincide with major examinations in school for many and this should be taken into account.

Treatment with 5 mg norethisterone (NET) two or three times a day for 3 weeks followed by a week off has been shown to reduce menstrual loss in adult women and appears to be effective in adolescents too. This is quite a large dose of an androgenic progestogen and whilst it gives good cycle control, can be associated with significant side effects such as acne, weight gain and particularly low mood. Courses of NET for less than 21 days are not effective. Medroxyprogesterone acetate (MPA, Provera®) 10 mg three times per day for 21 days followed by 7 pill-free days is an alternative to norethisterone.

We would not usually use depot-MPA (DMPA) injections in this group as first line due to the possible negative effect on bone mineral density. Implants seem to worsen cycle control. The levonorgestrel-releasing intrauterine system (IUS) is effective but requires a uterine cavity length of at least 6 cm (which can be measured at USS) for its insertion. Insertion is done under general anaesthetic in this population. It should be noted that it is difficult to insert a levonorgestrel-releasing IUS without damaging the hymen of a girl who has never been sexually active, even when using a small speculum. Patients and parents should be made aware of this when giving consent for the procedure. Levonorgestrel-releasing IUS are often not favoured by adolescent girls and reserved for difficult cases.

The desogestrel-only pill (Cerazette®) has some differences to the earlier POPs. In adults, it inhibits ovulation in 97% of users, has a 12 hour window for remembering to take it, and by 11 months of use 50% have infrequent bleeding or amenorrhoea compared to 10% in users of the older POPs [6]. The authors have experience of using the desogestrel POP and doubling the daily dose to control unpredictable bleeding in adolescent girls. It is a less androgenic progestogen and given in lower doses, so side effects are less than with NET and MPA .There are currently no studies in adolescents on the desogestrel-only pill regarding cycle control [7]. However, it can be given in peri-menarchal dysfunctional uterine bleeding (DUB) and may be useful where NET is not tolerated and oestrogen is contraindicated. There may be a case for starting therapy with NET to impose a cycle then continuing with the desogestrel POP. Studies need to be undertaken.

The UK Medical Eligibility Criteria (UKMEC) for contraception for age, states that treatment with POP is acceptable from menarche with a score of 1 [8]. This indicates that there is no restriction on use of the method and the benefits outweigh any proven or theoretical risk. Whilst it is appreciated that the indication for treatment in this group is not primarily contraception, a similar assumption of safety can be made.

There is sometimes a perception that treatment with the combined oral contraceptive is only for contraception and there may be reluctance to utilize these preparations especially in cultures which frown upon sex before marriage. It is important to be sensitive to the opinions of the girl and her parents.

The UKMEC for treatment with combined hormonal contraception (CHC) including the COC pill, the contraceptive patch and vaginal ring is acceptable from menarche with a score of 1 [8].

Before menarche, the Faculty of Sexual and Reproductive Healthcare (FSRH) advise condoms for contraception and levonorgestrel (Levonelle®) for emergency contraception [9]. They do not recommend hormonal methods are used before menarche.

Use of CHC usually imposes a cycle on the patient and gives lighter less painful withdrawal bleeds. Continuation of the method used will depend upon the side effects experienced. Delivery route is dependent upon individual preference. The authors have successfully used tricycling of the patch to reduce the number of withdrawal bleeds per year. Additional conditions should be taken into account. For example, if a young woman has PCOS with symptoms related to excess androgens it is appropriate to consider treatment with an anti-androgenic progestogen such as cyproterone acetate (Dianette®) or drospirenone (Yasmin®).

The most recent systematic review on COC use in under-18s notes that studies in young users are few, but that there is no indication of a negative impact on weight, body composition or height [10].

With regards to the future risk of breast cancer, features including duration of use, age at first use and dose and type of hormone used, had little additional effect when the recency of use had been taken into account. In particular, early use did not result in more cancers being diagnosed [11]. The effect on breast cancer in users of COC with *BRCA1* or *BRCA2* genes is unclear as the studies are inconsistent. This, therefore, may be a relative contraindication to COC use in girls who are known to carry the *BRCA* genes. It is rated UKMEC 3 (the risks outweigh the benefits of use). A family history of breast cancer without knowledge of gene status is UKMEC 1 (unrestricted use of the method).

The risk of ovarian cancer in COC users is reduced even in females with the *BRCA1* or *BRCA2* genes. The risk of endometrial cancer is also reduced in COC users. The risk of cervical cancer is said to be increased, but it is difficult to determine whether this is an associated or causative relationship. The use of the human papilloma virus (HPV) vaccination, condoms and the cytology screening programme, will reduce this risk.

There is a small increased risk of venous thromboembolism (VTE) with CHC use, but the absolute risk in young people is extremely small. There is no known increased risk of VTE with POP use.

Depression is listed as an undesirable effect of CHC or POP contraception as mood changes can occur, but there is no evidence that they cause depression. Premenstrual syndrome improves with COC use in some women but occasionally gets worse in others.

The return to fertility after COC is similar to other methods regardless of whether it is taken cyclically, continuously or for an extended period of time, and is not usually delayed, unless there is other pathology, e.g., PCOS.

In amenorrhoeic girls with eating disorders CHC can help improve bone mineral density, but is not a substitutre for normal nutrition.

Sometimes girls will continue to have heavy bleeding on CHC. A recent addition to treatment options is oestradiol valerate with dienogest (Qlaira®) with a license to treat heavy menstrual bleeding [12]. The authors have found it useful in the treatment of peri-menarchal DUB and also useful for young girls who find it difficult to tolerate oestrogenic side effects including headache and nausea. It is not a first line pill but it has the potential to improve the quality of life of a young woman enough to allow her to go to school, for example.

Studies have reported that up to 20% of sufferers of heavy menstrual bleeding have a blood clotting disorder, with von Willebrand's disease and thrombocytopenia or platelet function disorders being the most common causes [2]. The closer to the menarche that the heavy menstrual bleeding develops, the more likely there is an underlying haematological cause. Failure to respond to treatment should prompt investigation of blood clotting. Very often the treatment of menorrhagia is the same whether the girl has a blood clotting disorder or not, but it is essential that these disorders are diagnosed for future management.

Blood clotting disorders can occasionally present as catastrophic juvenile vaginal bleeding at menarche. This requires admission to hospital, transfusion of red cells and clotting factors and treatment with high doses of progestogens and intravenous tranexamic acid. In severe cases treatment with uterine artery embolization, recombinant factor VIIa and uterine packing has been used to prevent hysterectomy in young nulliparous girls.

Dysmenorrhoea is present in up to 85% of women and as such can almost be regarded as normal. In view of this it is considered acceptable to treat dysmenorrhoea with simple measures before investigating it. It is often associated with ovulatory cycles so may develop a year or two after menarche. The mechanism for its occurrence is increased levels of prostaglandins released from the menstrual endometrium causing increased uterine tone and uterine contractions. These are painful and occur as the uterus attempts to expel blood, endometrium and clots through the cervical os. The os can be pinhole size in a young nulliparous girl, resulting in higher amplitude or more frequent contractions. The cervix is innervated by the vagus nerve, which can cause a drop in blood pressure when stimulated. This can account for the pale washed out appearance, dizziness, fainting and vomiting experienced by girls during their period.

An extremely common theme in adolescent girls is the lack of attention to general health and wellbeing. For example, many of them do not drink enough fluid, or drink lots of fizzy drinks. They don't have breakfast or eat any fruit and vegetables and do not do any exercise outside of PE in school, which for many non-sporty girls involves a lot of standing around. This results in their bowels opening only once every two or three days with a type 2 or 3 (hard lumpy) stool on the Bristol stool chart. The rest of the bowel remains full and can cause spasms, which are painful. The combination of this with period pain or with peritoneal irritation from fluid or blood released with a ruptured follicle at ovulation can escalate their abdominal pain to a score of 7 or more and result in hospital admission. Girls need to understand that their bowels should open every day with a soft but formed stool. If they change their habits to drinking plenty of water, having breakfast, fruit and vegetables and exercising regularly they will very often eliminate all their pain, especially when done in combination with starting CHC or a POP contraceptive method, thus avoiding the need for further investigation such as laparoscopy.

Endometriosis is one of the differential diagnoses for dysmenorrhoea. It has been reported in girls as young as 10 years of age. It has been found that in girls who do not respond to hormonal treatment for dysmenorrhoea (we would try at least two different preparations for 2–3 months), the presence of endometriosis was 50–60% compared to 20% in asymptomatic women and 30% in subfertile women [2]. There are four stages of endometriosis. The more severe stages 3 and 4 should be apparent on USS with the presence of endometrioma or distorted anatomy due to adhesions. However, milder cases, stages 1 and 2 can only be diagnosed by laparoscopy. Laparoscopy has risk factors, although complications such as anaesthetic problems and damage to bladder, bowel and blood vessels in the pelvis is rare, and so should only be undertaken if there is no response to medical treatment. It is important to remember that early endometriotic lesions, such as those seen in the adolescent population may not have the classical powder burn appearance of those seen in adults. Clear vesicles are a common appearance of early endometriosis and must be actively sought at laparoscopy. Long-term prevention of progression of endometriosis is thought to be best with initial laparoscopic surgical management at diagnosis followed by medical hormonal treatment. This resulted in only 10% of patients progressing one stage at second-look laparoscopy. Medical hormonal treatment could constitute POP, MPA, levonorgestrel IUS or CHC. Gonadotrophin-releasing hormone analogues (GnRHa) can be used for a six-month course. With GnRHa, add-back hormone replacement therapy (HRT) is thought to reduce bone demineralization and hot flushes. Bone density returns to normal after cessation of therapy.

Duplications of the Müllerian system such as double uterus, cervix and vagina or accessory uterine horn with blockage of part of the double system and accumulation of menses (cryptomenorrhoea) are hard to diagnose as the girl will menstruate from the unblocked part of her system and present with dysmenorrhoea. Hence the importance of USS in the investigation of dysmenorrhoea that fails to respond to treatment. A blind horn of the uterus may be reported as an ovarian cyst or pelvic mass and may require further investigation with magnetic resonance imaging (MRI). The treatment is laparoscopic excision of the horn or surgical excision of the vaginal septum in the obstructed hemi-vagina. It is important to remember to investigate the renal tract of girls with Müllerian anomalies as 47% of them will have renal tract anomalies as well.

A special group of young girls are those with learning difficulties. Their parents sometimes wish to discuss the options for dealing with periods before the menarche, although we wait to see the first bleed before commencing treatment options [2]. The girls are often unable to understand the concept of periods and why they are bleeding. They sometimes cannot cope with sanitary protection, especially at school, which results in severe soiling. They may get premenstrual mood changes which result in very challenging behaviour. Many of them are epileptic and have an increase in seizures premenstrually. There may be drug interactions with hormonal treatments if their anti-epileptics are enzyme induction agents.

The aim in these girls is to induce amenorrhoea and DMPA is a useful treatment option. It will not induce amenorrhoea immediately, but should do so within one year of use. Interference with other medication is rare and it is not necessary to get the girl to swallow tablets.

The possibility of a reduction in bone mineral density or an increase in weight (side effects associated with use) needs to be balanced against the improvement in quality of life for the girl and her family.

We have recently started to use desogestrel POP down percutaneous endoscopic gastrostomy (PEG) tubes. It is an unlicensed use but the manufacturers have no contraindication to this as digestion only starts in the stomach and the tablets are small enough to be flushed in. We await the results of cycle control.

The levonorgestrel IUS can be inserted under general anaesthesia if the uterine cavity is at least 6 cm on USS. The USS can be difficult as the scan must be transabdominal and some of the girls are incontinent, cannot fill their bladder and therefore images are suboptimal. Levonorgestrel IUS may not induce amenorrhoea but it can make the bleeding more tolerable for the girl and her carers.

Oestrogen is relatively contraindicated in immobile girls due to the potential risk of VTE.

Combined hormonal contraceptives can be used in mobile girls and the extended regimen method of taking COCs is proving useful. Using a 20 μg COC continuously with 4 days off if there is 4 days of breakthrough bleeding is a good way of achieving minimal bleeds.

The case

Alex is a tricky case. She is obviously very distressed by her symptoms and is demonstrating this with behavioural difficulties. Being 13 is a difficult age anyway, but being overweight with acne and heavy menstrual bleeding can make it intolerable, especially if none of her friends are experiencing problems with their periods.

Social services will become involved in Alex's care if she misses too much school and management measures should aim to allow Alex to improve attendance by improving her mood and her self image as well as reducing her bleeding.

It is important to consider the psychological aspects of her care and it would appear that Alex is struggling with this. Referral to the local community adolescent mental health service (CAMHS) is indicated for Alex. Counselling with cognitive behavioural therapy may help her in dealing with her peers, her appearance and her weight reduction if she will engage with the service.

Although adolescent girls don't necessarily wish to have babies when they are young, they often worry excessively about whether they can conceive. Alex may be worried about this as her Mum needed clomiphene citrate to conceive. An explanation of what this involves and that it is different to in vitro fertilization (IVF) or test-tube babies may be reassuring to her.

As she already has acne (a symptom of hyperandrogenism) and oligomenorrhoea she only needs ultrasound evidence of PCOS to make the diagnosis. Remember that adolescent girls have multicystic ovaries anyway and that they should have more than 12 follicles to be classified as having polycystic ovaries. The family history of PCOS increases the likelihood of the diagnosis. Alex might be more likely to co-operate with the investigations if she doesn't have to go through a blood test, which can be quite traumatic at her age. Establishing a good rapport with Alex is essential to get her to co-operate with management, especially weight reduction and psychological intervention.

Unfortunately her increased BMI rules out several treatment options if she is diagnosed with PCOS. Her ideal treatment, if her BMI was less than 35, would be ethinyl oestradiol with drospirenone (Yasmin®) as this would regulate and lighten her periods, improve her acne and any hirsuitism and has a good effect on mood, particularly premenstrual mood changes. Cyproterone acetate (Dianette®) is the most potent anti-androgen but drospirenone (Yasmin®) has less of a negative effect on libido.

As Alex has a BMI of 42, the risk of VTE with oestrogen therapy would be too great.

In addition the adipose cells produce unopposed peripheral oestrogen in response to leptin production, which can result in endometrial hyperplasia. This condition over many years is a risk factor for endometrial cancer.

The key to management of PCOS is weight reduction. All symptoms will resolve or improve with this, and Alex could achieve a normal menstrual cycle if she normalizes her weight. If PCOS is diagnosed she should be investigated for insulin resistance with a glucose tolerance test, fasting insulin level and c-peptide. It is highly likely that she will have insulin resistance at this weight. Joint management by a gynaecologist and an endocrinologist is the ideal in these patients.

The other way to improve insulin resistance is lots of exercise and Alex needs to be convinced that this is worthwhile. Sadly in the UK, PE in school can be a very negative experience for many girls. If Alex is going to fully engage in exercise to become fit and healthy for life she needs to find something that she enjoys doing. For example, she might like Zumba if she had the opportunity to try it, or yoga or Pilates for less impact to start off with. It helps if a family member, such as her Mum, or a friend will go to the classes too. Some girls enjoy boxing or martial arts. Helping Alex to afford these sorts of classes such as providing gym vouchers or joining local fitness schemes will also be of help. Sometimes advice from a dietician or education regarding diet can be part of these schemes and Alex will need help with her diet. In particular good fluid intake, regular eating including breakfast, fruit and vegetables and avoiding long periods of time without eating, which encourage the body to retain fat in starvation mode, are essential.

We would probably avoid NET 5 mg three times per day for 21 days followed by a week off in Alex as there would be a concern that it could increase her appetite and worsen her mood and her acne.

Alex could try a levonorgestrel IUS inserted under a general anaesthetic if her uterus was greater than 6 cm long. This would lighten her bleeds and protect her against endometrial hyperplasia. Alex needs to have four bleeds per year to avoid overgrowth of the endometrium unless she is on hormonal treatment to avoid it. Then amenorrhoea is acceptable. A bleed can be induced with NET 5 mg tds for 10 days four times per year if necessary.

Lastly, regular appointments to support Alex initially can help her to achieve the changes she needs to make to take control of her condition and not allow it to control her.

Key learning points

- Menarche is usually one of the last events of puberty.
- The age of onset of menarche has decreased over the last 150 years, but this decrease has reversed in the last 20 years.
- Pubertal development before the age of 8 and menarche before the age of 9 should be investigated.
- Failure to menstruate in girls by the age of 14 where there is **no** secondary sexual development and in girls by the age of 16 where there **is** secondary sexual development should be investigated.
- Do not do pelvic or rectal examinations in young girls who are not sexually active.
- Blood clotting disorders can be present in up to 20% of young women with heavy menstrual bleeding. Consideration should be given to investigation of clotting factors.
- Dysmenorrhoea can be due to a blockage in the genital tract even if the girl is menstruating, due to the presence of a double system.
- Poor fluid intake, diet and lack of exercise are very common in young girls and can result in inefficient bowel function. This hugely exacerbates gynaecological pain and so should be addressed.
- Girls with learning difficulties commonly need help to manage menstruation and cyclical hormonal changes.

Less common conditions to watch out for

- **Imperforate hymen or transverse vaginal septum** – cyclical pain with no menstruation, diagnose with pelvic USS.
- **Obstructed hemi-vagina or functioning non-connecting uterine horn** – cyclical pain with menstruation, diagnose with pelvic USS.
- **Catastrophic juvenile vaginal bleed** – very heavy first menstruation, which does not stop, requires prompt hospital admission and transfusion with investigation of blood clotting.
- **Clotting disorders presenting as heavy menstrual bleeding** – suspect in young women with menorrhagia from menarche with little improvement despite treatment, enquire about family history of bleeding and refer to haematology.

References

1. Chang YT, Hayter M, Wu SC. A systematic review and meta-ethnography of the qualitative literature: experiences of the menarche. *J Clin Nurs* 2010; 19(3–4), 447–60.

2. Garden A, Hernon M, Topping J. *Paediatric and Adolescent Gynaecology for the MRCOG and Beyond.* London: RCOG Press, 2008.

3. Mann GS, Blair JC, Garden AS. *Imaging of Gynaecological Disorders in Infants*

and Children. London: Springer, 2012.

4. Rotterdam ESHRE/ASRM-Sponsored PCOS Consensus Workshop Group. Revised 2003 consensus on diagnostic criteria and long-term health risks related to polycystic ovary syndrome (PCOS). *Hum Reprod* 2004; 19(1): 41–7.

5. Karapanou O, Papadimitriou A. Determinants of menarche. *Reprod Biol Endocrinol* 2010; 8: 115–20.

6. Faculty of Family Planning and Reproductive Healthcare, Clinical Effectiveness Unit. Desogestrel-only pill. *J Fam Plann Reprod Health Care* 2003; 29(3): 162–4.

7. Faculty of Sexual and Reproductive Healthcare. *Clinical Guidance. Progestogen-only Pills*, November 2008 (updated June 2009). http://www.fsrh.org/pdfs/CEUGuidanceProgestogenOnlyPill09.pdf (accessed 28 February 2013).

8. Faculty of Sexual and Reproductive Healthcare. *UK Medical Eligibility Criteria for Contraceptive Use*, 2009. http://www.fsrh.org/pdfs/UKMEC2009.pdf (accessed 28 February 2013).

9. Faculty of Sexual and Reproductive Healthcare. *Clinical Guidance. Contraceptive Choices for Young People*, March 2010. http://www.fsrh.org/pdfs/ceuGuidanceYoungPeople2010.pdf (accessed 28 February 2013).

10. Warholm L, Petersen KR, Ravn P. The combined oral contraceptive pill's influence on weight, body composition, height and bone mineral density in girls younger than 18 years: a systematic review. *Eur J Contracept Reprod Health Care* 2012; 17(4), 245–53.

11. Collaborative Group on Hormonal Factors in Breast Cancer. Breast cancer and hormonal contraceptives. *Lancet* 1996; 22(347): 1713–27.

12. Ahrendt HJ, Makalová D, Parke S, Mellinger U, Mansour D. Bleeding pattern and cycle control with an estradiol-based oral contraceptive: a seven-cycle, randomized comparative trial of estradiol valerate/dienogest and ethinyl estradiol/levonorgestrel. *Contraception* 2009; 80(5): 436–44.

Chapter 10

Adolescence: contraception in the teenage years

Kathy French

This chapter will focus on the adolescence years, a time of change for young people when they are entering sexual relationships, dealing with peer pressure and the possible tensions from school and home.

Introduction

Young people learn about contraception from a variety of sources: family, friends, magazines, and from school-based sex and education lessons if they are lucky enough to get that input. It is well recognized that some young people are sexually active at a younger age than perhaps 50 years ago, and the media focuses much attention on teenage sexual activity and teenage pregnancy.

It is important to view teenage pregnancy through a sociological lens and understand how it becomes a 'problem' when other factors change.

Teenage sexual activity and reproduction continues to raise much interest in British policy, research and media arenas and it has become a topic for sociological research, public discourse and political discussion. This has intensified with the emergence of human immunodeficiency virus (HIV) in the early 1980s.

The UK is not alone in expressing concern about the issue of teenage conceptions; many other countries highlight how their teenagers compare to those of other countries. This is partly because of the potential political implications of morality discourses, but also the social and economic consequences to the young parent(s) and their children.

In the aftermath of the Second World War and in the 1960s it was both common and unremarkable for parenthood to begin in the teenage years [1]. The most important demographic change over the past 30 years and where most concern is expressed is the fact that teenage women choose other than the safety net of marriage to resolve their unintended pregnancy.

Whilst teenage pregnancy rates are considered high in the UK, the 1990s rates of teenage fertility were significantly below that of earlier decades. With the average age of first pregnancy in the UK now standing at 31 years, teenage parents become more visible than ever before.

Government solution to teenage pregnancy

The perceived problem with teenage conceptions led the British government to publish the Health for the Nation Strategy in 1992 [2], which highlighted the need for better services for young people. This was followed in 1999 by the Teenage Pregnancy Strategy (TPS) [3] with the ambition to reduce teenage pregnancies by 50% within 10 years. Latest data shows a sustained reduction in teenage pregnancy, and we have seen an increase in funding for contraceptive services and a greater access to emergency contraception over the past 10 years.

It was suggested in the Strategy that one way of reducing teenage conceptions was the provision of good sex and relationship education within schools and colleges; however, we do not have mandatory provision yet.

Many reasons were suggested regarding the cause of teenage pregnancy, ranging from poverty, low expectations and lack of knowledge about contraception and abortion services.

Whatever the political or demographic changes suggest, it is not generally in the 'best interest' of a young woman to have to deal with an unplanned/unintended pregnancy, when there are many methods of reliable contraception to choose from and contraceptive services are widely available. We know that for young people to access services they need knowledge, confidence and skills to negotiate a system that is not always welcoming to them. Young people live in a highly sexualized world, but at the same time when they express their sexuality at an increasingly earlier age, they are often demonized. These competing tensions may prevent or delay some young people from accessing help when they need it.

The contraceptive needs of young adolescents

Case scenario: Sophie

Sophie is a 15 year old who attends a walk in clinic.

During the sexual health assessment, Sophie tells you that she had her first sexual experience with a boy in her class when she was 14 years old. She admitted to being very drunk at the time and was not able to say whether he used a condom or not. This unexpected episode in her life was associated with her feeling anxious and depressed.

Sophie has a boyfriend now and her mother is aware of this and supportive of her having a reliable method of contraception.

She tells you that her friend has the 'rod' (subdermal implant) and she would like to have one fitted.

During the consultation she tells the doctor that she had her last normal menstrual period (LNMP) almost four weeks ago and she says that she has not had sexual intercourse since then. She is adamant about this when asked if there is any chance she could be pregnant. The doctor decides to perform a pregnancy test, which is negative.

She is counselled about the benefits and side effects of the subdermal implant, its mode of action and given the opportunity to ask any questions. She is sure this is the right method for her and being aware of her friend's and mother's approval of the method, she proceeds to have it inserted.

She did not return to the clinic as advised, but turned up six months later complaining of weight gain and feeling dizzy and generally unwell and requested that the implant is removed as she feels that this is responsible for her symptoms.

Before removal a pregnancy test was done and this proved positive and her pregnancy was estimated to be at least 28 weeks gestation.

This case history highlights the difficulty that clinicians sometimes encounter when making an assessment of a young person's needs. Some young people may not have developed the skills to recall when their last period was but also do not want to admit to sexual activity.

Self-esteem

Self-esteem is how a person feels about themselves. Someone with a positive self-esteem will generally approach things thinking they are a good person who deserves love and support and can succeed in life. On the other hand someone with low self-esteem will generally think the opposite; they're not good at things, don't deserve love or support and that situations will work out badly for them, in effect they are not deserving in any way, and this is equally true in relationships. The majority of young people, like adults, will have dips in their self-esteem as they go through different stages and challenges in life, but with support from family and friends they usually manage very well.

Communicating with young people

Communicating with young people may seem difficult, but it is important also to consider how this might feel for them. Seeing a nurse or doctor for contraception can be a brave step for some young people, especially if they feel they are being judged about being sexually active.

It is important to allow them time to express their needs and establish what they already know about contraceptive methods. Young people should be informed about all the methods available, their benefits, efficacy rates, side effects, how to use the method and how often they need to have further supplies. The information provided needs to be matched with the young person's willingness to engage in the consultation.

Young people differ in their needs: some may want a method which is invisible, for example the implant or the injectable, whilst others are happy to have supplies of the pill in their handbag. Part of the discussion should be around their lifestyle and home life, as it may be that contraceptive use in teenagers is frowned upon before marriage.

Alcohol

Drinking alcohol increases the chances of young people taking risks, including risks with their sexual health. There is a strong link between alcohol and sexual activity in our culture. If young people drink too much alcohol, they are unable to recall whether they had sex or not, thus inhibiting their ability to consent. Young people can get into very serious situations when very drunk and can fall prey to predatory adults resulting in rape or sexual assault.

Alcohol has the effect of making users more relaxed and less inhibited about choices they need to make. During any consultation around contraception, it is worth asking about alcohol and drug usage. Brook, a young person's charity, has published advice for young people on alcohol [4]:

- Your ability to think clearly will be reduced and you will tend to take more risks.
- You won't be quite so careful about how and when you have sex with someone.
- You will be less likely to use safe contraception and condoms if you have sex.
- You are more likely to regret it later.

Sexually transmitted infections in association with casual sex

Young people aged 16–24 years old are the age group most at risk of being diagnosed with sexually transmitted infections (STIs) because they are often lacking the confidence and skills to negotiate sexual relationships with partners. Data from the Health Protection Agency (HPA) [5] indicates a worrying increase in STIs, with 482 700 new cases in 2009, an increase of around 12 000 from the previous year. While better and more widespread testing plays a part in the rise, there are concerns about young people. Two thirds of the STI cases were in females aged 15–24.

Any contraceptive or abortion consultation/assessment with a young person should include a discussion on STIs. Regardless of contraceptive method, condom use should be discussed and encouraged.

Sexually transmitted infections are covered in Chapter 19.

Progestogen-only implants

Progestogen-only implants have been available for a long time in the UK. Norplant® was the first implant but it was discontinued in 1999. The current implant is called Nexplanon® and comprises a single subdermal rod and is licensed for three years. Each implant contains 68 mg of etonogestrel, which is released slowly over the 3 years.

The progestogen-only implant is highly effective at preventing a pregnancy, with serum concentrations sufficient to inhibit ovulation at eight hours post insertion. However, unless insertion takes place within the first five days of the menstrual cycle, a further seven days is required before the method can be relied on.

Young women should be advised that the pregnancy rate with the implant is very low, just less than 1 in 1000 women over 3 years. The clinician should take time to explain what this means in real terms.

The primary action of the implant is in the prevention of ovulation; additionally the progestogen alters the cervical mucus which prevents sperm penetration through the cervix and also inhibits endometrial development.

The implant is one of the four long-acting reversible contraceptive (LARC) methods, including the intrauterine device (IUD), intrauterine system (IUS) and the injectable. All these methods have the advantage of not needing user involvement once inserted.

Long-term use of the progestogen-only implant is highly cost-effective, and it is more cost-effective than the combined oral contraceptive (COC) even at one year of use [6].

Counselling of young women in relation to the implant

The counselling should be 2-fold: first to share/exchange information about all methods and specifically about this chosen method; and secondly to consider the issues of competency in the young person's ability to consent to the treatment. More importantly, counselling offers the opportunity to make an assessment about the relationship she is engaged in.

The clinical assessment

The clinician should take a full medical history, sexual history and enquire about any drug use, prescribed or otherwise. Additionally the clinician should be familiar with the recommendations of the Faculty of Sexual and Reproductive Healthcare (FSRH) and the UK Medical Eligibility Criteria (UKMEC) [7] in assessing a young woman's appropriateness for the contraceptive implant.

Table 10.1 lists what the clinician should discuss with a young person in relation to progestogen-only implants.

Young people can be assured that there is no delay in the return to fertility after removal of a progestogen-only implant.

All young people should be given written information about the progestogen-only implant and advised to use condoms as well to protect against STIs.

Table 10.2 lists the clinical situations when a progestogen-only implant should be inserted.

Table 10.1 The clinician should discuss the following with the young person in relation to the progestogen-only implant.

Side effects	Advice	Comments
Alteration in bleeding patterns	Young women should be advised that many women (20%) will have no bleeding whilst almost 50% may have frequent, irregular or prolonged bleeding and that this pattern is likely to remain	Explaining the possible changes in bleeding patterns is vital otherwise the young person will give up if this expectation is not managed at the onset. There are a number of potential treatment options for associated unscheduled bleeding including COCs, POPs or DMPA. Supporting the young woman during the first weeks and months of use is key to her ongoing use of the method. If the young woman is unable to accept the device after a reasonable time, the clinician should offer another method of contraception
Weight gain	Weight change is common with many young women during their adolescent years but they may blame the implant	The clinician can reassure the young woman that there is no evidence that the implant causes weight gain
Acne	Young women should be advised that acne may improve, get worse or occur during the use of the implant	Acne is an important issue for young women, but the clinician can reassure her that the use of any treatment for acne is not affected by the use of the implant
Liver enzyme-inducing drugs	The SPC recommends additional contraceptive protection whilst using a liver enzyme-inducing drug and for 28 days after stopping the drug If she is using a liver enzyme-inducing drug for less than 3 weeks, she can continue with the implant, but another method of contraception should be considered if she is using long-term liver enzyme inducers Non-liver enzyme-inducing antibiotics will **not** affect the efficacy of the implant	It is important to check with the young woman at subsequent visits if she has been prescribed any new medications or if she is taking any over-the-counter preparations Condoms should be offered

COCs, combined oral contraceptives; DMPA, depot-medroxyprogesterone acetate; POPs, progestogen-only pills; SPC, Summary of Product Characteristics.

Doctors who need training in the insertion of progestogen-only implants should follow the Faculty of Sexual and Reproductive Healthcare Guidance. Nurses can access the Royal College of Nursing (RCN) [9] criteria in the insertion of subdermal contraceptive implants.

Assessment of capacity to consent to sexual activity and treatment

It is important to understand that the majority of young people are in consenting relationships and clinicians will have no concerns about the possibility of the young person being coerced or exploited.

Table 10.2 When should a progestogen-only implant be inserted?

Clinical situation	When in the cycle?	Comments
Routine request early in cycle	Ideally inserted between day 1 and 5 of a cycle	No additional contraception needed
Later in cycle	Provided the doctor/nurse is reasonably certain the young person is not pregnant the progestogen-only implant can be inserted at any time (Think of Sophie in the case scenario)	Additional contraception (condoms) or abstinence should be used for 7 days
After a miscarriage or abortion	The progestogen-only implant can be inserted up to day 5 following a surgical abortion, second trimester abortion or miscarriage	No additional contraception needed unless inserted after day 5 (additional contraception is recommended for 7 days).
Postpartum	The progestogen-only implant can be inserted up to day 21 with immediate contraceptive cover	If inserted after day 21, additional contraception is needed for 7 days
Switching from one method to another, for example from COC, POP, injectable, etc.	See guidance from the Faculty of Sexual and Reproductive Healthcare on progestogen-only implant [8]	

COC, combined oral contraceptive; POP, progestogen-only pill.

Common law has recognized the principle that everyone has a right to have their bodily integrity protected against invasion from others.

Adults over the age of 18 years are presumed competent to give consent to treatment; however, some young people over 18 years of age may not be competent to consent. The common law does not exclude a young person under 16 years from giving consent, but to be valid, the consent has to be considered in the light of the well-documented Gillick case in 1984 [10]. Following the Gillick case, guidelines were given, known as the Fraser Guidelines, which stated that the doctor would be justified in proceeding with contraceptive advice without parental consent or even knowledge provided the doctor was satisfied that certain criteria were met and these are as follows:

- The young person understands the advice and has sufficient maturity to understand what is involved.
- The doctor could not persuade the young person to inform his/her parents, nor to allow the doctor to inform them.
- The young person would be very likely to begin or continue having sexual intercourse with or without contraceptive treatment.
- Without advice and treatment, the young person's physical or mental health or both would suffer.
- It would be in the young person's 'best interests' to give such advice or treatment without parental consent.

On a rare occasion the clinician will be concerned about the young person's ability to understand the nature of sexual activity and contraceptive use. In such situations it is important to discuss the case with a senior colleague in the first instance.

Table 10.3 List of presentations during the consultation/assessment which would concern any doctor/nurse providing care and treatment to young people within sexual health.

What?	Why?	Action
A 13-year-old attended the service with her boyfriend who is 25 years old (12 year age gap)	The age difference would suggest there is a power imbalance here Is she getting gifts, money or pressure from this man? Do her parents know about him? Where did they meet?	The clinician should discuss these concerns with the young person and discuss with the Safeguarding Children Team
A very immature 16-year-old girl from Romania attends the clinic and she is accompanied by a man who says she is pregnant and he wants her to get an abortion as soon as possible She looks concerned and anxious	The young person does not seem to have much to say about the situation Her English is poor She says the man says she must get back to 'work' Difficult to find out what her 'work' is? Could be trafficked into the sex industry?	The clinician should get an interpreter for her Discuss with the Safeguarding Children Team
A 14-year-old girl is taken to the clinic by her uncle who wants her to have the pill Her mother does not know about this request and her father is not in contact with the family. He says it is better that the mother does not know She is very vague about her 'boyfriend'	What is the relationship with the uncle? Why is he saying the mother must not know? Does she have a 'boyfriend'?	The clinician should see the young person on her own and try to find out whether or not she has a boyfriend Discuss with the Safeguarding Children Team

Table 10.3 lists the presentations during the consultation/assessment which would concern any doctor/nurse providing care and treatment to young people within sexual health.

If the doctor/nurse has concerns about the safety of any young person accessing their service they should be familiar with the Safeguarding Children Team who are skilled at dealing with these issues. The clinician should follow the Fraser Guidelines and document all actions taken. Greater harm can be done by inappropriate onward referral by clinicians who do not know where to refer to, and this can lead to lack of trust amongst young people and their sexual health provider.

Unplanned pregnancy

Unplanned/unintended pregnancy is unfortunate for women at any age, but can be more difficult for younger women, especially if they have not used contraception at all or used it incorrectly.

The reaction to the unplanned pregnancy will depend on the support or not of the partner, parents and friends and it can be a time of conflict for the young person.

Should a young person suspect she is pregnant, it is important to get that confirmed as soon as possible. If the test is negative but the history suggests that a pregnancy is possible a repeat test should be performed in a week, and offer condoms until then.

The doctor/nurse could have some discussion at this point about how the young person might feel if the test proved positive next week and who she might tell about it?

If positive, she has three options:

- Continue with the pregnancy and keep the baby.
- Have an abortion (not an option for Sophie as she was more than 24 weeks).
- Continue with the pregnancy and have the baby adopted.

If the test is positive and the young person opts for an abortion, she should be informed at this stage about the process, methods of abortion and aftercare. This is a good time to discuss ongoing contraception; however, this may need to be delayed if she is very upset about the pregnancy. Chapters 20 and 21 cover medical and surgical abortion.

Contraception following abortion

When a young person has an abortion, it might be the first real opportunity for her to discuss contraception and it is an opportunity to explore her views about methods with a health professional. Additionally, the doctor/nurse can dispel myths and misconceptions often gained from friends and family, as covered in Chapter 2. Depending on which method the young woman choses, she should ideally be given it immediately after the procedure, and follow-up care arranged with the local contraceptive/sexual health service or her general practitioner.

Looking to the future

In December 2012, '2020 health' published 'The Morning After: A Cross Party Inquiry into Unplanned Pregnancy' with many recommendations [11]. These recommendations invited the Department of Education, Department of Health, Clinical Commissioning Groups (CCGs), Public Health, National Institute for Health and Clinical Excellence (NICE), Local Authorities (LAs) and the Royal Colleges to work together. A robust national training programme for health professionals, statutory sex and relationship training for teachers and young people as well as equal access to all contraceptive methods including LARC are amongst the key recommendations. These recommendations should be seen as a real opportunity to empower young people, improve the skills of health professionals and improve the sexual health and wellbeing of the nation.

Conclusion

Young people may change their contraceptive method during their adolescent years and the role of the doctor/nurse is to ensure that they know about all the methods available. Helping them understand how the methods work and showing patience will go a long way in improving their ability to deal with potential side effects associated with the method chosen. The aim for the young person and the doctor/nurse is to reduce the risk of an unplanned pregnancy and the risk of an STI.

References

1. Furstenberg FF. Childbearing as a public issue and private concern. *Ann Rev Sociol* 2003; 29: 23–39.
2. Department of Health. *The Health of the Nation Strategy*. London: HMSO, 1992.
3. Department of Health. *The Teenage Pregnancy Strategy*. London: HMSO, 1999.
4. Brook. Alcohol and sex. http://www.brook.org.uk/sex-and-relationships/harmful-situations/alcohol-and-sex (accessed 28 February 2013).
5. Health Protection Agency. http://www.hpa.org.uk/ (accessed 2008).

6. National Institute for Health and Clinical Excellence. *Long-acting Reversible Contraception*, Clinical Guideline 30, October 2005 (modified June 2006). http://publications.nice.org.uk/long-acting-reversible-contraception-cg30 (accessed 28 February 2013).

7. Faculty of Sexual and Reproductive Healthcare. *UK Medical Eligibility Criteria for Contraceptive Use*, 2009. http://www.fsrh.org/pdfs/UKMEC2009.pdf (accessed 28 February 2013).

8. Faculty of Sexual and Reproductive Healthcare. *Clinical Guidance. Progestogen-only Implants*, April 2008 (updated January 2009). http://www.fsrh.org/pdfs/CEUGuidanceProgestogen OnlyImplantsApril08.pdf (accessed 28 February 2013).

9. Royal College of Nursing. *Inserting and Removing Subdermal Contraceptive Implants. RCN Accreditation and Training Guidance for Nurses and Midwives*, 7th edition, updated November 2012. http://www.rcn.org.uk/__data/assets/pdf_file/0003/412176/002_240_new.pdf (accessed 28 February 2013).

10. *Gillick v West Norfolk and Wisbech Area Health Authority* (1984) QB 581.

11. Beer G, James M. *The Morning After: A Cross Party Inquiry into Unplanned Pregnancy*, 20 December 2012. http://www.2020health.org/2020health/Publication-2012/Wellbeing-and-Public-Health/Unplanned-Pregnancy.html (accessed 28 February 2013).

Useful resources

Department of Health. *Best Practice Guidance for Doctors and other Health Professionals on the Provision of Advice and Treatment to Young People Under 16 on Contraception, Sexual Health and Reproductive Health*, 29 July 2004. http://www.dh.gov.uk/prod_consum_dh/groups/dh_digitalassets/@dh/@en/documents/digitalasset/dh_4086914.pdf (accessed 28 February 2013).

HM Government. *Working Together to Safeguard Children: a guide to interagency working to safeguard and promote the welfare of children*, March 2010 https://www.education.gov.uk/publications/eOrdering Download/00305-2010DOM-EN.pdf (accessed 28 February 2013).

Faculty of Sexual and Reproductive Healthcare for all methods of contraception at http://www.fsrh.org/

Contraception in the 20-somethings

Paula Briggs

Case scenario: Ana

Anastasia (Ana), a 22-year-old editor for a publishing company, attends a community sexual health service for advice regarding virtually constant vaginal bleeding for the previous 6 months in association with the use of hormonal contraception. This started when she was first prescribed hormonal contraception – initially a progestogen-only pill and then a combined oral contraceptive pill. She has no other symptoms.

She is currently using condoms for contraception, although a recent condom accident has highlighted that this is not a reliable method.

She is in her first sexual relationship and finds the constant bleeding annoying and embarrassing.

Ana's aunt died from cervical cancer in her early 30s and this has increased her anxiety regarding the vaginal bleeding she is experiencing.

This chapter will focus on the non-oral combined hormonal contraceptive options, including the patch and more specifically the vaginal ring, which are underused in the UK and Australia. These options are widely used in many European countries and the USA.

The above case scenario raises a number of important issues:

1. Which investigations should be undertaken in women complaining of unscheduled (breakthrough) bleeding?
2. The challenge of facilitating a contraceptive choice consultation with a woman who has had a bad experience, which may have resulted in a negative perception of hormonal contraception. She may be unaware that there remain many choices available to her, even within the method categories, which she has already tried, e.g., the progestogen-only pill (POP) and the combined oral contraceptive pill (COC).
3. The opportunity provided in routine consultations to discuss benefits and risks of hormonal contraception.
4. Unplanned pregnancy and abortion are significant in women between the ages of 20 and 24.

Management of unscheduled bleeding

The Clinical Effectiveness Unit of the Faculty of Sexual and Reproductive Healthcare developed a guideline to facilitate appropriate investigation of women presenting with unscheduled bleeding [1].

Contraception, eds Paula Briggs, Gabor Kovacs and John Guillebaud. Published by Cambridge University Press. © Cambridge University Press 2013.

This is common in the first few months of use of any hormonal method of contraception. Therefore reassurance is appropriate and important, particularly in view of Ana's anxiety about cancer.

A pregnancy test is important and simple to undertake. The urine sample provided for pregnancy testing can also be used for screening for chlamydia and gonorrhoea as long as the sample is first catch and the woman has not passed urine in the previous hour.

Regular screening for chlamydia for young people under the age of 25 is recommended by the National Chlamydia Screening Programme in the UK and is particularly important in any woman in whom there are symptoms, which may be indicative of infection. This is discussed in more detail in Chapter 19.

For women with breakthrough bleeding in association with the use of hormonal contraception, lasting longer than three months, it is important to view the cervix. Ideally this should be done during the consultation as younger women may fail to attend a further appointment. When doing a speculum examination, it may be appropriate to take the sample for chlamydia screening at the same time. Visualization of the cervix may detect the presence of an ectropion, polyps or an appearance suggestive of cancer. Referral to colposcopy is indicated if the cervix looks macroscopically suspicious. The National Cytology Screening Programme in England commences at the age of 25. This varies throughout the UK with screening in Scotland and Wales starting at 20. In Ana's case, therefore, a cervical smear test is not recommended at this stage.

A pelvic examination should be undertaken to exclude pelvic pathology including ovarian cysts, fibroids and gynaecological cancers. If an abnormality is detected an ultrasound examination should be arranged in the first instance.

Ana has screening for chlamydia and gonorrhoea, both of which are negative. Her cervix is grossly normal in appearance. A pelvic examination reveals no abnormality.

She is reassured by the tests undertaken and is willing to discuss the contraceptive choices available to her. Both she and her partner are fed up with using condoms and they are also concerned about the reliability of this method.

The challenge of facilitating a contraceptive choice consultation

Ana admits to forgetting pills. This may have contributed to the irregular bleeding which she experienced. You suggest the combined hormonal patch, as this will eliminate the need for daily activity. You explain to Ana that this method will deliver the same class of hormones as are used in some COC pills, but that delivery through the skin will promote more stable hormone levels which are more likely to lead to better cycle control. It also eliminates the need for daily pill taking and only has to be applied once a week. When Ana asks you how this is possible, you explain that the contraceptive patch enables the delivery of hormones directly to the blood stream via a 20 cm squared patch delivering 150 µg of norelgestromin and 20 µg of ethinyl oestradiol. She should apply a patch once a week for three weeks and then have a patch-free week, during which time she is likely to have a withdrawal bleed. There is a margin for error – application of a new patch does not have to be at the same time each week and in fact a patch can be left in place for nine days without any loss of efficacy or need for additional contraceptive cover. The patch is as effective as the combined pill if used as according to instruction [2].

She declines this option as she does not want a method which is potentially visible, and she has heard stories about patches coming off and leaving black sticky marks which are unsightly.

She is not interested in a progestogen-only implant as she has been advised that this might also result in unpredictable bleeding. Her friend Cindy has used the contraceptive injection and no longer has bleeding but has gained a considerable amount of weight. This is a particular concern for Ana and she asks if there are any other options?

You suggest intrauterine contraception but she is not keen on this as another friend Caroline had a bad experience with severe pain at the time of insertion. Despite the fact that the pain settled and Caroline is now very happy with her copper intrauterine device, Ana is too frightened to consider this option at the present time.

Her friend Kim has just returned from an elective in Spain and is using a combined vaginal ring. She is very enthusiastic about it. Is this a method that might be suitable for Ana?

Counselling for the combined vaginal ring, NuvaRing®

Ana is initially reluctant to consider the vagina as a route to deliver her contraception but with an opportunity to discuss her concerns, as listed below, she is reassured.

Will the ring stay in?

Expulsion is rare in terms of women-years of use, but between 4 and 20% of women who took part in studies reported at least one episode [3]. As long as this is recognized and the ring is re-inserted, it does not decrease efficacy. This needs to be covered in the counselling before the woman uses the method.

The upper part of the vagina where the ring will be located is angled, and in addition to this the vaginal muscles keep the ring in place. This is an opportunity to reassure Ana that the exact position of the ring is unimportant and to reinforce to her that she cannot fail to insert it correctly. If she is able to feel the ring in the vagina, then she needs to push it up a bit further. The upper part of the vagina has an autonomic nerve supply, which means that there will be no perception of a foreign body in this part of the vagina. She may also need assurance that removal of the vaginal ring will not be difficult for her.

Although the vaginal delivery of hormones is novel in the UK, the use of tampons is common and not associated with anxiety. This may be reassuring to some women considering using the vaginal ring.

Will the ring fit her?

There is only one size of ring available. The vaginal ring is made from synthetic material; it is transparent and measures 54 mm by 4 mm (Figure 11.1). It is soft and flexible and releases 15 µg of ethinyl oestradiol and 120 µg etonogestrel daily. It is important to tell all women requesting a vaginal ring that, 'one size fits all'.

How does it work?

The primary mode of action is inhibition of ovulation like the combined pill. However, a lower dose of ethinyl oestradiol is possible as absorption of the hormone through the vaginal mucosa is more efficient when compared with oral preparations and 'first pass' through the liver is avoided. This is because the vaginal rugae increase the surface area available for

- 1 ring per cycle
- Regimen:
  - −3 weeks of ring use
  - −1 ring-free week
- Daily release :
  - −15 µg ethinyl oestradiol
  - −120 µg etonogestrel

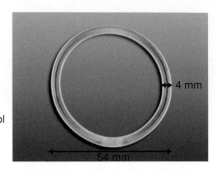

Figure 11.1 Ethinyl oestradiol/etonogestrel contraceptive vaginal ring.

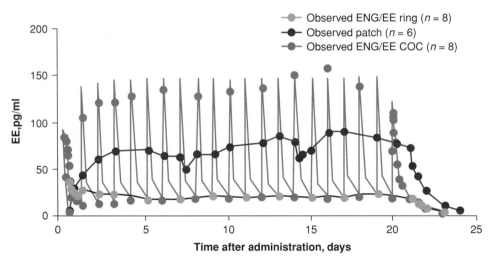

Figure 11.2 Consistent and low hormone levels versus COC or patch. (COC, combined oral contraceptive; EE, ethinyl oestradiol; ENG, etonogestrel.)

absorption and also as a result of the excellent blood supply to the vagina. The resulting level of ethinyl oestradiol in the systemic circulation is lower than that seen with the other combined hormonal contraceptive options, but the stable level achieved is associated with an improvement in cycle control [4] (Figure 11.2).

The failure rate is approximately 1%, which means that if 100 women used the method correctly for a year that one would become pregnant. Clearly imperfect use will increase the failure rate [5].

Ana is still concerned regarding the potential bleeding profile she should expect with the vaginal ring and she is worried about how to use it. She asks you the following questions.

What will happen regarding her 'periods'?

The vaginal ring should either be inserted immediately ('Quick Start' – seven days additional contraception required) or be inserted on day one of her period (no additional cover required). The ring should be left in the vagina for three weeks and then removed for one week, during which time she will be likely to experience a withdrawal bleed.

Are side effects common?

The vaginal ring has a similar side effect profile and contraindications to other combined hormonal contraceptive methods, namely the COC pill and patch. Use of the method is absolutely contraindicated for women who score a UK Medical Eligibility Criteria (UKMEC) category 4 and should be used only after careful consideration in women falling into UKMEC category 3, where the potential risks outweigh the benefits [6].

Side effects experienced include an increase in vaginal secretions and other oestrogenic side effects including nausea, headache and breast tenderness, although these are less marked due to the lower systemic levels of ethinyl oestradiol.

There is no delay in return to fertility on stopping the method.

How often will she need to attend the clinic to receive her rings?

A comprehensive medical history has been taken. During this several important points are covered. Ana has no history of migraine with aura, no family history of venous thromboembolism and she does not smoke. She is on no other medication, including herbal remedies. On examination, her blood pressure is 110/60 and her body mass index (BMI) is 22.

She is provided with three rings. You reinforce that she should insert one ring into her vagina for three weeks and then remove it for a week, during which time she is likely to have a withdrawal bleed. You advise her that NuvaRing® has a wide safety margin and can be left in place for four weeks followed by a ring-free week, with no loss of efficacy. You advise her that if she wishes to avoid a withdrawal bleed, she can insert the first ring for four weeks, followed by a further ring for four weeks without a break. She is really interested in a text messaging facility to help her remember to remove and reinsert her rings. Her life is 'ruled' by her smartphone and your ability to link her contraception to her lifestyle is valued [7].

You explain that NuvaRing® needs to be refrigerated until the point of dispensing, after which it can remain out of the fridge, but should be kept at a temperature less than 30°C. NuvaRing® has a shelf life of four to five months once dispensed. She will be reviewed in approximately 10 weeks time to ensure that she is happy with the method. Thereafter, she can be provided with pre-dated prescriptions to ensure that she does not need to attend the service any more frequently than other women using the combined pill.

Before she leaves, Ana requests an opportunity to allay her fears regarding cancer and other potential health risks associated with combined hormonal contraception. This is an opportunity for a discussion regarding benefits and risks associated with combined hormonal contraception.

Benefits and risks associated with combined hormonal contraception

Rather than start with potential risks, you start by reinforcing the potential benefits associated with combined hormonal contraception, particularly in a healthy young woman like Ana. You tell her that there is a reduction in the development of cancer of the bowel, ovary and endometrium (see Chapter 15), and that cancer of the cervix is caused by infection with certain oncogenic strains of human papilloma virus and that the use of combined hormonal contraception is a co-factor but not the primary cause. You explain that breast cancer is a common condition affecting one in nine women lifelong and that there is no contraindication to the use of combined hormonal contraception in young women who are not known to be carriers of the BRCA gene. You advise her that the most significant risk associated with the use of combined hormonal contraception is venous thromboembolism with a 2-fold increase over the background rate now thought to be 4.4 per 10 000 women [8]. You are able to reassure her that she has no factors in her personal history which will increase her risk of VTE above 9 per 10 000 women. This is discussed in detail in Chapter 6.

You also inform her about other potential benefits associated with combined hormonal contraception as a class effect, including a reduction in menstrual bleeding and pain, a reduction in premenstrual symptoms, a reduction in rheumatoid arthritis and an improvement in acne, more marked with some progestogens than others [9].

User satisfaction rates and the effect on unplanned pregnancy and abortion

Improvement in accessibility and method choice has resulted in pregnancy rates in women in their 20s reaching a plateau and stabilizing in the UK in the 10 years between 2001 and 2011. This is reflected in the number of women in that age category requesting abortion [10].

Satisfaction with method choice is likely to be associated with continuity and effectiveness. Satisfaction rates with NuvaRing® are high [11] with more than 90% of users continuing in clinical trials [12].

Take-home messages

1. In a woman in her 20s, breakthrough bleeding is unlikely to be due to significant pathology.
2. Missed pills are associated with significant side effects, including unplanned pregnancy and breakthrough bleeding. Therefore in a woman who admits to being a poor pill taker, other options should be considered.
3. Progestogen-only methods have the advantage of minimal contraindications but are not associated with regular withdrawal bleeds, which may be unacceptable to some women, like Ana.
4. All combined hormonal contraceptive methods have a similar side effect and risk profile.
5. In clinical trials, most users have been satisfied with the combined hormonal ring. The greatest barrier to this method is promoting the vagina as an ideal organ in which to place hormonal contraception and this remains a challenge to all providers of contraception.

References

1. Faculty of Sexual and Reproductive Healthcare. *Management of Unscheduled Bleeding in Women Using Hormonal Contraception*, May 2009. http://www.fsrh.org/pdfs/UnscheduledBleedingMay09.pdf (accessed 1 March 2013).
2. Faculty of Sexual and Reproductive Healthcare Clinical Effectiveness Unit. *New Product Review*, September 2003. http://www.fsrh.org/pdfs/ProductReviewEVRA.pdf (accessed 1 March 2013).
3. Milsom I, Lete I, Bjertnaes A, *et al*. Effects on cycle control and bodyweight of the combined contraceptive ring, NuvaRing, versus an oral contraceptive containing 30 mg ethinyl estradiol and 3 mg drospirenone. *Hum Reprod* 2006; 21: 2304–11.
4. Roumen FJ, Mishell DR. The contraceptive vaginal ring, NuvaRing®, a decade after its introduction. *Eur J Contracept Reprod Health Care* 2012; 17(6): 415–27.

5. Roumen FJ, Apter D, Mulders TM, Dieben TO. Efficacy, tolerability and acceptability of a novel contraceptive vaginal ring releasing etonogestrel and ethinyl oestradiol. *Hum Reprod* 2001; 16: 469–75.

6. Faculty of Sexual and Reproductive Healthcare. *UK Medical Eligibility Criteria for Contraceptive Use*, 2009. http://www.fsrh.org/pdfs/UKMEC2009.pdf (accessed 1 March 2013).

7. My NuvaRing Reminder Service. http://www.nuvaring.co.uk/ information-for-women/my-nuvaring/ Reminder-service (accessed 1 March 2013).

8. Dinger JC, Heinemann LA, Kühl-Habich D. The safety of a drospirenone-containing oral contraceptive: final results from the European Active Surveillance Study on oral contraceptives based on 142 475 women-years of observation. *Contraception* 2007; 75: 344–54.

9. Fraser IS. Added health benefits of the levonorgestrel contraceptive intrauterine system and other hormonal contraceptive delivery systems. *Contraception* 2013; 87: 273–9.

10. Department of Health. *Abortion Statistics, England and Wales: 2011*, May 2012. https://www.wp.dh.gov.uk/transparency/ files/2012/05/Commentary1.pdf (accessed 1 March 2013).

11. Dieben TO, Roumen FJ, Apter D. Efficacy, cycle control, and user acceptability of a novel combined contraceptive vaginal ring. *Obstet Gynecol* 2002; 100: 585–93.

12. Bjarnadóttir RI, Tuppurainen M, Killick SR. Comparison of cycle control with a combined contraceptive vaginal ring and oral levonorgestrel/ethinyl estradiol. *J Obstet Gynecol* 2002; 186; 389–95.

Chapter 12

Contraception in the 30-somethings

Anne Szarewski

Case scenario: Katie

Katie, a 34-year-old mother of two, presents for a further supply of her combined oral contraceptive pill. She does not smoke and has no medical contraindication to combined hormonal contraception, based on a risk assessment using the UK Medical Eligibility Criteria (UKMEC) 2009. She requests advice regarding running pill packs together to avoid a withdrawal bleed for a forthcoming family holiday.

The first thing to say is that age alone is not a contraindication to any method of contraception. A reasonably common scenario in the mid-30s is that women who reach the age of 35 and smoke have to stop taking the combined oral contraceptive (COC) pill. However, if she does not smoke and continues to have no other risk factors, there is no reason why a woman cannot stay on COC until she reaches the age of menopause.

Women in their 30s are a particularly disparate group. Some will already have one or more children and may be either spacing or have decided their family is complete. Others will not yet have children but may be thinking of having one soon; indeed, they may be worrying about their biological clock. A woman needs to consider whether to use a hormonal or non-hormonal method, whether she can commit to methods requiring daily, weekly, monthly or less frequent attention and which potential side effects she finds acceptable. Other considerations include her desired bleeding pattern, how she would feel about unscheduled bleeding and how discreet she wants her method to be.

Katie presents with a common scenario, that of not wanting to bleed during a holiday. Of course, running a couple of pill packs together is frequently done. However, a request such as this can provide an opportunity to educate women about the issue of periods, withdrawal bleeds and continuous COC use.

The concept of the regular, 28 day cycle is a relatively new phenomenon. Women in prehistoric times had far fewer periods than modern women, at around about 160 during their lives. They had a later menarche, at around the age of 16, and their first childbirth was at around 19.5 years. They were frequently pregnant – on average, women had six live births – and they breastfed for around two to three years, which helped them space their pregnancies. Such a pattern persists to this day in traditional hunter-gatherer societies in Africa and South America, where women are considered eligible for child-bearing once they have had their first period, and are then constantly either pregnant or breastfeeding for the whole of their reproductive lives.

By contrast, women in developed countries have an earlier menarche, at around 12.5 years, and have their first baby later, at about the age of 24. In general they only have

Contraception, eds Paula Briggs, Gabor Kovacs and John Guillebaud. Published by Cambridge University Press. © Cambridge University Press 2013.

two or three pregnancies, and breastfeeding is much less common and for a much shorter time. Since menopause also occurs later in these women, they are likely to have three times as many periods in their lives, at around 450.

When the COC pill was first developed in the late 1950s, Pincus and his co-workers felt that a monthly, cyclical pattern was optimal, for several reasons. They realized that very few women understood female reproductive biology and so would not understand how taking a daily pill could prevent pregnancy. In addition, it was important to reassure women they were not pregnant. The contraceptive methods used until then, mostly barriers, withdrawal and the rhythm method, were not very reliable, and there were no simple and quick pregnancy tests. Women were therefore accustomed to waiting for their monthly bleed for reassurance that they were not pregnant. This was especially important with the early high dose COCs, since some of the side effects in the early months of use – in particular nausea, breast tenderness, bleeding – were similar to those of early pregnancy. A further concern for one of the scientists, John Rock (who was a practising Catholic), was to try and offset potential objections from the Catholic Church. He hoped that monthly bleeding would be seen by the Vatican as being 'natural' and that this contraceptive would therefore be accepted. Regrettably, and to his dismay, he was wrong.

The seven day pill-free interval (PFI) was chosen to ensure that the majority of women would start to bleed before they were due to start their next packet. The high doses used (100 µg ethinyl oestradiol (EE)) meant that it took several days before the hormone levels fell sufficiently to cause the bleed. Nowadays, with much lower doses of hormones being used, the seven day pill-free week is clearly too long, with increasing evidence of follicular activity and even ovulation despite accurate pill taking. In addition, over the years, awareness has increased regarding problems specifically related to the PFI, such as premenstrual symptoms, headaches and painful bleeds [1].

Reducing the length of the PFI to 4 days has proved effective in preventing ovulation and there are now several 24/4 regimen COCs on the market, though not yet in the UK. Another approach is to reduce the number of PFIs. Tricycling (taking three packets of 21 pills before having a break) has become accepted practice for women who suffer headaches, painful bleeds or premenstrual symptoms in the PFI. This has also become standard practice for women in whom PFIs are positively detrimental, for example those with endometriosis or epilepsy. For maximum benefit, tricycling is often coupled with a shortened (four day) PFI. Eliminating the PFI altogether is another option, and continuous use pill regimens are licensed in countries other than the UK (as are tricycle pills).

The greatest barrier to eliminating the PFI is psychological. Although it is already common practice to run packets together for special occasions, such as holidays and weddings, there seems to be a feeling (not just among women, but also some healthcare professionals) that this is acceptable sometimes, but surely not on a regular basis – indeed, this would undoubtedly be one of the questions Katie would ask. There is also the issue that the more packets are run together, the greater the risk of unpredictable breakthrough bleeding (BTB), which is very poorly tolerated by women, much less well than amenorrhoea in the long term.

Nevertheless, there are a growing number of women who find withdrawal bleeding a nuisance and, indeed, a recent survey in Europe, USA, Canada and Brazil showed that around a third of women would like to bleed only every two to three months while on the pill [2]. In fact, in the UK 40% of women favoured this option. Approximately a fifth of women said they would like to eliminate their bleeding completely using a COC. Women aged over 40 were more likely to prefer this option than women aged under 25, perhaps because younger women believe monthly or at least regular bleeding demonstrates they are fertile.

Clearly, different women want different length cycles, so the solution is to tailor the length of COC use to the individual woman. The woman should be advised to take her pill continuously until such time as she gets BTB. If she bleeds for more than three days, she should take a break of four days. The advantage of this is that, for an individual woman, on a particular COC, once she establishes how long she can take the pill without bleeding, the bleed-free duration for her, on that COC, will generally be the same. So, for example, if a woman finds she can take her pill for 14 weeks continuously before she starts to get BTB, she now knows that it is likely to always be 14 weeks. This means she can plan ahead; if, for example, she realizes that her holiday is booked for 14 weeks after her last withdrawal bleed, she can elect to stop her pill after 12 weeks in order to ensure she does not bleed while on holiday. The same principle could apply to other important events, whether work or leisure related. In effect, it puts a woman in control of when she bleeds. It has been shown that this practical approach deals effectively with the BTB and results in greater patient satisfaction. A similar approach has proved successful using the NuvaRing® [3], which is in fact licensed for extended use (though the licence is only for two cycles).

A disadvantage of the tailored continuous approach has been that it is off-licence, which often makes both health professionals and women uneasy about safety. However, in 2012, a COC with a flexible extended regimen received a European licence. The formulation is 20 μg EE combined with 3 mg drospirenone and the licence allows women to have a monthly bleed, or to extend the length of tablet intake as they wish. They are advised to have a four day break if they experience three days of BTB.

Efficacy studies were carried out in both the USA and Europe and showed Pearl Indices of 0.64 (95% CI 0.28–1.26) in Europe and 1.65 (95% CI 0.96–2.65) in the USA. Efficacy is always lower in the USA than in Europe, due to compliance issues. Comparisons between the extended regimens and a conventional 24/4 regimen showed both fewer bleeding days and less dymenorrhoea with the extended regimens. The safety profile of the flexible extended regimens was similar to that seen in general in COC studies [4–7].

An exciting development accompanying the new licensed regimen is that it comes with a palm-sized dispenser that records usage, notices when a tablet has been missed and provides an alert that alternative contraception must be used. Currently called Yaz Flex® in Australia, where it has already been launched, the pill cartridge, containing 120 tablets, fits into the bottom of the dispenser (in Europe it may be called Flexyess®). The Clyk® digital tablet dispenser can be programmed to sound a daily alarm to remind women to take the pill. Because the studies had to include a PFI after 120 days, the instructions tell women they should have a break after 120 days, if they have not had one before [8] (Box 12.1).

It must be remembered that there will be certain groups of women who do not wish to decrease the frequency of their bleeds, and who have extremely low tolerance of irregular bleeding. It is important to be culturally sensitive, while nevertheless making women aware of their options.

One thing that should be remembered, and needs to be checked in Katie's case, is that continuous, flexible COC use can only be undertaken using monophasic pills. As women get older, they may be attracted to newer COCs containing oestradiol – as opposed to EE – which they may perceive as being 'more natural'. One such, already available, is Qlaira®, a four-phasic COC, containing varying doses of oestradiol valerate (E_2V) and dienogest (DNG) in a 26/2 regimen, i.e., there are only 2 hormone-free days (with placebo tablets included in the packet). Studies have confirmed that Qlaira® is as effective as COCs containing EE. Qlaira® has received regulatory approval for use in the treatment of heavy menstrual bleeding, for

> **Box 12.1** How to take Yaz Flex®
>
> **Follow all directions given to you by your doctor or pharmacist carefully.** They may differ from the information contained in this leaflet. The information contained in this leaflet tells you how you should take the pill.
>
> A separate set of instructions is enclosed with the Clyk tablet dispenser; please follow these instructions carefully on how to use the Clyk tablet dispenser.
>
> The Clyk tablet dispenser is a dispensing system for Yaz Flex; it tells you when it is time to take your pill. It will also allow you to determine the status of your intake regimen.
>
> If you do not understand the instructions printed on the pharmacist label, ask your doctor or pharmacist for help.
>
> **How to take it**
>
> Take your first Yaz Flex tablet by dispensing the pill from the Clyk tablet dispenser. Insert the narrow end of the cartridge into the dispenser so that the window of the dispenser (as well as the tablets in the cartridge) can be seen
>
> **Preparing the Clyk tablet dispenser for use**
>
> Unpack and insert the cartridge on the day you want to start taking your pill.
>
> Make sure the day and time you release your first pill is convenient for you.
>
> The dispenser will automatically record when the first tablet is released by setting this time as the reference time.
>
> Press the two soft sides of the dispenser at the same time to release the tablet.
>
> Take one tablet daily at about the same time every day. You must take Yaz Flex every day even if you do not have sex very often. It will also help you remember when to take it. Take the tablets for the first 24 days (fixed phase) without a tablet-free break.
>
> A 4 day tablet-free break can be taken between the flexible phase – days 25–120. A tablet-free break should not be longer than 4 days.
>
> A 4 day tablet-free interval must be taken after taking the pill for 120 consecutive days.
>
> After each 4 day tablet-free interval, a new cycle of pill taking starts with a minimum of 24 days and a maximum of 120 days.
>
> **Swallow the tablets whole with a glass of water.** It does not matter if you take this medicine before or after food. If you see an exclamation mark symbol (!) on the Clyk tablet dispenser screen, this means you must use additional barrier contraceptive precautions (e.g., condoms, diaphragm) until this symbol (!) disappears. If you do not understand the instructions provided, ask your doctor or pharmacist for help.
>
> Adapted from [8].

which it is certainly effective; however, it does not lend itself to flexible continuous use for elimination of withdrawal bleeds.

Another natural oestradiol COC is due to be launched in the UK in 2013. Zoely® contains 1.5 mg 17β oestradiol, combined with 2.5 mg of the progestogen nomegestrol acetate (NOMAC). This is a monophasic 24/4 preparation (24 active tablets and 4 placebo tablets). Unlike Qlaira®, flexible continued use should be possible with Zoely®. Although cycle control with Zoely® was not quite as good as with Yasmin® in a comparative trial, the bleeds were shorter and lighter – possibly due to the shorter hormone-free interval (four as opposed to seven days). Efficacy of the two preparations was similar [9]. Although it is hoped that COCs containing natural oestradiol will have fewer health risks, such as venous thromboembolism, actual confirmation of this awaits the results of large post-marketing studies, due to be available in the next few years.

In the context of postponing periods (as opposed to withdrawal bleeds), it is worth noting that new information has been incorporated into the Summary of Product Characteristics of Primolut N®, a commonly prescribed formulation of norethisterone 5 mg, used for the postponement of periods in women not using COCs. High dose norethisterone is metabolized to EE; 1 mg orally administered norethisterone metabolizes to 4–6 μg EE, a fact that should be considered when prescribing to women at high risk of venous thromboembolism [10].

References

1. Szarewski A. Sisters doing it for themselves. *J Fam Plann Reprod Health Care* 2009; 35(2): 71–2.

2. Szarewski A, von Stenglin A, Rybowski S. Women's attitudes towards monthly bleeding: results of a global population-based survey. *Eur J Contracept Reprod Health Care* 2012; 17(4): 270–83.

3. Kerns J, Darney P. Vaginal ring contraception. *Contraception* 2011; 83(2): 107–15.

4. Strowitzki T, Kirsch B, Elliesen J. Efficacy of ethinylestradiol 20 mg/drospirenone 3 mg in a flexible extended regimen in women with moderate-to-severe primary dysmenorrhoea: an open-label, multicentre, randomised, controlled study. *J Fam Plann Reprod Health Care* 2012; 38(2): 94–101.

5. Jensen JT, Garie SV, Trummer D, Elliesen J. Bleeding profile of a flexible extended regimen of ethinylestradiol/ drospirenone in US women: an open-label, three-arm, active-controlled, multicenter study. *Contraception* 2012; 86(2): 110–18.

6. Klipping C, Duijkers I, Fortier MP, *et al.* Contraceptive efficacy and tolerability of ethinylestradiol 20 μg/drospirenone 3 mg in a flexible extended regimen: an open-label, multicentre, randomised, controlled study. *J Fam Plann Reprod Health Care* 2012; 38: 73–83.

7. Klipping C, Duijkers I, Fortier MP, *et al.* Long-term tolerability of ethinylestradiol 20 mg/drospirenone 3 mg in a flexible extended regimen: results from a randomised, controlled, multicentre study. *J Fam Plann Reprod Health Care* 2012; 38: 84–93.

8. Mydr.com.au. How to take Yaz Flex. http://www.mydr.com.au/medicines/cmis/yaz-flex-tablets (accessed 3 March 2013).

9. Mansour D, Verhoeven C, Sommer W, *et al.* Efficacy and tolerability of a monophasic combined oral contraceptive containing nomegestrol acetate and 17β²-oestradiol in a 24/4 regimen, in comparison to an oral contraceptive containing ethinyloestradiol and drospirenone in a 21/7 regimen. *Eur J Contracept Reprod Health Care* 2011; 16: 430–43.

10. Mansour D. Safer prescribing of therapeutic norethisterone for women at risk of venous thromboembolism. *J Fam Plann Reprod Health Care* 2012; 38: 148–9.

Contraception in the 40-somethings

13

Sunanda Gupta and Ali A. Kubba

Case scenario: Alison

Alison is 42 years old and has two grown-up children. Her husband had a vasectomy and therefore she has not had to consider contraception for many years. She has suffered from heavy painful periods for most of her life and she is currently being treated for anaemia. Her general practitioner did suggest using an intrauterine system to manage her bleeding, but she was reluctant to consider this. She and her husband have separated and she has met a new partner. She is very concerned about becoming pregnant as she feels that she has spent most of her life looking after her husband and children and she now wants some time for herself. She has retrained and is now working as a yoga teacher. Her heavy menstrual bleeding is affecting her job as she has recently had a very embarrassing episode where she flooded in public. She has always considered hormones to be 'bad'.

Alison's situation is far from unusual for this age group, where the risk of relationship break-down is high. It is apparent that Alison's first priority is a highly effective contraceptive method. However, she requires much more from her method: effective control of bleeding and dysmenorrhoea; restoration of menstrual predictability and/or amenorrhoea; and in the future possible help with peri-menopausal symptoms.

History

The first step would be to obtain a comprehensive medical, gynaecological, obstetric, family, social and sexual history.

A medical history will ensure that prescribing is in line with evidence-based WHO/UK Medical Eligibility Criteria for safe and effective contraceptive provision.

The following areas are of particular importance:

Bleeding pattern

- Duration and amount of bleeding, including flooding and clots.
- Length and possible change in cycle.
- Date of last menstrual period.
- History of social 'accidents' and impact on quality of life.
- Any tendency to bruising easily and/or excessive bleeding after tooth extraction/surgery and family history of bleeding disorders would be relevant.
- Any associated symptoms of intermenstrual and/or post-coital bleeding. Suspicion of possible malignant causes for the bleeding should trigger referral under the two-week rule.

Contraception, eds Paula Briggs, Gabor Kovacs and John Guillebaud. Published by Cambridge University Press. © Cambridge University Press 2013.

Associated pain

- Ascertain whether the dysmenorrhoea is premenstrual and/or menstrual. Dysmenorrhoea that is relieved with the onset of menses is generally not associated with organic pathology. Have the periods always been painful? Has she sought help in the past? What relieves the pain and what makes it worse?
- Bowel or urinary symptoms and dyspareunia and pelvic pain, may indicate underlying problems.
- Does she suffer from menstrual migraine or premenstrual symptoms?
- What medication has been tried for this problem to date and is she taking any other drugs that would have the potential to interact with a contraceptive method or exacerbate symptoms?

Sexual history

- Sexual history with a risk assessment for sexually transmitted infections (STIs) including human immunodeficiency virus (HIV) is essential. (This is covered in detail in Chapter 19.)
- Lifestyle risk factors such as smoking, recreational drug use and alcohol consumption.
- Exploring any potential psychosexual issues.
- Establishing Alison's past contraceptive experiences prior to her husband's vasectomy may give an indication for the reason behind her reluctance to consider hormonal contraception.
- Her cervical screening history needs documenting.

What are Alison's preferences and expectations from her contraceptive method?

- Does she wish to retain personal control and be able to discontinue the method without having to return to a healthcare professional?
- Would she wish to consider a long-acting reversible (LARC) method as she may forget a daily/weekly/monthly preparation?
- How does she feel about monthly withdrawal bleeds? Would she welcome light/ infrequent bleeds and/or amenorrhoea?
- How important is it for Alison to use a highly effective contraceptive method?

Examination

- A general examination should be performed including blood pressure measurement.
- An abdominal examination should be performed for any abdomino-pelvic masses and/or tender areas.
- A speculum examination should be undertaken to visualize the cervix and vagina to exclude any local pathology.
- A bimanual examination is undertaken to assess for uterine enlargement (fibroids, adenomyosis), uterine mobility and adnexal masses and/or tenderness.

Investigations

- Full blood count
- Thyroid function tests and/or clotting screen are not required unless clinically indicated.

- A cervical smear should not be routinely performed unless clinically indicated.
- Pregnancy should be excluded if this is suspected.
- A pelvic ultrasound is indicated if Alison has intermenstrual bleeding (IMB), an abdomino-pelvic mass, an enlarged uterus on bimanual examination or failure to respond to previous medical treatment for heavy menstrual bleeding (HMB).
- An endometrial biopsy, to exclude endometrial cancer or atypical endometrial hyperplasia is advisable in women with risk factors including obesity, diabetes, polycystic ovarian syndrome, a family history of endometrial or bowel cancer, persistent intermenstrual bleeding (IMB), or where treatment has been ineffective [1].
- Hysteroscopy is indicated if intrauterine pathology is suspected on ultrasound.
- STI screening for chlamydia and gonorrhoea by dual polymerase chain reaction (PCR)/nucleic acid amplification tests should be offered.

Contraceptive options

Having established Alison's priorities and concerns with a working diagnosis in hand (dysfunctional uterine bleeding), Alison will be advised that, although a natural decline in fertility occurs with increasing age, effective contraception is still required. Her age does not restrict her contraceptive choices.

The levonorgestrel-releasing intrauterine system (Mirena®)

The levonorgestrel-releasing intrauterine system (LNG-IUS) would be an ideal option if the uterine cavity is not more than 10 cm deep and reasonably regular (distortion of the uterine cavity is associated with a higher expulsion rate of devices). Small fibroids and those that are intramural or subserous are generally not a problem as they do not result in any significant distortion of the uterine cavity and the associated bleeding is controlled by the LNG-IUS.

Other contraindications to the use of this method include a current history of breast cancer (five years) and/or acute or severe liver disease. The intrauterine system (IUS) does not have prothrombotic effects and could safely be used even if Alison has a history of deep venous thrombosis (DVT) or pulmonary embolism (PE).

Contraceptive efficacy

As prevention of unintended pregnancy is important for Alison, the IUS is ideal with a pregnancy rate of 0.2% during the first 12 months of use and a cumulative gross pregnancy rate of 0.5–1.1 per 100 users at 5 years. As the progestogen is directly released from the IUS at the site of action, the efficacy would not be diminished if Alison is taking enzyme-inducing drugs.

Other non-contraceptive benefits

In idiopathic or fibroid associated menorrhagia, there is the additional benefit of a 96% reduction in menstrual blood loss (MBL) at year one with an associated improvement in haemoglobin and haematocrit levels. This effect on menorrhagia is endorsed by the Royal College of Obstetricians and Gynaecologists (RCOG) Guidelines [2] and the National Institute for Health and Clinical Excellence (NICE) *Heavy Menstrual Bleeding* Clinical Guidance released in 2007 [1]. Long-term use of the LNG-IUS has been known to be associated with prevention of fibroid growth in many but not all users. Barrington and Bowens-Simpkins [3] showed an 80% improvement in dysmenorrhoea on the basis that the atrophic endometrium is likely to produce less prostaglandins, which may help with painful periods.

If Alison has endometrial hyperplasia without atypia, the risk of progression to endometrial cancer in the absence of treatment is 1 : 100. Long-term use of the IUS is likely to induce regression of endometrial hyperplasia. If Alison has adenomyosis, her heavy painful periods are likely to improve with a concomitant improvement in quality of life at one year. This effect has been shown to last for up to three years. If Alison has disorders of haemostasis (von Willebrand's disease, platelet disorder or specific coagulation deficiencies), she is likely to respond favourably to treatment with the LNG-IUS.

Counselling

Alison will be advised about how the LNG-IUS works by profound endometrial glandular and stromal suppression, cervical mucus changes and a foreign body effect within the endometrium. Most women ovulate, though in some women ovulation suppression is likely during the first year. Though licensed for 5 years for contraception, if Alison was over the age of 45, she could retain the device for contraception until the menopause is confirmed or until contraception is no longer required and for as long as it continues to work to control heavy painful periods.

She should be informed about possible progestogenic side effects including headache, breast tenderness and acne. Most of these symptoms are likely to settle down with time due to the known decline in levonorgestrel (LNG) levels.

Menstrual disruption is not uncommon during the first few months following insertion, with frequent and prolonged bleeds in up to 35% of women in the first 3 months, decreasing to 6% by the end of the first year. A proportion of women become amenorrhoeic by 9–12 months. Informing Alison about the menstrual side effects is likely to be associated with acceptance of the menstrual pattern, improved satisfaction and retention of the device.

Alison should be advised about the small risk of pelvic infection associated with the introduction of intrauterine contraception, with an increase in infection in the first few weeks following insertion. Risk of pelvic inflammatory disease (PID) is reported to be lower with the LNG-IUS compared to the copper intrauterine device (IUD) and is under 1 : 100 in women assessed as being at low risk of STIs.

The risk of displacement of the LNG-IUS is 4–5% particularly if Alison has a heavy bleed or if she has a large uterine cavity.

The incidence of uterine perforation is 0.5–1.0 per 1000 insertions and is highly dependent on the skill of the operator.

A previous ectopic pregnancy does not contraindicate use of the method and the risk of ectopic pregnancy is reduced when compared with copper IUDs.

Some 10–12% of LNG-IUS users develop functional ovarian cysts which are essentially harmless, self limiting and do not require intervention.

Insertion

The IUS should be inserted up to day seven of a normal cycle. It can be inserted at other times in the cycle if there has been no unprotected sex, but a further week of protection after insertion will be required.

Insertion is generally not a painful procedure, but there may be difficulties with insertion if Alison is unduly anxious, she has a history of Caesarean sections and/or a past history of laser/loop treatment of the cervix with subsequent scarring. A local anaesthetic gel or intracervical block can facilitate the procedure. This may be required in a small number of women. Prior use of misoprostol has not been shown to improve the patient experience with insertion, but some clinicians do use it.

Safety issues

- As most women using the LNG-IUS have ovulatory cycles and oestradiol levels remain within the follicular range of a normal menstrual cycle, there is no adverse effect on bone mineral density (BMD).
- The LNG-IUS is not known to increase the risk of venous thromboembolism (VTE) as evidenced by many studies including a recent large Danish cohort study of 1.5 million women, which concluded that LNG-IUS users have the lowest relative risk (RR) of VTE, followed by the implant and combined hormonal contraception (CHC) users.
- Studies do not show an increase in risk of stroke in LNG-IUS users compared to non-users.
- Recently, Dinger et al. published a study which demonstrated that current or ever use of the LNG-IUS compared with copper IUD was not associated with an increase in risk of breast cancer [4].
- If Alison has a history of breast cancer with no recurrence in the last five years, use of the LNG-IUS is not contraindicated. However, if Alison developed breast cancer whilst using the device, one recent study showed a higher risk of recurrence, of borderline significance and a higher risk of nodal involvement [5].

CHC options

If Alison is not keen on the IUS and does not smoke, is not overweight, does not take enzyme-inducing drugs, does not have a history of migraine with aura, pulmonary hypertension, liver disease, breast cancer, DVT/PE, myocardial infarction (MI), stroke, hypertension, diabetes with vascular complications and multiple risk factors for cardiovascular disease, low dose CHC methods are an option.

Efficacy of CHC

The combined oral contraceptive (COC) pill has come a long way since it was introduced in the 1960s and is an effective contraceptive method. With perfect use the failure rate is less than 1%; however, with typical use it increases to 8%. The transdermal patch Evra® and vaginal ring NuvaRing® have similar efficacy to COCs.

Counselling

Alison should be advised about the mode of action of CHC-suppression of ovulation, induction of cervical mucus changes and alteration of the endometrium. Combined oral contraceptives, transdermal patch and combined vaginal ring are best started on days 1–5 of the cycle with immediate effect, but can be 'Quick Started' any time in the cycle provided there has not been unprotected sex, and back-up contraception is used for the following seven days.

The hormone-free interval (HFI) is traditionally seven days, but tricycling is common and further extended regimens can be used (see Chapter 12). Packs containing 84 pills (Seasonale®) or 365 pills (Lybrel®) are available in the USA as extended regimen pills.

Missed pill guidelines are issued and regularly updated by the Faculty of Sexual and Reproductive Healthcare and the reader is directed to the Faculty website for current information.

Breakthrough bleeding (BTB) and breast tenderness are more common with the patch compared to COCs. Cycle control is better with NuvaRing® compared to COCs and may be an option for Alison as long as she has no deficiency of her pelvic floor caused by childbirth as this might increase the risk of expulsion.

Side effects such as headaches, nausea, bloating, breast tenderness, mood changes and BTB are not uncommon and often settle with time.

Newer COCs

There are two newly licensed pills containing natural oestrogens, Qlaira® and Zoely®. The oestrogen component is covered in Chapter 5. In addition to the novel oestrogen component, both these pills have shorter HFIs and are associated with a reduction in bleeding. Qlaira® contains oestradiol valerate and the hybrid progestogen dienogest which is anti-androgenic and in a variable dosing regimen is associated with good cycle control. It is taken for 28 consecutive days with the last 2 pills being placebo. After a few months use menstrual blood loss is significantly decreased. It could be used as an alternative to the LNG-IUS. Alison may continue to use it up to the age of 50 in the absence of contraindications.

Zoely® is a monophasic COC containing nomegestrol acetate 2.5 mg (NOMAC), oestradiol 1.5 mg (24 active pills) and 4 placebo tablets. Alison may experience shorter, lighter or absent bleeds with Zoely®.

Yaz® the 24/4 COC regimen containing 20 μg ethinyl oestradiol and drosperinone, is approved in the USA for contraception, premenstrual dysphoric disorder (PMDD) and acne. It is not available in the UK.

Other non-contraceptive benefits of CHCs

- A Cochrane systematic review/ meta-analysis of six randomized controlled trials (RCTs) concluded that COCs may reduce menstrual prostaglandin release, which is likely to reduce uterine cramps and blood loss [6].
- Reduction in MBL of 43% was seen in a small study [7]. However, a Cochrane systematic review of the pill and HMB found insufficient evidence for the reduction of MBL [8].
- The use of COCs can increase haemoglobin concentration but there is no significant reduction of iron deficiency anaemia [9]. Combined oral contraceptives may also be useful for HMB associated with fibroids. NICE supports the use of COCs for treatment of HMB and to improve bleeding pattern. The level of improvement in blood loss is less with COCs compared to the LNG-IUS, as evidenced by a recent RCT [10]. Newer formulations like Qlaira® are proving better at reducing HMB.
- Alison should be counselled about the other non-contraceptive benefits of the combined pill with evidence of significant protection against endometrial cancer with a 40% reduced risk after 1 year of use and 80% reduction after 10 or more years of use. Combined oral contraceptives reduce the risk of ovarian cancer by 20% for every 5 years of use, with up to 50% reduction in incidence after 15 years of use. Protection persists for 30 years after discontinuation. Women with BRCA1 and BRCA2 mutations may benefit from the COCs' chemoprophylactic effect against ovarian cancer but could be left with a risk of breast cancer. Combined oral contraceptive use is classified as a UK Medical Eligibility Criteria (UKMEC) 3 in the presence of BRCA1 and BRCA2 mutations.
- Improvements in acne occur by a reduction in serum-free testosterone concentrations. Suppression of ovulation may treat premenstrual syndrome (PMS).

- There is an 18% reduction in the risk of colon cancer among current/ever users of COCs compared with never users as evidenced by a meta-analysis.
- Vasomotor symptom relief is possible with COCs and there is a reduction in risk of benign breast disease with CHC use.

Safety

The lower impact of oestradiol-based COCs may equate to an improved safety profile, but epidemiological studies are not yet available. Exposure to systemic hormones is greatest with the transdermal patch followed by COCs and the least with the ring. Extended use of a COC is safe; there is no known medical benefit to routine monthly bleeding. Risks of VTE, stroke and MI increase with age. Alison should be advised that the risk of VTE is increased 2 to 6-fold in COC users compared to non-users. The risk is similar for all CHC methods. The risk of MI increases with age, but is not increased in pill users who do not smoke and do not have multiple risk factors for cardiovascular disease. Hypertension and smoking increase the risk 3 to 10-fold respectively over that of non-users – safe prescribing guided by the World Health Organization/UKMEC confers negligible risks. In a recent study:

- The absolute RR of MI was increased by a factor of 1.3–2.3 with COCs, 2.5 with the contraceptive vaginal ring and 3.2 with the patch.
- The risk of ischaemic stroke increased by 1.5 and there was a slight increase in risk of haemorrhagic stroke.
- The annual risk of breast cancer increased with age irrespective of hormone use, but there was a small additional risk of breast cancer in COC users (RR 1.24) which reduced to no risk 10 years after stopping COCs. This is further discussed in Chapter 15.

Progestogen-only pill

Progestogen-only pills (POPs) would be an option for Alison if she has contraindications to taking oestrogens. The desogestrel pill (Cerazette®) is anovulant and likely to prove useful if Alison suffers from dysmenorrhoea.

With the desogestrel pill there is a greater tendency towards infrequent bleeding and amenorrhoea by the end of the first year of use, compared to the traditional POP. It also has a 12-hour window before efficacy is affected, in contrast to other POPs (3 hours).

Ovulation is inhibited in under 40% of cycles with traditional POPs, and in 97% of cycles with the desogestrel pill.

Injectable progestogens

Depo-Provera® (depot-medroxyprogesterone acetate) is an option for women with HMB with or without fibroids. Altered bleeding patterns are usual, with about 80% of women becoming amenorrhoeic within one year of use. Increase in haemoglobin levels and reduced fibroid volume have been known to occur with six months use. With typical use, the contraceptive failure rate is 3%. There is an association with weight gain and Alison may be worried about this and also initial irregular bleeding. If she does choose this method, she should stop at 50 years of age. There is a recognized association with a reduction in BMD and prolonged use may increase her risk of osteoporosis. There is little or no increase in risk of VTE, stroke and MI.

Progestogen-only implants

If Alison does not suffer from breast cancer, active liver disease, benign or malignant liver tumours and does not take enzyme-inducing drugs, the contraceptive implant Nexplanon® would be an option. It is a highly effective method with an overall pregnancy rate of under 1 per 1000 over 3 years. An advantage of an implant over the injection is that as a result of continued oestradiol production, BMD is not affected. Menstrual disturbances are common and 50% of women suffer from frequent, infrequent or prolonged bleeding episodes and 20% are amenorrhoeic. Three per cent of women request removal due to weight gain. Insertion and removal is a simple procedure, removal problems are rare and deep and impalpable implants should be located by ultrasound, in the first instance. If the implant cannot be located with high frequency ultrasound, an X-ray should be arranged to determine whether an implant is present.

Barrier methods with tranexamic acid

As Alison is in a new relationship, it is good practice to recommend the additional use of condoms. Several reviews have shown effectiveness of condoms in minimizing transmission of herpes, HIV, genital warts, chlamydia and gonorrhoea.

If she opts for a diaphragm, retention could prove difficult if she suffers from any degree of utero-vaginal prolapse. Diaphragm use requires concomitant spermicide usage. It is becoming more difficult to access supplies, which limits the use of this method of contraception.

Tranexamic acid is not considered a long-term treatment option for heavy periods.

Female/male sterilization with endometrial ablation

- Female sterilization is an option, but will not help with heavy periods, unless combined with an endometrial ablation, and will require a hospitalization with associated risks. Sterilization is covered in detail in Chapter 16.
- Vasectomy is a safe, simple and effective procedure and can be performed under local anaesthetic. The failure rate is 1 : 2000, but discussion of this method is not appropriate for couples in a new relationship and it is covered in detail in Chapter 17. It also would not influence Alison's abnormal bleeding.

Key points

- The LNG-IUS is a safe effective option for painful heavy periods and contraception.
- Combined hormonal contraceptives may be considered in the absence of risk factors and in line with UKMEC prescribing. The delivery route – oral, transdermal or vaginal – depends on the woman's preference.
- Shortened hormone-free interval, extended cycle regimens and newer natural oestradiol formulations could prove useful if the LNG-IUS is not desired or is contraindicated.
- The POP Cerazette® is an option and may help with heavy painful periods as it is anovulant and is associated with amenorrhoea after a few months of use.
- Depo-Provera® can help with HMB and painful periods, but is not recommended beyond the age of 50 and side effects may preclude its usage.
- Nexplanon® is an option for contraception but may not offer additional benefits with regards to heavy menstrual bleeding in particular.

Following the consultation and consideration of all benefits and risks, Alison has a LNG-IUS inserted for both contraception and to control her heavy menstrual bleeding.

Twelve months later, Alison and her partner win the lottery and decide to try for a baby. They are very pleased that they opted for a reversible form of contraception.

References

1. National Institute for Health and Clinical Excellence. *Heavy Menstrual Bleeding.* Clinical Guidelines 4, January 2007. http://guidance.nice.org.uk/CG44 (accessed 30 October 2012).

2. Royal College of Obstetricians and Gynaecologists. *The Initial Management of Menorrhagia.* Evidence-based Clinical Guideline No.1. London: RCOG Press, 1998.

3. Barrington JW, Bowens-Simpkins P. The levonorgestrel intrauterine system in the management of menorrhagia. *Br J Obstet Gynaecol* 1997; 104: 614–16.

4. Dinger J, Bardenheuer K, Minh TD. Levonorgestrel releasing and copper IUDs and the risk of breast cancer. *Contraception* 2011; 83: 211–17.

5. Trinh XB, Tjalma WA, Makar AP, *et al.* Use of the levonorgestrel releasing system in breast cancer patients. *Fertil Steril* 2008; 90: 17–22.

6. Wong CL, Farquhar C, Roberts H, Proctor M. Oral contraceptive pill for dysmenorrhea. *Cochrane Database Syst Rev* 2009; 2: CD002120.

7. Fraser IS, McCarron G. Randomised trial of two hormonal and two prostaglandin-inhibiting agents in women with a complaint of menorrhagia. *Aust NZJ Obstet Gynecol* 1991; 31: 66–70.

8. Farquhar C, Brown J. Oral contraceptive pill for heavy menstrual bleeding. *Cochrane Database Syst Rev* 2009; 4: CD000154.

9. Milman N, Clausen I, Byg KE. Iron status in 268 Danish women aged 18–30 years: influence of menstruation, contraceptive method and iron supplementation. *Ann Hematol* 1989; 77: 13–29.

10. Shabham MM, Zakherah MS, El-Nashar SA.The levonorgestrel IUS compared to low dose COC for idiopathic menorrhagia. *Contraception* 2011; 83: 48–54.

Contraception in the 50-somethings

Marie-Odile Gerval, Nicholas Panay and Paula Briggs

Case scenario: Janice

Janice is 51 years old. She is married and has a daughter aged 26. She has not used contraception recently as she and her husband have been having a stressful time with relationship issues and work pressures. Janice had an ectopic pregnancy in her late 40s and this unexpected pregnancy was a shock and a warning to her of the continued need for contraception, despite infrequent sex.

She has had very heavy and irregular periods recently and the fatigue associated with this has further reduced her libido. She has not been sleeping well as a result of night sweats.

She has a high powered job and is feeling emotional all the time, which has resulted in some difficulties with her boss and she is concerned regarding the possibility of redundancy.

Janice is fit and well and a non-smoker. She has no significant family history.

The fear of an unplanned pregnancy and her exhaustion have brought things to a head and the couple attend together to seek help.

Janice's husband is having difficulty sustaining an erection.

Introduction

According to the Office of National Statistics, data compiled from the 2011 Census shows that there are 3.9 million women aged 50–59 years in the UK (about 12% of the female population). The older woman may wish to have greater sexual freedom without the risk of pregnancy. Some women may fear the possibility of pregnancy and the problems that this may bring to otherwise settled lives. Others may feel that contraception is no longer a consideration due to proximity to the menopause.

In order to offer Janice the best possible medical care, these considerations, amongst others should be taken into account. Contraceptive choices available to younger age groups are increasingly being taken up by older women, albeit with clinicians having to keep in mind some factors unique to this population, and in this chapter we will review these. Added to this, the menopausal symptoms that Janice is presenting with can lead to a host of additional problems that can be easily remedied by the administration of oestrogen, progesterone and possibly testosterone hormone replacement therapy (HRT).

Of course, sex also requires the willing participation of an able partner with an adequate libido. However, this age group also sees a dramatic increase in the incidence of impotence and associated depressive symptomatology. With a range of treatment options now available, clinicians should seek to identify these psychosocial or additional medical problems in male partners and manage them appropriately.

Contraception, eds Paula Briggs, Gabor Kovacs and John Guillebaud. Published by Cambridge University Press. © Cambridge University Press 2013.

The peri-menopause

Typically, a woman's fecundity ends with the menopause, which by definition is 12 consecutive months without having a period. The peri-menopause is defined as the transition before the menopause and starts in a woman's 40s with impaired ovarian function that continues until she is post-menopausal. During this 'menopause transition', periods become irregular and eventually stop altogether. Even when periods are still regular, the egg quality of women in their 40s is typically lower than that in younger women, making the likelihood of conceiving a healthy baby dramatically lower.

The average duration of the peri-menopause is 5 years, with an average age of onset around the 46th year. The stages in reproductive ageing have recently been re-defined through a collaborative consensus [1].

The average monthly probability of conception declines by 50% at age 43. However, up to 80% of women aged between 40 and 43 are still able to conceive [2]. During this time intermittent unpredictable ovulation will occur.

The oldest verified mother to conceive naturally is Dawn Brooke from the UK. She gave birth to a son at the age of 59 years in 1997 [3].

Statistics show that the actual number of pregnancies in the over-40s is relatively low (25 500 compared with 870 000 total conceptions in England and Wales in 2006). However, this age group are much more likely to end their pregnancies with a termination; data reveals that 32% of the over 40 age group compared to 21% of the under 40 age group opt for termination. Even if the pregnancy is continued, maternal and perinatal outcomes are much worse. Maternal mortality is increased, as well as complications such as miscarriage, gestational diabetes, placenta praevia and Caesarean section, placental abruption, preterm birth, low birth weight and chromosomal abnormalities [4].

This reveals that there is a potential health promotion need that is not currently being met, and that both patients and scarce National Health Service (NHS) funds could be protected by improving the education of both this age group and the clinicians who manage them, to avoid unplanned pregnancy.

Therefore, the woman presenting for contraceptive advice in her 50s is in a different position to younger women. Although the peri-menopause is a stage of life when a woman has lowered fertility, the consequences of an unplanned pregnancy are serious, and contraception is still important, particularly when the additional associated non-contraceptive benefits of hormonal use are considered. For some women the peri-menopause is associated with menstrual dysfunction as well as menopausal symptoms and a contraceptive method that has the potential to manage these additional problems is ideal.

When can a woman in her 50s stop using contraception?

The Faculty of Sexual and Reproductive Healthcare (FSRH) recommends that women using non-hormonal methods can stop contraception after 1 year of amenorrhoea if over 50 (2 years if under 50) [5]. However, women who use exogenous hormones cannot depend on amenorrhoea as an indicator of the cessation of ovarian activity. Furthermore, a single elevated blood level of follicle stimulating hormone (FSH) is not a reliable indicator of the menopause, as these levels can oscillate and ovulation may still occur subsequent to a post-menopausal level of FSH. This is especially so for women using hormonal contraception, even if measured in the hormone-free period. In order to have an accurate indication as

Table 14.1 Contraceptive advice on stopping contraception method.

Non-hormonal contraception: stop contraception after 1 year of amenorrhoea

CHC and DMPA: stop CHC and DMPA at 50 years and choose from:

- A non-hormonal method, and stop after 1 year of amenorrhoea, *or:*
- Switch to the POP, implant or LNG-IUS and follow advice below

Implant/POP/LNG-IUS: can be continued until the age of 55

If amenorrhoeic:

- Check FSH levels (no need to discontinue contraceptive method) and stop method after 1 year if serum FSH is > 30 IU/L on 2 occasions 6 weeks apart, *or:*
- Stop at age 55 years when natural loss of fertility can be assumed for the vast majority of women

If not amenorrhoeic:

- Consider investigating any abnormal bleeding or changes in bleeding pattern, and continue contraception beyond age 55 years until amenorrhoeic for 1 year

Modified from [5].
CHC, combined hormonal contraceptive; DMPA, depot-medroxyprogesterone acetate; FSH, follicle stimulating hormone; LNG-IUS, levonorgestrel-releasing intrauterine system; POP, progestogen-only pill.

to whether ovarian activity has genuinely ceased, hormone levels should be measured six weeks after stopping combined hormonal contraception on two separate occasions six weeks apart. A reliable alternative method should be provided. The use of progestogen-only contraception should not affect the reliability of the FSH level, although the use of depot-medroxyprogesterone acetate (DMPA) can make values difficult to interpret.

The advice given by the FSRH is shown in Table 14.1.

The ideal contraceptive

Methods which have an unacceptably high risk of failure at younger ages become a reasonable option for the 50-something women. So, what would be the ideal contraceptive up to and during the menopause transition? The choice of method should be tailored to a woman's symptoms, medical history and her personal preferences and requirements. Janice's symptoms are as a result of hormonal fluctuation and resulting abnormal uterine bleeding. Therefore in her case, the use of HRT and treatment for heavy menstrual bleeding (HMB) both need to be considered in addition to her contraceptive requirements. Consultations with women like Janice provide the opportunity to improve quality of life and reduce certain risk factors for disease. The interaction with a health professional provides a platform to discuss other important lifestyle topics, which influence morbidity.

In general, the ideal contraceptive would fulfil all of the following criteria. It should:

- Offer sufficient efficacy – it will work, keeping in mind decreased fertility.
- Have minimal health risks and systemic side effects.
- Help with the control of menopausal symptoms.
- Manage HMB, and subsequently decrease the likelihood of surgical intervention.
- Offer a reduction in the rates of gynaecological pathology including cancer of the endometrium and ovary.
- Not impede sexual activity/intercourse as this can limit spontaneity and reduce compliance.

Contraceptive options

A woman in her 50s, or during the menopause transition, may need her contraceptive options re-evaluated. As is the case with other areas of modern medical practice, the choice of method should be tailored to a woman's preference with particular reference to her medical history. In practice, this includes a range of options from the progestogen-only pill (POP), the progestogen-only subdermal implant, the levonorgestrel-releasing intrauterine system (LNG-IUS) or a copper intrauterine device (IUD) for women who do not have problems with HMB.

Whilst combined hormonal contraception has a theoretical appeal as it could provide contraception, management for HMB and menopausal symptoms, its use is contraindicated by the Clinical Effectiveness Unit (CEU) of the FSRH which does not recommend the use of combined hormonal contraceptive (CHC) beyond the age of 50 years [5].

In the following sections we outline the various suitable methods for the over 50s.

Four types of progestogen-only contraception are available:

* Progestogen-only pill
* Levonorgestrel-releasing intrauterine system
* Progestogen-only subdermal implant (Nexplanon®)
* Injectable DMPA (Depo-Provera®). As the use of DMPA is supported by the FSRH only up to the age of 50, it will not be considered further in this chapter.

In contrast to CHC, which controls and regulates bleeding, all progestogen-only contraceptive methods disrupt the menstrual cycle. The bleeding pattern is unpredictable with the most widely used POP containing desogestrel (Cerazette®) and also with progestogen-only subdermal implants. This can deter women from trying these methods. Potential users of all progestogen-only methods need to be warned about the likelihood of irregular bleeding.

There are very few absolute contraindications to progestogen-only methods of contraception. Current breast cancer or a diagnosis within the previous five years is an absolute contraindication to the use of progestogen-only contraception. Where there is a history of ischaemic heart disease, cerebrovascular accident or transient ischaemic event, the use of progestogen-only contraception is relatively contraindicated. Progestogen alone has not been demonstrated to have any significant effects on coagulation, nor has it been associated with venous thromboembolism (VTE) in epidemiological studies. This is of particular relevance considering that the most significant risk associated with CHC is VTE.

The POP

The POP has a negligible effect on haemostasis, lipid and carbohydrate metabolism. Side effects are infrequent and include unscheduled bleeding, breast tenderness and skin changes. There is no effect on body weight. The older POPs prevent pregnancy by thickening of the cervical mucus, preventing sperm penetration, and do not result in anovulation, unlike the newer preparations containing desogestrel only. The POP is taken every day with no break, which makes it easier to remember.

Having established the clear advantages, there still remain problems with the POP. Unscheduled bleeding in women approaching the menopause may lead to unnecessary investigations including transvaginal ultrasound scanning, endometrial biopsy and hysteroscopy in order to exclude underlying pathology. This potentially costs both the NHS and the patient time and money.

The mode of action of the different POPs should be explained to women so that they understand the reason for the alteration in their bleeding pattern. Desogestrel-only POPs generally result in amenorrhoea, although this can take an average of 11–13 months to develop. Contraceptive efficacy is equivalent to that of CHC in compliant women with a Pearl Index of 0.14 [6].

The POP is not licensed for HRT, whether alone or as part of another regime.

The LNG-IUS (Mirena®)

The LNG-IUS is one of the long-acting reversible methods of contraception (LARC) which has the benefit of being highly effective whilst requiring minimal compliance once inserted by a trained practitioner. The LNG-IUS offers specific benefits in the 50-something age group. First, it can cause 'periods' to become lighter or even stop completely. Trials show that 80% of women treated with the LNG-IUS are satisfied with the resulting improvement in their bleeding. It is recommended first line by the National Institute for Health and Clinical Excellence (NICE) for the management of HMB in women with a normal sized or mildly enlarged uterus. Furthermore, it is licensed for use as endometrial protection in conjunction with the delivery of oestrogen for up to four years in the UK and up to five years in other countries.

Where the device is being used to control HMB there is no limit to the licence. For women who require contraception over the age of 45, the device can be left in situ for 7 years, and over age 52 reinsertion of a new device should be negotiated dependent upon need.

Overall, the LNG-IUS provides an ideal method of contraception in the older woman offering particular advantages where management of HMB and HRT is required. The LNG-IUS is a novel method of delivering contraception in that it is placed by a trained clinician where it needs to act, at the endometrium so it has an end-organ effect. For the majority of women, introduction of intrauterine contraception is not associated with significant or enduring pain. Bradycardia and cervical shock are uncommon complications of IUD insertion. Analgesia can be delivered orally, by the administration of local anaesthetic gel (Instillagel®) or as a cervical block, dependent upon need – this should be negotiated with the patient. Only hospital gynaecologists recommend general anaesthesia for insertion, though some women do request this!

The LNG-IUS was developed by Leiras in Finland, in conjunction with the Population Council in the USA. It has a polyethylene frame, which is surrounded by a cylinder containing 52 mg of levonorgestrel, which releases approximately 20 μg of hormone every 24 hours after a settling in period lasting on average 6 weeks. It is inserted into the uterus using a simple introducer, which has recently been modified to make insertion even easier. Removal is usually straightforward and conducted by pulling on the threads present at the external cervical os.

Insertion of the LNG-IUS results in circulating systemic levels of levonorgestrel in the region of 100–200 pg/ml (much lower levels than those seen with combined oral contraceptive pills containing levonorgestrel (2000–6000 pg/ml) or the POP containing levonorgestrel (up to 1000 pg/ml) and even the progestogen-only implant, Norplant® (200–400 pg/ml).

Nonetheless, some women who are severely progestogen intolerant might still suffer with premenstrual syndrome (PMS)-type emotional and physical side effects. These are usually transient lasting for 6–12 weeks when systemic levonorgestrel levels are at their highest. Appropriate counselling avoids the need for removal during this time in the majority of women.

Table 14.2 Administration of systemic HRT. What is appropriate?

Without uterus or with Mirena® in situ: oestrogen alone can be administered
With an intact uterus:
• LMP > 12/12 ago: continuous combined HRT usually is accompanied by amenorrhoea
• LMP 12/12 ago: sequential HRT will give better cycle control
Review at 3 months and reassess
HRT, hormone replacement therapy; LMP, last menstrual period.

The LNG-IUS's action is on the endometrium, preventing proliferation, as well as the progestogenic effect on the cervical mucus. In addition, in some women the circulating progestogen suppresses the luteinizing hormone (LH) peak and inhibits ovulation. Furthermore, within the endometrium a weak foreign body reaction is also achieved, which has an anti-implantation effect.

Whilst the LNG-IUS is excellent for managing HMB, it can be associated with persistent spotting and bleeding in some women, especially during the first three to six months of use. As the endometrium thins, under the influence of concentrated levonorgestrel within the endometrial cavity, there is a significant reduction in bleeding (approximately 90%) and approximately 50% of women become amenorrhoeic.

Complications of use include infection, expulsion and perforation at insertion (very rare). Occasionally the threads cannot be seen at the external cervical os and the presence of the IUS has to be confirmed by ultrasound examination. If the endometrial cavity is empty, an X-ray should be performed to detect the presence of the IUS in the peritoneal cavity as a result of perforation or to confirm expulsion of the device.

For the vast mast majority of women, there are no contraindications to using an LNG-IUS, even for the older women in her sixth and subsequent decades. Cardiovascular disease is a relative contraindication and pulmonary hypertension an absolute contraindication due to the inability to increase cardiac output in the event of a vasovagal episode during insertion. Breast cancer is also an absolute contraindication within the first five years following diagnosis.

Hormone replacement therapy

For concurrent HRT, therapeutic doses of oestrogen can be administered orally, transdermally by patch or gel or subdermally (Table 14.2). The LNG-IUS provides the progestogenic arm of HRT in this situation, with the high concentration of levonorgestrel in the endometrial cavity offering superior endometrial protection against endometrial proliferation and cancer than any other delivery route. The combination of an LNG-IUS and oestrogen in a woman still having some bleeding is likely to provide a reasonable bleeding profile and endometrial protection. In fact, this is the only continuous combined HRT regimen recommended in women with ongoing menstruation/bleeding in the peri-menopause. Most women in their 50s have had enough of bleeding and welcome a reduction or no bleeding. In peri-menopausal women using traditional oral or transdermal HRT, oestrogen is typically used in combination with 12–14 days of sequential progestogen for at least a year before a switch to a continuous combined regimen is attempted. Introduction of a continuous combined regimen before this is commonly associated with breakthrough bleeding due to the effect of ongoing endogenous hormone fluctuations.

The use of transdermal oestrogen is associated with a lower, typically neutral, risk of VTE. This is the most significant risk associated with the use of oral HRT, although for many women, their main concern is the risk of breast cancer. The initial interpretation of the Women's Health Initiative (WHI) and Million Women Study (MWS) caused considerable inappropriate anxiety, not only among potential users of HRT but also amongst the medical profession.

The results have since been questioned, particularly as the MWS was a questionnaire survey and the WHI data were not relevant to the age group typically using HRT in their 50s [7].

Recent data from modern trials such as the Kronos Early Estrogen Prevention Study (KEEPS) and a long-term Danish Osteoporosis Trial reaffirm the belief of many health professionals in menopause medicine that early treatment (up to mid-50s) with HRT during the 'Window of Opportunity' seems to confer many benefits for osteoporosis and cardiovascular disease and has very few risks. The Danish trial reported a neutral impact on breast cancer risk after 16 years of follow-up, though it was not originally powered to study this outcome [8].

Despite a favourable re-evaluation and new HRT trials, many women and medical professionals still think that HRT should be avoided if possible. This is an unhelpful situation for women, like Janice, who are suffering as a result of numerous physical and emotional menopause-related symptoms, with a knock-on effect on their relationship with their partner and other family members.

The British Menopause Society have recently issued a series of recommendations which represent a substantial position statement on how menopausal women's health should be optimized including the appropriate use of HRT [9].

Assessing symptoms of menopausal hormone deficiency

There is wide variation in symptoms that women suffer as they pass through the menopause transition, menopause and post menopause. The main factor is a **deficiency of oestrogen** manifest by four groups of symptoms; vasomotor, muculoskeletal, urogenital and psychogenic. On the other hand, peri-menopausal HMB is caused by anovulatory cycles resulting in **progesterone deficiency**, with the unopposed oestrogen causing excessive endometrial proliferation.

Measuring hormone levels (oestrogen or FSH) are of no benefit in assessing which women should be treated with HRT, and women should be assessed on their symptoms. Several semi-quantitative questionnaires have been designed to document the severity of symptoms. A therapeutic trial of HRT can be provided to see if the woman's symptoms improve. Higher than average doses of oestrogen e.g., 100 μg patches or 4 doses of Oestrogel are often required to adequately supress hormone fluctuations in the peri-menopause if psychological PMS symptoms are to be ameliorated as well as menopause symptoms. If psychogenic symptoms persist despite HRT, assessment for psychotropic medication should be undertaken. It is helpful if these women are co-managed with a psychologist or a psychiatrist [10].

Fibroids and the LNG-IUS

Fibroids are the most common tumour in women during reproductive life. They are symptomatic in 50% of women who have them and the majority are currently treated by surgical interventions. Many women are often not keen on these interventions due to the possibility of complications. The LNG-IUS is recognized as being effective in reducing menstrual blood loss in women with fibroids, albeit to a lesser extent than in women for whom HMB or fibroids are not a problem. The IUS prevents endometrial proliferation and consequently reduces both the duration and amount of bleeding, resulting in significant potential increases in haemoglobin levels.

If the fibroids have a significant submucus component (> 20%), it is recommended that these are resected before the LNG-IUS is inserted.

Over 75% of women using the LNG-IUS may have amenorrhoea or light bleeding, yet they continue to ovulate. It is recommended that women who have an LNG-IUS fitted after the age of 45 may continue to use this method for 7 years if their bleeding pattern is acceptable. If bleeding/spotting occurs even at age 52, this suggests ovarian activity, and the device should be replaced.

A novel approach to managing fibroids with a LNG-IUS is with pre-treatment with ulipristal acetate, a selective progesterone receptor modulator, in a dose of 5 mg daily for up to 3 months [11]. Ulipristal acetate, marketed as Esmya®, is licensed as a pre-surgical treatment to reduce fibroid size, to facilitate surgical intervention. This 'proof of concept' pilot study suggests that the use of ulipristal acetate significantly reduces fibroid size, as measured by cross-sectional ultrasound, and with the subsequent insertion of the LNG-IUS, reduces bleeding to such a degree that many women may be prevented from having to have a surgical procedure. Many of these women would have been otherwise unable to have a Mirena® fitted or have been at a significant increased risk of expulsion of the device due to the size of the fibroid. This study reported an average reduction in fibroid size of 47% at 3 months post treatment.

Progestogen-only implant: Nexplanon®

This is an effective LARC that is particularly useful in any age group which has found progestogen-only contraception to be effective. Nexplanon® contains the progestogen etonogestrel which is metabolized to desogestrel. It has a similar side effect profile to the POP containing desogestrel. Fitting is straightforward with training. The implant is licensed for three years but can be removed at any time during that period. Removal is a simple process if the implant has been inserted correctly in the inner aspect of the non-dominant arm, 8–10 cm from the medical epicondyle in a subdermal location. It has the advantage that oestrogen levels are maintained despite suppression of ovulation as with the desogestrel POP. Data on its use as the progestogenic component of HRT are lacking, though this is a theoretical possibility.

Intrauterine devices

The copper IUD is a suitable method of contraception for the older women, although it offers none of the advantages associated with the IUS. Bleeding is generally heavier and more painful, but this can settle after a few months.

Prevention of sexually transmitted infections

Age is not a barrier to acquiring sexually transmitted infections (STIs); therefore, the safer sex message remains equally important during contraceptive choice counselling, regardless of the final method of contraception settled upon.

Women in their 50s should be advised about the use of condoms to decrease the risk of transmission of various STIs. This is discussed in detail in Chapter 19.

Psychosocial considerations and erectile dysfunction

Requests for contraception in the older woman may not always be as simple as they first appear. For example, it may in fact be a way of seeing a practitioner to try and discuss a psychosexual problem, or a problem with intercourse that is difficult to broach. This can include male sexual dysfunction and even depression in the woman herself, or a decline in libido. The astute practitioner should be vigilant for cues in the consultation and have a low threshold for bringing up such issues in a non-judgemental manner.

Depression

Depression is a highly prevalent illness, with studies reporting that women are 1.5–3 times as likely as men to report a history of depression. Mid life, generally defined as 45–55 years, for most women both coincides with the menopause and numerous life changes. These may include physical health problems, changes in family and professional roles, changes in relationships and sexual functioning and new care giving roles (e.g., aged parents or ill partners). These changes place women in this age category at a significantly increased risk of depression. Studies demonstrate that depressive symptoms are common during the menopause, and that women with negative attitudes towards the menopause will in general report more symptoms during the menopause transition. This is confounded by the fact that depressive symptoms such as sleep disturbance and fatigue in mid-life women may be difficult to distinguish from menopausal symptoms and therefore may not always reflect mental illness.

Erectile dysfunction

It is equally not uncommon for women to come for contraceptive advice when they really want to know why their husband has become disinterested in sex, or why he cannot maintain an erection (often perceived as the same). Where these are related, the issue of erectile dysfunction (ED) is potentially easily remedied. It is defined by NICE as the inability to achieve or maintain an erection sufficient for satisfactory sexual performance and is the most common sexual problem in men, with incidence increasing with age. The prevalence is around 12% in men under the age of 59 years, 22% in those 60–69 years of age and 30% in those older than 69 years, representing a significant factor in the quality of the lives of many couples as they age. However, since a number of interventions are available for the treatment of ED (including psychological interventions, oral medication, intraurethral drug delivery, local injection and vacuum devices), its presence should be sought early before it becomes an entrenched problem.

Older men have a high prevalence of cardiovascular and metabolic diseases with the potential to impact negatively on sexual functioning. The opportunity to engage with men suffering from ED may facilitate the diagnosis of significant underlying medical conditions which have the potential to respond to appropriate treatment.

The phosphodiesterase type 5 inhibitors (PDE5) sildenafil (Viagra®), tadalafil (Cialis®) and vardenafil (Levitra®) are an effective treatment for ED caused by age-related vascular insufficiency, diabetes, drug therapy or prostatectomy. These drugs are contraindicated for use in conjunction with nitrates, for example glyceryl trinitrate (GTN) spray and isosorbide mononitrate. This combination can lead to significant arterial hypotension. The PDE5 inhibitors should be used with caution with alpha-blockers. Typical side effects include headache, flushing and dizziness.

The menopause, testosterone and declining sexual interest

Some women may present with concerns over reduced libido during the menopause. Previously sexually active women may have valid concerns, and this may cause or exacerbate depressive symptoms. In early studies on the relationship between menopausal symptoms and interest in sexual activity, data on hot flushes and plasma oestradiol and testosterone levels yielded significant negative associations between hot flush ratings and the regularity of sexual intercourse. This early study has since been confirmed, concluding that a close association exists between increasing irregularity of menstrual cycles, hot flushes, declining oestradiol levels and declining frequency of intercourse during the peri-menopause.

In all patients this association will need to be discussed, but in select sub-groups, there may be a role for testosterone therapy. Testosterone replacement can have a huge impact on general quality of life as well as the sexual desire of women such as Janice in the menopause. Women with reduced sexual desire should be counselled about the possible benefits of testosterone as well as oestrogen. Recent studies have shown that the benefits of testosterone can be achieved not only in women with a surgical menopause but also in those with a natural menopause and in women using testosterone without oestrogen [12, 13].

Unfortunately, it has recently been announced that due to profitability decisions, both testosterone implants and patches have been withdrawn. Off-license use of testosterone gel can be used as an alternative – Testim® and Testogel® can both be used at a dose of 0.5–1.0 ml/day such that each tube/sachet lasts for approximately 1 week (a large pea-sized blob applied to the lower abdomen) or Tostran® gel, 1 pump every 2–3 days. As with any off-label prescribing, responsibility lies with the health professional rather than the manufacturer/supplier. Androgenic side effects are uncommon with these female physiological doses and reversible if they do occur, with dose reduction or cessation.

Livial® (tibolone) has an androgenic effect and can also be used as an alternative to implants (though not in peri-menopausal women due to problems with breakthrough bleeding).

It should be kept in perspective that oestrogen/progestogen HRT, started soon after menopause, appears safe and relieves many of the symptoms menopausal women face as well as improving mood and markers of cardiovascular risk [14].

According to a multicentre, randomized study presented at the North American Menopause Society (NAMS) Annual Meeting, data showed improvements in cognition, mood, menopausal symptoms and sexual function in younger women. In addition, some measures showed slight evidence that hormone therapy might be cardio-protective in this age group. The KEEPS, a four-year randomized, double-blinded, placebo-controlled clinical trial of low-dose oral or transdermal (skin patch) oestrogen and cyclic monthly progesterone in healthy women also found many favourable effects of HRT in newly menopausal women. Together the results provide reassurance for women who are recently menopausal and taking HRT for the short-term treatment of menopausal symptoms. It again needs to be stressed that HRT is not necessarily a contraceptive, and this needs to be addressed as well as Janice's problem of HMB.

Given her symptoms and desire for highly effective contraception, the LNG-IUS would be an excellent contraceptive choice for Janice. If Janice opts to have a LNG-IUS fitted for contraception and to control her HMB, the device will provide endometrial protection, and if she wishes to take HRT for her menopausal symptoms she will require oestrogen only, with delivery route dependent upon her preference.

With regards to the associated psychosocial aspects of her presentation, it may be best to follow a 'wait and see' policy with regards to her mood as the combination of HRT and the LNG-IUS may resolve these. However, should her mood continue to be an issue, alternative treatments should be offered in line with best practice on depression.

In summary, women in their 50s requesting contraception often have additional needs, particularly regarding the management of menopausal symptoms. Consultations such as this offer the opportunity to provide balanced information regarding contraception, management of the menopause, relationship issues and ED.

There are very few absolute contraindications to HRT and the Menopause Matters and British Menopause Society websites provide a valuable resource for all potential providers and users of hormone therapy [15, 16, 17]. For the busy general practitioner, it is important to check blood pressure and ask about a history of VTE. The key recommendation of the British Menopause Society is that all women in the peri-menopause should have the opportunity to have a consultation in primary care about how to optimize their immediate and long-term health. There is a window of opportunity with maximal benefit in the peri-menopause, long before consistent elevation of FSH levels. Therefore, rather than repeatedly measuring blood tests, it is important to take a detailed history and offer women current information to support them to make appropriate choices.

References

1. Harlow SD, Gass M, Hall JE, *et al.* STRAW + 10 Collaborative Group. Executive summary of the Stages of Reproductive Aging Workshop + 10: addressing the unfinished agenda of staging reproductive aging. *Climacteric* 2012; 15(2): 105–14.

2. Toner JP, Flood JT. Fertility after the age of 40. *Obstet Gynecol Clin North Am* 1993; 20: 261–72.

3. Guinness World Records. Oldest mother to conceive naturally. http://www.guinnessworldrecords.com/records-12000/oldest-mother-to-conceive-naturally-/ (accessed 11 August 2012).

4. Cleary-Goldman J, Malone FD, Vidaver J, *et al.* FASTER Consortium. Impact of maternal age on obstetric outcome. *Obstet Gynecol* 2005; 105: 983–90.

5. Faculty of Sexual and Reproductive Healthcare. *Clinical Guidance. Contraception for Women Aged Over 40 Years,* July 2010. http://www.fsrh.org/pdfs/ContraceptionOver40July10.pdf (accessed 1 March 2013).

6. Collaborative Study Group on the Desogestrel-containing Progestogen-only Pill. A double-blind study comparing the contraceptive efficacy, acceptability and safety of two progestogen-only pills containing desogestrel 75 μg/day or levonorgestrel 30 μg/day. *Eur J Contracept Reprod Health Care* 1998; 3: 169–78.

7. Shapiro S, Farmer RD, Mueck AO, Seaman H, Stevenson JC. Does hormone replacement therapy cause breast cancer? An application of causal principles to three studies: Part 3. The Women's Health Initiative: unopposed estrogen. *J Fam Plann Reprod Health Care* 2011; 37(4): 225–30.

8. Schierbeck LL, Rejnmark L, Tofteng CL, *et al.* Effect of hormone replacement therapy on cardiovascular events in recently postmenopausal women: randomized trial. *BMJ* 2012; 345: e6409.

9. British Menopause Society Council. Modernizing the NHS: observations and recommendations from the British

Menopause Society. *Menopause Int* 2011; 17(2): 41–3.

10. Studd J, Panay N. Are oestrogens useful for the treatment of depression in women? *Best Pract Res Clin Obstet Gynaecol* 2009; 23(1): 63–71.

11. Briggs P. The role of ulipristal (Esmya, PregLem SA) in the treatment of fibroids associated with heavy menstrual bleeding in a community gynaecology setting. A 'proof of concept' pilot study. Fifteenth World Congress of Human Reproduction, 2013, in press.

12. Davis SR, Moreau M, Kroll R, *et al.* Testosterone for low libido in postmenopausal women not taking estrogen. *N Engl J Med* 2008; 359(19): 2005–17.

13. Panay N, Al-Azzawi F, Bouchard C, *et al.* Testosterone treatment of HSDD in naturally menopausal women: the ADORE study. *Climacteric* 2010; 13(2): 121–31.

14. Panay N, Currie H, Morris E. What really matters is the menopausal woman! *J Fam Plann Reprod Health Care* 2012; 38(2): 136–7.

15. Menopause Matters. http://www.menopausematters.co.uk (accessed 20 March 2013).

16. The British Menopause Society. http://www.thebms.org.uk (accessed 20 March 2013).

17. Women's Health Concern. http://www.womens-health-concern.org (accessed 20 March 2013).

Chapter 15

What is the risk of cancer with hormonal contraception?

Philip C. Hannaford and Lisa Iversen

Introduction

Over the past 50 years, there have been hundreds of clinical studies investigating whether hormonal contraception changes the risk of cancer among users. Most of the epidemiological evidence comes from observational case control and cohort studies examining cancer risk among users of combined oral contraceptives (COCs). Interest in any carcinogenic effects arises from the recognition that hormonal contraception is used by a very large number of women around the world, often for prolonged time periods, to prevent pregnancy not treat a disease. Currently an estimated 100 million women use COCs, and 40 million use injectable preparations, mostly progestogen-only products containing depot-medroxyprogesterone acetate (DMPA). Thus, even a small change in risk among users could have important public health consequences, especially since cancer is a major cause of death and morbidity in all parts of the world.

Determining with certainty whether hormonal contraception affects cancer risk has been difficult for a number of reasons. There is a long latent period between exposure (contraceptive use) and putative outcome (diagnosis of cancer). This can make the accurate recall of exposure problematic in case-control studies, and requires the prolonged follow-up of women in cohort studies. Women tend to use a variety of contraceptive methods during their reproductive lives, and different methods may have opposite effects (e.g., hormonal contraceptives may increase the risk of cervical cancer, whereas barrier methods are probably protective). There have been important changes within methods over time, such as the lowering of the oestrogen content and the introduction of new progestogens in COCs. It has been difficult to know whether these changes in composition have altered cancer risk, because COC users tend to use several brands during their lifetime and it is impossible to know whether an association is due to the preparation used nearest to the cancer diagnosis, or lingering effects from previously used formulations. Cancer risk may also be influenced by when in a user's reproductive life a contraceptive is used (e.g., before first full-term pregnancy), duration of use or time since last use. Some studies have been unable to look closely at these issues. Others have categorized exposure-related variables in different ways, hampering comparisons between studies.

All observational epidemiological studies are prone to confounding, the distorting effect of a third factor related to both exposure and outcome, which is the real explanation for an apparent association between exposure and outcome. There are many potential reproductive (e.g., number of pregnancies or children, breastfeeding and number of sexual partners) and

Contraception, eds Paula Briggs, Gabor Kovacs and John Guillebaud. Published by Cambridge University Press. © Cambridge University Press 2013.

non-reproductive (e.g., smoking, social class and use of screening services) confounding factors that might explain, at least partially, cancer associations with hormonal contraception. Some studies have had low statistical power to detect an altered cancer risk because they had few women exposed to the contraceptive of interest, or a short length of follow-up.

These challenges mean that results from epidemiological studies of cancer and hormonal contraception must be interpreted cautiously. Nevertheless, clinicians have a duty to provide women with good information about whether these popular methods of contraception are likely to alter a user's chances of cancer, so that informed choices can be made. When considering the epidemiological evidence attention should focus on the totality of data, rather than concentrating on the findings from one or a few studies. Consistent patterns of risk, across many studies using different designs and conducted among different populations, increase confidence in conclusions that a real cause-and-effect association exists.

Breast cancer

Breast cancer is the most common cancer in women around the world, including those living in the UK where 46 458 new cases and 12 122 deaths occurred in 2008.

Our understanding of a possible association between breast cancer and hormonal contraception advanced greatly in 1996 when the Collaborative Group on Hormonal Factors in Breast Cancer published a re-analysis of individual data about 53 297 women with and 100 239 without the tumour [1]. This represented 90% of the global data, from 54 studies undertaken in 25 countries. An assessment of what is known about the missing studies did not suggest that the re-analysis had been adversely affected by their omission. Compared with non-users, ever users of COCs had a small increased risk of being diagnosed with breast cancer (relative risk (RR) 1.07, 95% confidence interval (CI) 1.03–1.11). The increase was due to an elevated risk whilst women used COCs (RR 1.24, 95% CI 1.15–1.33) and for a few years after stopping (1–4 years after stopping: RR 1.16, 95% CI 1.08–1.23; 5–9 years after stopping: RR 1.07, 95% CI 1.02–1.13). The risk among users had disappeared by 10 years after stopping (RR 1.01, 95% CI 0.96–1.05). Cancers diagnosed in COC users were more likely to be localized to the breast than in non-users. The pattern of risk was not materially affected by a family history of breast cancer, country where the study was conducted, study design used, reproductive history, duration of use, oestrogen content of formulations used, or most other factors assessed. Slightly higher risks during current or recent use were found among women who started using COCs before the age of 20 years (current: RR 1.59, 95% CI 1.41–1.77; within 5 years of stopping: RR 1.49, 95% CI 1.31–1.67). The overall pattern (of onset during current use, no relationship with duration of use, disappearance with time after stopping and localization to the breast) is unusual for cancer epidemiology. It suggests a hormonal promotion of tumours which have already started to develop or the earlier detection in some way of tumours among COC users (or a mixture of both), rather than the initiation of new cases of cancer.

Although extensive and carefully conducted, the re-analysis had some important limitations. Biases and confounding arising from problems with the original studies included in the re-analysis could not be corrected for. There was little information available about any consequences after stopping hormonal contraception more than 20 years previously. Much of the data related to women who started using older formulations of COCs containing 50 μg or more of oestrogen after their teens, for relatively short durations, often after their first pregnancy. Women today are more likely than earlier generations of users to use COCs at a younger age, perhaps for longer durations, often before a first full-term pregnancy. Thus, more women are using hormones at a time when less differentiated breast tissue may be particularly sensitive to any carcinogenic effects of exogenous hormones.

In order to examine whether oral contraceptive use before first full-term pregnancy is important, Kahlenborn and colleagues undertook a meta-analysis of 34 case-control studies of pre-menopausal women or those aged less than 50 years, conducted in 17 countries in or after 1980 [2]. The authors had to rely on published data so were only able to estimate crude pooled odds ratios (OR). Other limitations included a lack of detailed information about the hormonal content of the oral contraceptive preparations used and the inability to examine relationships with current or recent use. Ever use of oral contraception was associated with an increased risk of breast cancer (OR 1.19, 95% CI 1.09–1.29), with a higher OR among parous women who used this method before their first full-term pregnancy (OR 1.44, 95% CI 1.28–1.62) than afterwards (OR 1.15, 95% CI 1.06–1.26). All women in this meta-analysis were pre-menopausal and so closer to current or recent use than women in the Collaborative Group's re-analysis (where two thirds of women were older than 45 years). This may explain the higher risk estimate for ever use of oral contraception found in the meta-analysis of pre-menopausal women than in the Collaborative Group's re-analysis.

The collective evidence suggests that COCs are associated with an increased risk of a diagnosis of breast cancer during current and recent use, an effect which *might* be greater among women who start using them at a young age or before their first full-term pregnancy. Since any effects disappear within 10 years of cessation, the absolute number of women affected depends on the age when oral contraception is stopped. Most users stop when the background incidence of breast cancer is low (i.e., before their mid-30s), so the extra number of users affected is small. For example, it has been estimated that 5 extra cases of breast cancer will accumulate by the age of 40 among every 10 000 North American or European women who cease oral contraception before 30 years of age [1]. Even if use at a young age or before first full-term pregnancy is associated with a higher relative risk than that found in other oral contraceptive users, there will be few additional cases *if* these higher risk women stop at an age when breast cancer is still rare. On the other hand, because of the greater background risk of breast cancer, oral contraceptive use near the menopause is associated with a larger number of extra cases (e.g., 32 in the following decade among every 10 000 North American or European women stopping at age 45) [1].

Several large cohort studies have looked at whether ever users of oral contraception have an increased risk of dying from breast cancer; none have found such an effect, even after prolonged (up to 41 years) follow-up. Other studies have looked at whether previous oral contraceptive use affects survival after a diagnosis of breast cancer, with no clear picture of poorer survival emerging.

Women who have a family history of breast cancer, especially among first-degree relatives, have an increased lifetime background risk of the disease. Those with such a history, however, can be reassured that there is no reason to preclude them from using hormonal contraception, or require them to undergo extra screening if they wish to use this method of contraception. This is because the relative risk of breast cancer among hormonal contraceptive users with a family history of breast cancer appears to be similar to that of users without such a history. Compared with non-carriers, women with *BRCA1* and *BRCA2* gene mutations have an enhanced risk of both breast and ovarian cancer, often occurring at a young age. A number of studies have examined whether such carriers have an even greater risk of breast cancer if they use oral contraceptives, with conflicting results. Virtually all of the studies have been small and so lacked statistical power to definitively answer this important clinical issue. Several have suggested an enhanced risk, especially in some sub-groups with the genetic mutation (e.g., those with *BRCA2* who use oral contraception before first full-term pregnancy for long durations). Some clinicians recommend that *BRCA1/2* carriers use oral contraceptives to reduce their risk of ovarian cancer, even if such usage increases the chances of breast cancer, although robust evidence to support this advice is lacking. Others feel that they should wait for more substantial evidence before they can make such a recommendation.

In spite of its widespread use, there is a paucity of information about the cancer risks, including breast cancer, associated with progestogen-only contraceptives. The Collaborative Group's re-analysis found a similar pattern of breast cancer risk among users of progestogen-only contraceptives (mostly pills and injections) as that among COC users [1]. Findings consistent with the pattern have also been found in some, but not all, of the subsequent studies, although several had limited power to examine the risk. Until more empirical evidence becomes available, clinicians should assume that progestogen-only contraceptives, and combined contraceptive patches, rings and injections, have the same breast (and other) cancer risk as combined oral preparations.

Cervical cancer

Globally cervical cancer is the second most frequent cancer in women, although 8th in the UK where 2729 new cases and 1111 deaths occurred in 2008. The cancer is caused by persistent infection with oncogenic types of human papillomavirus (HPV), in conjunction with necessary co-factors such as cigarette smoking, high parity and, possibly, hormonal contraception.

A re-analysis of individual data about 16 573 women with cervical cancer (approximately two thirds invasive, the rest grade 3 cervical intraepithelial neoplasia or carcinoma-in-situ) and 35 509 without was published in 2007 [3]. The 24 included studies were conducted in 26 countries, half in less developed parts of the world. The authors were unable to include approximately 15% of the known data about cervical cancer and COCs. Published results from the missing studies, however, were broadly compatible with the main findings of the re-analysis. Compared with never users, current users of COCs had an increased risk of cervical cancer; an association which got stronger with duration of use (7%, 95% CI 5–8% increase for each year of use). The risk decreased after stopping and had disappeared by 10 years after cessation. For example, among women with 5 or more years of use- whilst using and within 1 year of stopping: RR 1.9, 95% CI 1.7–2.1; 2–9 years after stopping: RR 1.3, 95% CI 1.1–1.4; 10 years or more after stopping: RR 0.9, 95 CI 0.8–1.1. The pattern of risk was broadly unaffected by type of cancer (invasive or in-situ), high risk HPV status, study design or characteristics of the women studied.

Within the limitations of data collected for the original studies, the re-analysis allowed for potential confounding by age at first intercourse, number of sexual partners, smoking, number of full-term pregnancies, screening status and age. These adjustments had only a minor effect on the risk estimates, and did not change their statistical significance. It is possible, however, that at least part of the elevated relative risk during current and recent use was due to residual confounding from variables that had not been measured or were imperfectly allowed for. Furthermore, observed differences between users and non-users of oral contraceptives may be due to a protective effect of barrier methods used by the non-user group rather than an adverse effect of hormones in the user group. Theoretical mechanisms by which oral contraceptives might exert a carcinogenic effect include: enhancing the processes through which HPV exposure results in cervical infection, changing the clearance or persistence of HPV infections, or reducing the regression of pre-invasive changes.

The re-analysis had insufficient data to examine the effects of oral progestogen-only contraceptives. Although based on small numbers, progestogen-only injectable contraceptives were associated with an increased risk of cervical cancer with prolonged duration of use, albeit at a lower level than that seen for COCs. The effect declined after injectables were stopped. A similar pattern was seen in a more recent study of black South African women.

Overall, the evidence suggests a causal relationship between hormonal contraceptives and cervical cancer. The absolute number of women affected depends both on duration of use and the age when women stop using hormonal contraceptives. For example, if women use oral contraception for 10 years between the ages of 20 and 30 years, it is estimated that by age 50 the cumulative incidence of cervical cancer will increase from 73 to 83 per 10 000 such users in less developed countries and from 38 to 45 per 10 000 such users in more developed countries [3]. In many countries users of hormonal contraceptives can minimize the adverse consequences of an increased cervical cancer risk by participating in screening programmes. Empirical evidence so far does not suggest that hormonal contraception accelerates progression from pre-invasive to invasive cancer. The age at starting, and frequency of, screening among users of these contraceptives, therefore, should be the same as that of women using other methods.

Liver cancer

Liver cancer is uncommon in areas of the world with a low prevalence of hepatitis B infection. In the UK, there were 1348 new cases and 1316 deaths attributed to this cancer among women in 2008. Survival rates are poor.

Most epidemiological studies investigating a possible association between oral contraception and hepatocellular cancer have been small, conducted in areas with a low prevalence of hepatitis B (USA, UK and other parts of Europe), and adjusted, to a varying extent, for important confounders such as hepatic infections, diabetes and alcohol use. They have also tended to examine effects in the first generation of COC users, taking formulations with 50 μg or more of oestrogen. Twelve case-control studies were included in a meta-analysis published in 2007 [4]. Compared with never users, ever users of oral contraception had a modest, statistically non-significant, elevated risk of hepatocellular cancer (age and sex-matched summary OR 1.57, 95% CI 0.96–2.54). Although prolonged use was defined differently in the various studies (more than 5, 6 or 8 years, between 5–9 years), longer use was associated with significantly higher odds ratios than shorter use. Thus, the odds ratio for longer durations ranged between 2.0 and 20.1, compared with 0.3 and 2.6 for shorter durations. Two studies conducted in countries where hepatitis B is endemic did not find a relationship between ever use of oral contraception and hepatocellular cancer, regardless of duration or recency of use. This suggests that oral contraception does not magnify the already higher background risk of hepatocellular cancer among women living in these areas. There have been very few cases of liver cancer reported in cohort studies with prolonged follow-up, with no indication of a risk emerging many years after stopping oral contraception.

Although incomplete, the evidence indicates a possible association between prolonged use of combined oral contraception and hepatocellular cancer. The incidence of this cancer, however, is low and there is no evidence of a persisting effect after stopping oral contraception. This means that the public health implication of any association is very small.

Oral contraceptives may also be associated with an increased risk of benign liver tumours, such as hepatocellular adenoma and focal nodular hyperplasia. Trends of increasing risk with longer periods of use have been found, although not in every study. There is no evidence of persisting risk after oral contraception is ceased. More recently introduced, low-oestrogen dose combinations may have a smaller effect. The rarity of benign liver tumours means that the public health implications of a possible association will be very small.

Thyroid cancer

Thyroid cancer is also uncommon, accounting for 1655 new cases and 219 deaths among women in the UK in 2008.

A re-analysis of individual data from 13 case-control studies of thyroid cancer and oral contraception found a modest elevated risk of borderline significance among ever users, compared with never users (OR 1.2, 95% CI 1.0–1.4) [5]. Current users had a slightly higher risk (OR 1.5, 95% CI 1.0–2.1), which disappeared within 10 years of stopping. There was no relationship with duration of use, age at starting, use before first full-term pregnancy, country of study or type of control group. Slightly stronger associations were found for papillary cancers than follicular tumours. Subsequent studies have not found a consistent pattern of elevated risk among COC users.

The low incidence of thyroid cancer, and lack of persistence of risk after stopping, means that the public health implications of any relationship with hormonal contraception will be minimal.

Ovarian cancer

Ovarian cancer is the 7th most frequent cancer worldwide, and 6th in the UK, where 6747 new cases and 4254 deaths occurred in 2008. The cancer has a poor survival rate, because many women have advanced disease when first diagnosed.

Individual data from 45 studies conducted in 21 countries concerning 23 257 women with ovarian cancer and 87 303 without were re-analysed and published in 2008 [6]. Three studies could not be included, but omission of their data is unlikely to have affected materially the findings of the re-analysis. Ever users of oral contraceptives (almost entirely combined preparations) had a lower risk of ovarian cancer than never users (overall RR 0.73, 95% CI 0.70–0.76). The protection strengthened the longer women used COCs, so that overall there was a 20% reduction for every 5 years of use. Thus, the risk of ovarian cancer among women who had used oral contraceptives for 15 years or more was halved. Although there was a diminution in protection with time since stopping, statistically significant reductions among ever users were still seen more than 30 years after stopping (last use 10–19 years previously: RR 0.67, 95% CI 0.62–0.73; last use 20–29 years previously: RR 0.76, 95% CI 0.71–0.81; last use 30 or more years previously: 0.86, 95% CI 0.76–0.97). The results were essentially unchanged by adjustments for numerous potential confounding factors, including ethnic group, education, age at first birth, age at menarche, menopausal status, use of hormone replacement therapy, height, weight, body mass index, alcohol use and smoking. Similar effects were seen for most histological subtypes of epithelial and non-epithelial cancers, except mucinous lesions where the protective effect was smaller and not statistically significant. The authors did not have precise information about preparations used, so analysed their results by mid-year of use as a proxy for oestrogen dose: before 1970 corresponding to use of preparations with 100 μg of oestrogen; 1970–79, formulations with 50 μg of oestrogen; and 1980 or later, combinations with 30 μg or less of oestrogen. Similar protective effects were seen among ever users in the different calendar periods. These results, and those from a small number of other studies, suggest that more recently introduced, low-oestrogen dose COCs continue to protect against ovarian cancer.

Although derived from observational studies, and so subject to possible bias and confounding, the collective evidence suggests a substantial real effect. The mechanism(s) by which COCs produce this benefit is unknown. It has been estimated that since their introduction 50 years ago, COCs have already prevented 200 000 ovarian cancers and 100 000 deaths worldwide [6]. Women with a higher than average background risk of ovarian cancer, such as carriers of *BRCA1/2* gene mutations or nullips, will enjoy a greater absolute risk reduction.

Limited data about progestogen-only contraceptives (mostly DMPA-containing injectables) suggest that they also protect against ovarian cancer, especially among longer-term users.

Endometrial cancer

Cancer of the corpus uteri (endometrial cancer) is the 6th most frequent cancer globally, but has a higher ranking (4th) in the UK, where 7468 new cases and 1554 related deaths occurred in 2008.

A meta-analysis of epidemiological studies published up to 1997 found that, compared to never users, ever users of COCs had a reduced risk of endometrial cancer, a benefit which increased with longer durations of use [7]. Thus, the risk was estimated to decrease by 56% with 4 years of use, 67% with 8 years of use and 72% with 12 years of use. Although the benefit attenuated after stopping oral contraception, it persisted for more than 20 years: 67% reduction in risk at 5 years after stopping, 59% at 10 years and 49% at 20 years. Subsequent studies have generally found a similar pattern of benefit. The different studies have adjusted, to varying degrees, for potential confounding factors, such as parity, body mass index and smoking. These adjustments did not tend to change the statistical significance of any risk estimates. Limited data suggests that more recently introduced, low-oestrogen dose COCs continue to protect against endometrial cancer.

As with ovarian cancer, the persisting protection enjoyed by previous users of COC to an age when endometrial cancer becomes more common, means that a large number of women will avoid experiencing this tumour.

Although the evidence is sparse, progestogen-only injectable contraceptives also appear to reduce the risk of endometrial cancer, especially with prolonged use.

Colorectal cancer

The third most frequent cancer in females throughout the world, colorectal cancer accounted for 18 030 new cases and 7606 deaths among women in the UK in 2008.

Almost all of the studies examining the risk of colorectal cancer among ever users of COCs have found a reduced risk compared with never users, although some studies were small and so underpowered to detect a statistically significant effect if it exists. Taken together, ever use of combined oral contraception appears to reduce a woman's chance of being diagnosed with colorectal cancer by nearly 20% (RR 0.82, 95% CI 0.69–0.97) [8]. Similar benefits were found among studies which examined colonic and rectal cancer separately, and among case-control and cohort studies. The reduction was not related to duration of use. Few studies have examined colorectal cancer risk after stopping oral contraception, although there is a suggestion that the reduction diminishes with time (<10 years since stopping: RR 0.51, 95% CI 0.35–0.74; ≥ 10 years since stopping: 0.77, 95% CI 0.60–0.99). Given the high incidence of this cancer, especially among older women, it will be important to ascertain in future studies how long the reduced risk of colorectal cancer persists after stopping oral contraception.

Virtually nothing is known about whether other forms of hormonal contraception also protect against colorectal cancer.

Lung cancer

Worldwide, lung cancer is the fourth most frequent cancer in women. In the UK, it is now the 3rd most common cancer in women, accounting for 17 974 new cases and 15 349 deaths in 2008. It is associated with poor survival rates.

Data about whether combined oral contraception increases the risk of lung cancer are sparse [9]. None of the few studies examining this issue, including several large cohort studies with prolonged follow-up, have found an increased risk among oral contraceptive users. This argues against a major association existing.

Other cancers

A number of studies have investigated whether oral contraception is associated with cutaneous malignant melanoma, with inconsistent findings. A re-analysis of original data from 10 case-control studies gave an overall OR for oral contraceptive use of one year or longer, compared with never use or use for less than one year, of 0.86, 95% CI 0.74–1.01 [9].

Other studies have considered neuroblastoma, lymphoma, and renal, oesophageal, gastric, pancreatic and gallbladder tumours [9]. None have produced convincing evidence of an important association with oral contraception.

Overall balance of cancer risks and benefits

A Working Group for the International Agency for Research on Cancer recently concluded that COCs should be classified as carcinogenic to humans (Group 1) [9]. It felt that there was sufficient evidence of an increased risk of breast and cervical cancer in current and recent users, and of liver cancer in populations with a low prevalence of hepatitis B infection. The Group also concluded that there was convincing evidence of protective effects against ovarian and endometrial cancer.

A key question is whether the increased risk of some cancers among COC users is off-set by a reduced risk of other malignancies, particularly in the long-term. If the persisting protection extends to an age when cancer becomes common, substantial public health benefits might accrue. Several researchers have constructed mathematical models to examine this issue. Empirical data about any long-term effects, however, has come mainly from two large cohort studies established in the UK in the late 1960s: the Royal College of General Practitioners' (RCGP) oral contraception study and the Oxford/Family Planning Association (Oxford/FPA) contraceptive study. The larger RCGP study examined the balance of all incident cancers reported to 2004 among ever and never users of oral contraception,

Compared with never users, ever users had a statistically significant 12% reduced risk of any cancer (RR 0.88, 95% CI 0.83–0.94). A later mortality paper reporting on 39 years of follow-up, observed a 15% reduction in cancer-related deaths among ever users (RR 0.85, 95% CI 0.78–0.93); and a 12% reduction in all-cause mortality (RR 0.88, 0.82–0.93) [10]. Similar mortality results were found after prolonged (41 year) follow-up of the Oxford/FPA contraceptive study cohort cancer-related deaths among ever users versus never users: RR 0.90, 95% CI 0.8–1.0; all cause mortality: RR 0.87, 95% CI 0.79–0.96. Older women benefit from the greatest reductions. For example, in the RCGP study there was an estimated 14 fewer deaths per 100 000 woman-years at age 40–49 years; 86 per 100 000 woman-years at age 50–59; 122 per 100 000 woman-years at age 60–69 years and 308 per 100 000 woman-years above age 70 years [10]. Continued follow-up of these cohorts is needed to determine whether these benefits increase further with time.

The experience of women living in the UK may not reflect that of women residing elsewhere, where patterns of oral contraception usage, duration of use, age at stopping and incidence of cancer are different. A study of 259 000 Chinese textile workers recruited between 1989 and 1991, and followed up to 2000, found no association between oral contraceptive use and overall risk of 12 cancers (breast, colon, gallbladder, liver, lung, ovary, pancreas, rectum, stomach, thyroid, uterine cervix and uterine corpus: RR 0.94, 95% CI 0.88–1.01). This result is reassuring, although an important limitation of the study was the low prevalence of oral contraceptive use and relatively short duration of follow-up.

There have been few studies examining the balance of cancer risks and benefits among users of other hormonal contraceptives. The Chinese cohort study of textile workers also examined the combined risk of 12 cancers associated with monthly combined injectable contraceptives. Although the statistical power of the study was low, there was no suggestion of an altered risk of all cancers combined among users of the monthly injection (RR 0.91, 95% CI 0.81–1.03).

Summary

After nearly half a century of extensive study, users of COCs can be reassured that their family planning choice does not lead to a substantial cancer risk. Although women may be at increased risk of several cancers (breast, cervix, liver and possibly thyroid) whilst using this contraceptive method, the effects appear to be transient, disappearing within a few years of stopping. Conversely, COCs protect against several other cancers (ovary, endometrium and colorectum), with the benefits persisting for many years after stopping (at least for ovary and endometrium). This sustained protection may produce major public health benefits over time, through reduced overall cancer incidence and mortality. Until more evidence becomes available, it would be prudent to assume that women exposed to combined hormonal contraception supplied via a non-oral route experience the same pattern of cancer risks and benefits as those using oral preparations. Limited data suggests that users of progestogen-only contraceptives (especially injectables and implants) experience a similar pattern of cancer risks and benefits as COC users.

References

1. Collaborative Group on Hormonal Factors in Breast Cancer. Breast cancer and hormonal contraceptives: collaborative re-analysis of individual data on 53 297 women with breast cancer and 100 239 women without breast cancer from 54

epidemiological studies. *Lancet* 1996; 347: 1713–27.

2. Kahlenborn C, Modugno F, Potter DM, Severs WB. Oral contraception use as a risk factor for premenopausal breast cancer: a meta-analysis. *Mayo Clin Proc* 2006; 81: 1290–302.

3. International Collaboration of Epidemiological Studies of Cervical Cancer. Cervical cancer and hormonal contraceptives: collaborative re-analysis of individual data for 16 753 women with cervical cancer and 35 509 women without cervical cancer from 24 epidemiological studies. *Lancet* 2007; 370: 1609–21.

4. Maheshwari S, Sarraj A, Kramer J, El-Serag HB. Oral contraception and the risk of hepatocellular carcinoma. *J Hepatol* 2007; 47: 506–13.

5. La Vecchia C, Ron E, Franceschi S, *et al.* A pooled analysis of case-control studies of thryoid cancer. III. Oral contraceptives, menopausal replacement therapy and other female hormones. *Cancer Causes Control* 1999; 10: 157–66.

6. Collaborative Group on Epidemiological Studies of Ovarian Cancer. Ovarian cancer and oral contraceptives: collaborative re-analysis of data from 45 epidemiological studies including 23 257 women with ovarian cancer and 87 303 controls. *Lancet* 2008; 371: 303–14.

7. Schlesselman JJ. Risk of endometrial cancer in relation to use of combined oral contraceptives. A practitioner's guide to meta-analysis. *Hum Reprod* 1997; 12: 1851–63.

8. Bosetti C, Bravi F, Negri E, La Vecchia C. Oral contraceptives and colorectal cancer risk: a systematic review and meta-analysis. *Human Reprod Update* 2009; 15: 489–98.

9. IARC Working Group. *IARC Monographs on the Evaluation of Carcinogenic Risks to Humans. Volume 91. Combined Estrogen–Progestogen Contraceptives and Combined Estrogen–Progestogen Menopausal Therapy.* Lyon, France: International Agency for Research on Cancer, 2007.

10. Hannaford PC, Iversen L, MacFarlane TV, *et al.* Mortality among oral contraceptive users: cohort evidence from the Royal College of General Practitioners' Oral Contraception Study. *BMJ* 2010; 340: c927.

Chapter 16

New developments in female sterilization

Gabor Kovacs and Paula Briggs

Case scenario: Fatima

Fatima is 38 years old. She and her husband have three girls aged 10, 7 and 4. She does not want any more children as she wants to resume her legal practice full time. Her husband still dreams that one day they will have a son. She is 'sick of taking the pill', and she finds the thought of having something like a 'coil' inside her repulsive. She does not want to use a progestogen-only method, as she has heard that they result in irregular bleeding. Her husband does not want to have a vasectomy as he thinks it is 'too final'. She comes to see you asking about the 'reversible sterilization'.

Sterilization should be viewed as the irreversible loss of fertility. Women who undergo sterilization should be 100% certain that they do not want to become pregnant again. Otherwise the use of a long-acting reversible method of contraception (LARC) should be advised. In the case of Fatima and her husband there may be regret in the future that they did not try for a boy. The fact that she is asking about 'reversible' sterilization gives an indication that she is not 100% committed.

In females, sterilization can be achieved by hysterectomy or tubal occlusion. If hysterectomy is performed for some gynaecological reason, the result will be that the woman will be 'sterile', but such a major operation should never be performed purely for the purpose of contraception. A method of tubal occlusion should be used. The approach used for tubal occlusion is usually laparoscopic, but mini-laparotomy and a transvaginal approach have also been used.

Recently some hysteroscopic approaches have been developed, although these do have some limitations and this will be discussed later in the chapter.

Transvaginal sterilization should not be performed because of the unacceptable rate of post-operative complications. These include bleeding and infections.

Prevalence of female sterilization

In 2011 it was estimated that 150 million women worldwide have been sterilized [1].

In the UK, 10 000 women each year are sterilized under the National Health Service (NHS), with many others being operated on privately. However the rate of female sterilization surgery in the UK is decreasing. Even in China, there has been a move away from sterilization towards intrauterine devices [2].

In the USA, female sterilization is the second commonest method of contraception overall, and the most common method used by married women and women aged over 30 [3].

Counselling prior to sterilization

Prior to deciding on a sterilization operation, the woman or preferably the couple should be given information about alternatives, especially LARC and also vasectomy. They should understand that vasectomy has a lower failure rate and fewer complications than tubal sterilization. The permanency of the procedure also needs to be explained, but they should still be informed about the feasibility and possible success rates for reversal operations, and the possible alternate use of subsequent in vitro fertilization (IVF). The couple should also understand that there is a failure rate for all methods of tubal occlusion. The most commonly used method, the application of Filshie® clips, has a failure rate of 2–3 per 1000 operations [4].

Mini-laparotomy should only be considered in rare circumstances if laparoscopy is contraindicated. The option of a hysteroscopic approach, if available, should be discussed.

The woman can be reassured that there is no evidence that periods will get heavier after a sterilization procedure. However, women who have got used to a reduction in bleeding in association with the use of hormonal contraception will go back to natural menstruation, which often results in heavier bleeding.

It has been noted that women who have been sterilized have a higher rate of subsequent hysterectomy, but no causative association has been demonstrated.

Counselling needs to include the risks and complications of the procedure:
- Anaesthetic complications
- Gas embolism
- Trauma to organs such as bowel or ureters
- Bleeding due to vessel injury
- Infection in the wound or Fallopian tube
- Inflammation and pain
- Failure (there is a very small chance of the tubes becoming unblocked)

Post-operatively it is normal to experience some pain and nausea in the first 4–8 hours and some abdominal discomfort for 24–36 hours from the gas used during laparoscopy.

No test of efficacy is required after laparoscopic sterilization, but hysteroscopic methods should have confirmation of tubal blockage three months post-operatively with a hysterosalpingogram (HSG).

Special care and possibly legal advice should be taken if there is any question about a person's ability or mental capacity to consent to sterilization.

Various approaches to tubal occlusion

When a laparoscopic approach is used, the application of Filshie® clips has evolved as the preferred method. This is as effective as tubal coagulation, but avoids the risk of burning other organs. Laparoscopic diathermy also has a higher incidence of ectopic tubal pregnancy post-operatively. Clips are the least destructive to the Fallopian tubes, making the success of reversal more likely.

Laparoscopic Filshie® clips

This has been the preferred method of sterilization for the last three decades. There were however a spate of pregnancies when some of the applicators that were used lost calibration, resulting in inadequate application of the clips. Two strategies to prevent this happening have been developed. First the use of a gauge, which ensures appropriate application, and secondly the introduction of a single use disposable applicator which is provided with each set of clips.

Performing tubal occlusion transcervically has the advantage that no abdominal scars result and the procedure can be performed without general anaesthesia in an outpatient setting. The approach can be achieved either blindly or by direct vision (hysteroscopic) or indirect visualization (radiological) techniques. Once the isthmus has been located, occlusion can be achieved by chemical, mechanical or thermal techniques.

Chemical occlusion is achieved with quinacrine and is only used in the developing world and will not be discussed further.

Hysteroscopic procedures have recently been developed and deserve detailed description.

Hysteroscopic approach

There is only one method currently available for hysteroscopic female sterilization, Essure®.

It is dependent on the placement of devices into the proximal Fallopian tube. Other devices have been developed, but are no longer commercially available. The Adiana® device was approved by the US Food and Drug Administration (FDA) in 2009. Its method of action is a combination of controlled thermal damage to the lining of the Fallopian tube followed by insertion of a non-absorbable biocompatible silicone elastomer matrix within the tubal lumen. This resulted in a fibroblast ingrowth, acting as a scaffold for the matrix. Over the next few weeks, scar tissue developed and acted as a permanent stopper. However the device has now been withdrawn, and is no longer available for clinical use.

The Essure® microinsert (Essure® Permanent Birth Control System, Conceptus Inc., San Carlos, CA, USA)

The Essure® microinsert (Figure 16.1) grew out of the transiently popular practice of 'Falloposcopy' developed in the early 1990s by the Imagyn/Conceptus companies under the guidance of the late Dr John Kerin [5].

It requires the hysteroscopic transcervical placement of a microcoil (STOP) device into each of the tubal ostia. The device consists of an inner coil of stainless steel and polyethylene terephthalate (PET) fibres and an outer coil of nickel–titanium (nitinol). The device is placed in the proximal Fallopian tube in the wound-down state and then deployed and allowed to expand, so it anchors the insert along a segment of the tube. After placement, the PET fibres stimulate a benign tissue response that elicits a foreign body reaction. Placement is critical, as the device has to be anchored for some weeks, during which time an inflammatory response results in extensive fibrosis and consequent tubal blockage. The device was approved by the FDA in 2002 as a method of permanent birth control. Over 600 000 women have since had the devices inserted.

The technique has a sharp learning curve, and its proper placement requires excellent hysteroscopic vision of the tubal ostia. Accurate placement is essential. Sufficient loops need to be placed inside the Fallopian tube to anchor the microcoil, and sufficient left within the uterine cavity to prevent the coil's expulsion along the tube.

In 2012, Povedano et al. reported on 4306 women who underwent the Essure® sterilization procedure from 2003 to 2010 [6]. A total of 4108 (96.8%) women completed the

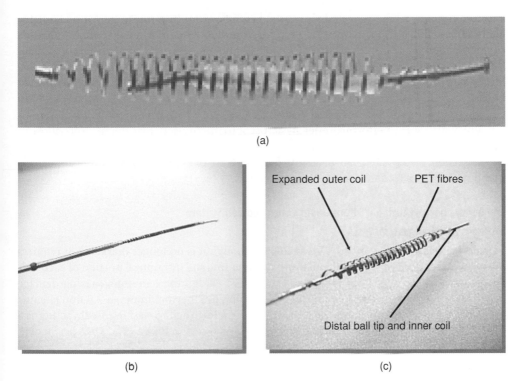

Figure 16.1 (a) The Essure® microinsert. (b) Microcoil device wound down. (Device made from materials successfully used in cardiac surgery for decades.) (c) Proprietary device expansion.

3 month follow-up visit. There were 115 (out of 4306; 2.7%) recorded complications, none of which resulted in the need for hospitalization. Vasovagal syncope at the time of the procedure was the most frequently encountered adverse event, occurring in 85 (2.0%) of 4306 cases. In 19 cases, one device was expelled, with most expulsions (14 out of 19) being detected before or during the 3 month follow-up. They concluded that outpatient hysteroscopic sterilization using the Essure® system is safe, with a low rate of complications.

A review by Smith in 2010 [7] concluded that after 6 years of use, the real-world experience demonstrated an efficacy of 99.74% with a low risk of adverse effects and risks. The procedure was associated with high patient satisfaction. The ability to perform the procedure in an outpatient setting offsets the relatively high cost of the device.

Levie and Chudnoff carried out an interesting study to try and dispel that learning the insertion technique for Essure® (ESS 305) is difficult [8].

They assessed the placement rates for the new ESS 305 delivery catheter for the Essure® microinsert via hysteroscopy in experienced users versus newly trained physicians in a multicentre prospective cohort study by 37 newly trained and 39 experienced gynaecologists. A total of 578 insertions were performed, with 98% successful placement rate for experienced versus 96.1% for novice clinicians. Average procedural time was 9 minutes (±7 standard deviation (SD)), with experienced clinicians and 10.7 minutes (±8.3 SD) for novices. There was no significant adverse association between successful placement with patient characteristics such as body mass index, surgical history, parity or prior vaginal deliveries observed. They concluded that the Essure® procedure can be performed quickly and safely with high bilateral placement rates regardless of clinician experience or patient characteristics.

One of the disadvantages of the Essure® device is the necessity to ensure that the tubal lumen is adequately occluded. An HSG is recommended three months after the insertion of the microcoils ('Essure® confirmation test').

The need for such follow-up has been confirmed by a recent study of 240 HSG examinations which were performed after hysteroscopic microinsert placement procedures in 235 women [9].

They confirmed that HSG is necessary because 6.3% of examinations showed abnormalities requiring an alternative form of contraception.

The Adiana device (Adriana® Permanent Contraception System (Hologic, Inc., Bedford, MA, USA)

This device was approved by the FDA in 2009, although it is no longer marketed. It requires the hysteroscopic placement of the delivery catheter into the intramural portion of each Fallopian tube, where it delivers radio-frequency (RF) energy for 1 minute, causing damage to the lumen for a 5 mm segment of tube. Following the thermal injury, a 3.5 mm silicone polymer matrix is injected down the catheter. This results in a fibroblast ingrowth, acting as a scaffold for the matrix. Over the next few weeks, scar tissue develops and acts as a permanent stopper.

The US Collaborative Review of Sterilization Study and other published reports documented the efficacy of established permanent sterilization procedures. They concluded that the efficacy of the Adiana® system for pregnancy prevention is similar to other permanent sterilization methods.

Comparison of Essure® and Adiana®

Palmer and Greenberg compared Essure® and Adiana® as the two options available for transcervical sterilization, at the time of their study [10]. They concluded that the transcervical approach offers women the option of a less invasive hysteroscopic procedure. There is a decreased potential for complications with sterilization performed in an outpatient or even a community setting. They found that the bilateral placement rate for Essure® was 94.6% and for Adiana® it was was 94%.

Both Essure® and Adiana® reduce procedural discomfort and increase patient satisfaction when compared with laparoscopic tubal occlusion. The potential for outpatient delivery of transcervical female sterilization also gives these methods a favourable cost profile when compared with other methods.

They emphasized that the effectiveness data for both methods are based on proper placement and confirmation of tubal occlusion including:
- Confirming proper device placement during the procedure.
- Confirming tubal occlusion at 90 days (HSG).
- Understanding the risk of pregnancy for women who do not attend for follow-up.

In contrast to the Essure® system, after the Adiana® matrix has been deployed, nothing remains in the endometrial cavity. This could be of benefit in the future if endometrial ablation or IVF are to be undertaken.

Laparoscopic or hysteroscopic approach?

An evidence-based clinical decision analysis to estimate the probability of successful sterilization after a hysteroscopic or laparoscopic procedure was undertaken by Gareipy and colleagues [11].

They concluded that the proportion of women having a successful sterilization procedure on the first attempt is 99% for laparoscopic sterilization, 88% for hysteroscopic sterilization in the operating theatre and 87% for hysteroscopic sterilization in the outpatient setting.

Consequently, women choosing laparoscopic sterilization are more likely to have a successful procedure. Approximately 5% of women who have a failed hysteroscopic attempt declined further sterilization.

The National Institute for Health and Clinical Excellence (NICE) supports the use of hysteroscopic sterilization provided that normal arrangements are in place for clinical governance and audit. As discussed above, the recommendations include ensuring that patients understand that additional contraception must be used until appropriate imaging confirms satisfactory tubal occlusion. Women should be advised, as with any method of contraception, that there is a small risk of pregnancy.

Sterilization reversal

Although counselling is aimed at preventing sterilization procedures on people who may regret their decision, circumstances can change and there will always be women requesting sterilization reversal. If, for example, Fatima's financial circumstances improve, she may be in a position to have another child, to placate her husband.

To minimize regret, one should be especially careful in women aged under 30, and those who are making decisions at a time of stress, such as in combination with a termination of pregnancy or in the immediate post-partum period.

The options for women who have been sterilized and wish to restore fertility are to undergo sterilization reversal or to attempt IVF.

Sterilization reversal by laparotomy versus laparoscopy

La Grange and colleagues reviewed the efficacy of sterilization reversals by laparotomy versus laparoscopy [12].

One hundred and eighty-four patients were studied, 88 and 96 respectively undergoing laparoscopy and laparotomy. Pregnancy rates achieved by laparoscopy ranged from 65 to 80% (mean 74%) and by laparotomy from 70 to 80% (mean 71%). They concluded that there is no difference between the two approaches to tubal re-anastomosis when regarding overall pregnancy rates.

If hysteroscopic sterilization was undertaken, tubo-uterine implantation would need to be performed rather than tubal re-anastomosis. Pregnancies have been reported after both Adiana® and Essure® using this technique.

There is also a theoretical concern about the effect of Essure® microcoils if IVF is attempted, but there have been reports of successful pregnancies with the devices still in situ [13].

In conclusion, the ultimate decision on the method of sterilization to be undertaken will depend on the skills and training of the operator, the availability of the equipment required, the cost of the various methods and the sources of funding for the procedure and, ultimately taking into consideration all these factors, the preference of the patient.

References

1. Delvin D. Sterilisation for women. http://www.netdoctor.co.uk/sex_relationships/facts/sterilisation_women.htm#ixzz2H7VkxWMr (accessed 1 March 2013).
2. Tan L, Ren Q, Cui Z, *et al.* Trends in contraceptive patterns and behaviors during a period of fertility transition in China: 1988–2006. *Contraception* 2012; 86: 204–13.
3. Bite N, Borrero S. Female sterilisation in the United States. *Eur J Contracept Reprod Health Care* 2011; 16: 336–40.
4. Kovacs GT, Krins AJ. Female sterilisations with Filshie clips: what is the risk failure? A retrospective survey of 30 000 applications. *J Fam Plann Reprod Health Care* 2002; 28: 34.
5. Valle RF, Carignan CS, Wright TC; STOP Prehysterectomy Investigation Group. Tissue response to the STOP microcoil transcervical permanent contraceptive device: results from a prehysterectomy study. *Fertil Steril* 2001; 76(5): 974–80.
6. Povedano B, Arjona JE, Velasco E, *et al.* Complications of hysteroscopic Essure® sterilisation: report on 4306 procedures performed in a single centre. *BJOG* 2012; 119: 795–9.
7. Smith RD. Contemporary hysteroscopic methods for female sterilization. *Int J Gynaecol Obstet* 2010; 108: 79–84.
8. Levie M, Chudnoff SG. A comparison of novice and experienced physicians performing hysteroscopic sterilization: an analysis of an FDA-mandated trial. *Fertil Steril* 2011; 96: 643–8.
9. Lazarus E, Lourenco AP, Casper S, Allen RH. Necessity of hysterosalpingography after Essure® microinsert placement for contraception. *Am J Roentgenol* 2012; 198: 1460–3.
10. Palmer SN, Greenberg JA. Transcervical sterilization: a comparison of Essure® permanent birth control system and Adiana® permanent contraception system. *Rev Obstet Gynecol* 2009; 2(2): 84–92.
11. Gariepy AM, Creinin MD, Schwarz EB, Smith KJ. Reliability of laparoscopic compared with hysteroscopic sterilization at 1 year: a decision analysis. *Obstet Gynecol* 2011; 118: 273–9.
12. la Grange J, Kruger TF, Steyn DW, *et al.* Fallopian tube reanastomosis by laparotomy versus laparoscopy: a meta-analysis. *Gynecol Obstet Invest* 2012; 74(1): 28–34.
13. Kerin JF, Cattanach S. Successful pregnancy outcome with the use of in vitro fertilization after Essure® hysteroscopic sterilization. *Fertil Steril* 2007; 87: 1212.

Male sterilization

Tina Peers and Tony Feltbower

Introduction

Vasectomy is a simple surgical procedure which results in male sterilization and, as such, is a permanent method of birth control.

The procedure was first developed as early as 1822 by Sir Ashley Cooper at Guys' Hospital London, when he performed an operation on a dog's testicles and noted that spermatogenesis continued for the rest of the dog's life. However it wasn't until the Second World War that it became popular as a method of contraception. The first National Vasectomy Programme was in India in 1954.

The technique involves severing or blocking of the vas deferentia which prevents sperm from entering the seminal stream (ejaculate), and as such is irreversible. Apart from the use of condoms, it is the only method of birth control that is the responsibility of the man. Vasectomy is more cost effective, less invasive and has a lower failure rate than sterilization in women. It also has a much lower instance of post-operative complications. In spite of this, in the USA, vasectomies are half as common as female sterilization. However, in New Zealand, the UK, Canada, Bhutan and the Netherlands the uptake is very high with 16% of all men and 25% of married men opting for a vasectomy as their chosen method of contraception.

The failure rate for non-scalpel vasectomy is 1 : 2000. The failure rate for female sterilization is 1 : 2–300 [1]. The early failure rate for vasectomy is 1 : 500. Pregnancy results typically from unprotected sexual intercourse too soon after the procedure and before a negative sperm sample has been confirmed. In rare cases it can also occur after spontaneous rejoining of the vas tubes, or the growth of a new tube. Late failure rate results from re-canalization of the vas resulting in pregnancy and has been reported [2]. A systematic review of 28 studies in 2005 showed a failure rate of 0.4% (183 failures out of 43 642 vasectomies) and 20 studies showed 60 pregnancies in 92 184 vasectomies, a rate of 0.07% [3].

Vasectomy counselling

The general practitioner (GP) plays a very important role when a couple or an individual consults them about a vasectomy referral. There are a number of important considerations that must be covered before the referral is made, and it is vitally important that there is sufficient time for questions to be answered and worries to be addressed.

Contraception, eds Paula Briggs, Gabor Kovacs and John Guillebaud. Published by Cambridge University Press. © Cambridge University Press 2013.

Pre-vasectomy counselling

- Alternatives to vasectomy
- Irreversibility
- Regret/relationship break-up
- Sperm storage
- Operative techniques used
- Complications
- Long-term effects

Alternatives to vasectomy

It is particularly useful if both partners are present for this discussion. It is essential to inform the couple about alternative methods of contraception, especially the long-acting reversible contraceptive (LARC) methods which are so effective. These include:

- Depo-Provera® injection
- Intrauterine contraception – especially the Mirena® intrauterine system (IUS)
- Implants

It is important to cover all the non-contraceptive benefits of these reversible, highly effective methods, so that the couple/patient can make a fully informed decision about using an irreversible method of sterilization.

Irreversibility

A vasectomy should be considered irreversible [4, 5]. However, it can be reversed with some success if the reversal is performed within 10 years of the vasectomy, giving a 55% success rate. This reduces to 25% if the procedure is more than 10 years after the original sterilization. At this point in the counselling session it is useful to discuss the possibility of regret. Forty per cent of all marriages are re-marriages and, whilst it may be difficult to imagine the loss of a child or partner, or improved finances, or indeed a change of circumstances such as a relationship breakdown [6], it is important that these are considered and discussed.

One should also point out that the cost of reversal would be borne by the couple/man. In the UK vasectomy reversal is not usually available on the National Health Service (NHS) and would cost over £6000, while in the USA the cost may be as high as $10 000.

Sperm storage

Bearing in mind the poor pregnancy rate of vasectomy reversal and the potential cost, some men may want to have information about sperm storage. Cryo-storage would allow artificial insemination of their current partner or of a new partner [6]. It is useful to have the details of some local clinics where sperm storage can be arranged (privately). When considering this the cost of the artificial insemination must also be borne in mind.

Intracytoplasmic sperm insemination (ICSI) using in vitro fertilization technology is also possible and may be a cheaper option. This procedure involves aspiration of sperm from the testicles or epididymis under local anaesthetic, and usually results in sufficient sperm to allow ICSI.

Vasectomy methods

At this point in the consultation it is useful to give the man some idea of the different methods of vasectomy performed locally. In the UK, the method recommended by the Royal College of Obstetricians and Gynaecologists and the Faculty of Sexual and Reproductive Healthcare is the No-Scalpel technique because of the lower incidence of complications and lower failure rates. This is also known as the 'key-hole' vasectomy, as a small 3 mm opening is made in the scrotal skin (after local anaesthetic has numbed the skin!) and the whole operation is performed through this single tiny aperture. It is worth pointing out that the procedure is performed under a local anaesthetic.

The vas deferentia are identified, a small section is removed, at least one end is cauterized and the vas are returned to the sac. The tiny opening results in less bruising and means that there is a reduced risk of haematoma, discomfort, infection and post-vasectomy pain syndrome. It heals very quickly and requires no stitching.

Most men will find this description somewhat reassuring; however, be sensitive in your approach, as some men do not want to hear about the details of the operation!

Other vasectomy operative techniques available include:

1. Open-ended vasectomy. This is where the testicular portion of the vas is left open allowing sperm produced to spill into the scrotal sac. This is considered to potentially reduce the incidence of post-operative testicular pain, caused by increased pressure in the epididymis [7] and thus reduce the risk of post-vasectomy pain syndrome (PVPS).
2. Fascial imposition helps to reduce the chances of recanalization of the vas deferens [8]. The fascia is a sheath that surrounds the vas. The testicular end is left inside the sheath, whilst the prostatic end is not, both being cauterized intraluminally.
3. A new clip device, Pro-Vas®, is available to put on the vas. Theoretically this technique should mean that reversal should be easier. However, this method has an unacceptably high failure rate, as did the previously available Vasclip®, which is no longer on the market.

Complications

Explain that the man may experience a small amount of pain and discomfort during and after the procedure and that usually paracetamol is sufficient for pain relief. As with any operation, there is a risk of complications. These include swelling, bruising, infection, development of chronic PVPS and even, very rarely, testicular atrophy (this can occur if the blood supply to the testicle is inadvertently interrupted resulting in the testicle dying). It is important to emphasize that it is very unlikely that any of them will be severe.

Immediate complications

Bruising – Some men will have no bruising at all, whilst others may experience dramatic bruising of the surface of the skin in the area of the operation. In some cases, the bruising may not be evident for a couple of days. There is usually no swelling associated with this bruising.

Haematoma – This is where a small vessel damaged at the time of the operation leaks blood into the scrotal sac. The swelling can be very dramatic and look very purple and black. It is prudent to refer such cases back to the surgeon who performed the operation, who may, in extremely rare cases, admit them to hospital for exploration or observation. Thankfully, the risk of post-operative bleeding and haematoma formation has a very low incidence with the No-Scalpel technique – 1% in most centres.

Infection – This is very uncommon and is usually over diagnosed. Sometimes between days 7 and 10 post-operatively, as a result of increased activity and the general healing process, there can be an increase in discomfort and this can be inappropriately diagnosed as an infection without any evidence of swelling or discharge.

Late complications

Sperm granulomas – These can occur at the testicular end of the vas, presenting as a tender lump. If necessary it can be excised, although reassurance and anti-inflammatories for a few days should normally be sufficient.

Congestive epididymitis – This is also a recognized complication, again treated with simple analgesics and reassurance. Some evidence suggests that leaving open the testicular end of the vas may reduce the incidence.

Blood in the ejaculate – This may be seen in the first couple of weeks post operation. Reassurance is all that is required, unless it continues beyond two weeks when it would require full investigation.

Testicular atrophy – This is extremely rare and could occur if there is an aberrant arterial supply to the testicle. If it is supplied by only one artery, and not the three that usually exist, and that artery is damaged during the operation, then avascular testicular atrophy could occur.

Post-vasectomy pain syndrome – Quoted rates can be anything from 6 to 1%. Most surgeons and GPs rarely see a case. It has been described in various forms ranging from very mild, to moderate and, only very rarely, severe enough to interfere with normal life thus requiring treatment. Usually, the cases of PVPS are mild to moderate, intermittent and self-limiting. It is thought to be due to scar tissue formation and, rather bizarrely, severe cases sometimes respond to vasectomy reversal.

It is extremely useful to give the man a copy of the Patient Information Leaflet that is recommended by the British Association of No Scalpel Vasectomists (BANSV), now part of the Association of Surgeons in Primary Care (ASPC) (see Appendix 1).

This allows the couple to read all about the vasectomy and enables them to make a fully informed decision. Once they have an appointment with the local service provider the likelihood is that they will have an appointment on a 'see and do' basis, i.e., a 'one-stop clinic'.

It is also good practice for the surgeon to send a copy of the consent form to the patient with the appointment. This enables the couple to read all about the potential risks and have a full discussion prior to their appointment. They can then take any questions they may have with them for clarification before going ahead with the procedure.

A copy of the consent form suggested by BANSV is shown in Appendix 2. Appendices 1 and 2 can be downloaded from the ASPC/BANSV website (http://www.aspc-uk.net/BANSV.htm).

Case scenario

Rebekah and Richard have been married for 10 years. They have two sons and have been trying for a third child for several years.

Rebekah is 34 years old. She is a non-smoker and is overweight with a body mass index (BMI) of 32. She has just been discharged from hospital following a period in the intensive treatment unit (ITU) as a result of a pulmonary embolus.

Richard took time off work to care for the children while she was ill and has just been made redundant. The couple have had to review their priorities and have decided that their family is complete.

They consult you to discuss sterilization. Richard feels that after everything that Rebekah has been through, he should have a vasectomy.

Possible points for discussion

1. Irreversibility
2. Regret/relationship break-up
3. His possible anxieties
4. Methods used
5. Complications
6. Long-term effects
7. Sperm storage
8. Reversibility
9. Costs

It sounds as if this poor couple have had considerable stress recently with Rebekah's life-threatening illness and Richard's job loss.

With Rebekah's history and BMI she could safely consider using the progestogen-only pill or the IUS. She would, no doubt, be on an anticoagulant and therefore the intrauterine contraceptive device would not be a suitable option.

It would be important to ask the couple how they would feel if Richard managed to get a new job in the near future, and whether this would make them change their minds about not trying for a third child.

Appendix 1

Example of Patient Information Leaflet as written and recommended by the British Association of No Scalpel Vasectomists

What is vasectomy?

Vasectomy or male sterilization is a simple, safe, effective and permanent method of surgical contraception for men. In vasectomy, the vas deferens, which is the tube that takes the sperm from the testes to the penis, is cut. Sperm are made in the testes and once the tube is cut, sperm can no longer get into the semen that is ejaculated during sex.

How can I be sure that I need a vasectomy?

If you are absolutely sure that you don't want to have any more children

If you want to enjoy sex without worrying about pregnancy

If you don't want to use any other form of birth control

If pregnancy poses a risk to the health of your partner

If you want to save your partner from a tubal ligation which has a higher rate of failure and complications

When should I not consider a vasectomy?

Vasectomy is a lifetime decision. Consider the possibility of unforeseen changes in life – divorce, death of a spouse or child, or just the likelihood of you and your partner changing your mind about your desired family size.

A vasectomy might not be right for you if:

You are young

You have few, if any, children

Your current relationship is not stable

You are pressurized by your partner or by circumstances

You are under a lot of stress

Vasectomy is performed during time of personal crisis

You have a religious affiliation prohibiting vasectomy

You are counting on being able to reverse the procedure later

You hope vasectomy will solve sexual and marital problems

Your partner is expecting, especially if a planned pregnancy

How is a No-Scalpel vasectomy different from a conventional vasectomy?

In a conventional vasectomy, the scrotum is numbed with an injection of local anaesthetic into the skin on either side above the testes. A small cut is then made in the numbed area with a scalpel and the vas deferens on each side dissected out in turn. The tube is then cut and the cut ends tied. The small cuts in the skin are then stitched.

In the case of a No-Scalpel vasectomy, after anaesthetizing the skin and the vas, the doctor holds the vas deferens under the skin and secures it in place with a special ring clamp. Instead of making two incisions, a tiny puncture is made in the skin and the vas delivered and blocked with a special cautery instrument called the Hyfrecator. This effectively pushes the blood vessels and the nerves aside instead of cutting across them. No stitches are needed to close the small opening which heals quickly with no scar.

This technique was developed first in China by Dr Shunqiang in 1974. It was introduced into the USA in 1988. In the UK, doctors have been performing this operation since 1995.

What are the advantages of No-Scalpel vasectomy over conventional methods?

Less discomfort

One small opening in the skin instead of two incisions

No stitches

Faster procedure

Faster recovery

Less chance of bleeding and other complications

More effective (Although probably the most important factor is the competence and experience of the surgeon!)

Does No-Scalpel vasectomy work?

Yes. This is a very reliable procedure. However it is estimated that there is a 1 in 2000 chance that the man might become fertile again at some point in the future. Rarely, the two cut ends of the vas deferens can reunite. Serious problems are very rare; less than 3 in 100 cases even have a minor problem

Is No-Scalpel vasectomy painful?

This is an almost painless procedure. You will experience mild discomfort when the local anaesthesic is administered. However, once it takes effect you should feel no pain. Some men feel a slight 'tugging' sensation as the tubes are manipulated and some sense of pressure.

Will it hurt after No-Scalpel vasectomy?

After surgery you may be a little sore for a few days. You might need to take a painkiller.

How long will the whole procedure take?

The whole procedure will take on average about 30 minutes.

Is No-Scalpel vasectomy safe?

Yes. It is safe and simple and most men do not have any problems. However, like any surgical procedure, it has some risks. There are no life-threatening complications associated with No-Scalpel vasectomy. The minor complications are generally short-lived and resolve with rest, ice, anti-inflammatories and time.

So, what are the possible complications?

Mild discomfort: Some men report a mild aching sensation to the scrotum for a few hours to a few days after the procedure.

Bleeding: Bleeding into the scrotum causing a small painful swelling and bruising for a few days. A major bleed can cause a grapefruit-sized scrotum which can take months to heal, but this is very rare with No-Scalpel vasectomy.

Infection: Redness and pus from the healing site opening.

Epididymitis: Tender swelling of the epididymis, the tube connecting the vas deferens and the testes.

Sperm granuloma: Sperm can leak from the cut end of the vas deferens and form a potentially uncomfortable small nodule in the scrotum. Most cases are asymptomatic.

Post-vasectomy pain syndrome: An uncommon complication of a persisting pain in the testicle where the inflammation does not settle down. It may resolve on its own or persist and require further specialist treatment.

Failure: Because one or both tubes have rejoined.

When can I go back to work?

Generally, two or three days rest is enough time for recovery before men can return to work and most normal, non-strenuous physical activity. If your job involves heavy work, you should take a full week off.

When can I start having sex again?

Sex can usually be resumed seven days after the procedure when you feel comfortable.

Will I be sterile right away?

No. After a vasectomy there are always some active sperm left in your system. Some sperms survive in the 'upstream' part of the vas deferens for several weeks after a vasectomy and these can get into the semen for a while after the operation. It takes about 25 ejaculations to clear them. You and your partner should use some other form of birth control until your semen has been tested and confirmed free of sperm.

When would I have the semen test?

We do a single test 16 weeks after the procedure. Further tests at monthly intervals may be required if any sperm are still seen in the semen.

Will it affect my long-term health in any way?

No. Studies have shown conclusively that vasectomized men are no more likely to get heart disease, cancer, arthritis or any other disease. Disabling post-vasectomy pain syndrome is extremely rare.

Will vasectomy change me sexually?

The only thing that will change is that you will not be able to make your partner pregnant. Your penis and testes are not altered in any way. Your body will continue to produce the hormones that make you a man. The operation has no impact on the man's ability to perform sexually. Vasectomy does not change your beard, your muscles, your sex drive, your erections or climaxes.

Furthermore most men report that sex is better after vasectomy because they no longer need to worry about an accidental pregnancy. With the security and peace of mind permanent contraception brings, sex can be more relaxed and spontaneous.

What happens to the sperm after a vasectomy?

Sperms are still made as before in the testes. The sperm cannot get past the blocked vas deferens and are reabsorbed internally. Sperm make up about 1% of the ejaculate, so there will be no detectable difference in the volume. Vasectomy does not reduce the amount of semen you ejaculate during sex as most of it is made in the seminal vesicles and prostate upstream.

Will it protect me from getting sexually transmitted diseases or AIDS?

No. A vasectomy cannot protect you from sexually transmitted diseases including AIDS. Condoms are still the best protection against these diseases.

What if I were to change my mind after the vasectomy?

A vasectomy should be considered permanent. Reversal operations to reattach the cut ends are expensive and often unsuccessful. If you are asking this question, perhaps a vasectomy is not right for you.

Why not a tubal ligation for my partner?

Vasectomy is preferable to a tubal ligation because tubal ligation:

Carries a greater potential health risk for a woman
Requires general anaesthesia
Is an intra-abdominal procedure

Post-operative recovery is longer
Failure rate is more common
More difficult to confirm the efficacy
If pregnancy occurs, it could be an ectopic one

© 2012 Association of Surgeons in Primary Care. Design by ASGBI.

Appendix 2
Consent to treat – vasectomy

Being an adult, I .... hereby consent to undergo the operation of VASECTOMY under local anaesthetic, the nature and effect of which has been explained to me by Dr .... I have been counselled regarding alternative forms of long-term *reversible* contraception, e.g., coils/implants and have read and understood the information leaflet.

I also consent to such further alternative measures as may be found necessary or advisable during the course of the operation and to the administration of a local anaesthetic for any of these purposes.

I have been told that the object of the operation is to render me sterile and incapable of further parenthood and I understand that the effect of the operation may be irreversible. Further I confirm that I acknowledge there is a rare but accepted failure rate associated with Non-Scalpel vasectomy reported to be in the order of 0.05% (1 in 2000) and therefore a small risk of pregnancy in the future even after being given the 'all clear'.

No assurance has been given to me that the operation will be performed by a particular surgeon and I understand that no guarantees can be given that the operation will be successful or that it will be free from side effects.

I acknowledge that there is a small risk of significant complications like severe infection and excessive bleeding/bruising (common to any surgical procedure – for non-scalpel vasectomy, 1%), a small risk of developing chronic testicular pain and extremely rarely: testicular atrophy. Any complication may require further medical treatment, hospitalization or further surgery.

I understand that I should not abandon other methods of contraception prior to receipt of notification that at least one sperm count at least four months after my vasectomy has proved negative, or special clearance has been given after seven months.

I understand that I can change my mind at any time and decide not to proceed with the vasectomy.

Date of procedure: ....
Past medical history: ....
Allergies: ....
Current medication: ....
Contraception currently used: ....
Alternatives to vasectomy discussed: ....
Children: ....
Procedure: ....
Risks: ....   all explained as above

Failure rate: . . . .

Irreversibility: . . . .

Questions: . . . .

Doctor's confirmation

I confirm that I have explained to the patient/and partner* the nature and effect of vasectomy as detailed above. Further, I confirm that the patient has read (or had read to him) the above form and I am satisfied that he understands what is proposed, has no further questions and is happy to proceed with a vasectomy.

Signature of doctor: . . . .

Date: . . . .

I confirm that I have read (or had read to me) and understand the above form and I am satisfied with the conditions stated therein.

Signature of patient: . . . .

Date: . . . .

Any additional signature (e.g., interpreter): . . . .

Date: . . . .

Name: . . . .

Role: . . . .

References

1. Royal College of Obstetricians and Gynaecologists. *Sterilisation for Women and Men: what you need to know*, January 2004. http://www.rcog.org.uk/files/rcog-corp/ Sterilisation%20For%20Women%20and% 20Men.pdf (accessed 1 March 2013).

2. Philp T, Guillebaud J, Budd D. Late failure of vasectomy after two documented analyses showing azoospermic semen. *BMJ* 1984; 289(6437): 77–9.

3. Griffin T, Tooher R, Nowakowski K, Lloyd M, Maddern G. How little is enough? The evidence for post-vasectomy testing. *J Urol* 2005; 174 (1): 29–36.

4. Abdelmassih V, Balmaceda JP, Tesarik J, Abdelmassih R, Nagy ZP. Relationship between time period after vasectomy and the reproductive capacity of sperm obtained by epididymal aspiration. *Hum Reprod* 2002; 17(3): 736–40.

5. Sukcharoen N, Ngeamvijawat J, Sithipravej T, Promviengchai S. High sex chromosome aneuploidy and diploidy rate of epididymal spermatozoa in obstructive azoospermic men. *J Assist Reprod Genet* 2003; 20(5): 196–203.

6. Murphy C. 'Divorce fuels vasectomy reversals'. *BBC News*, 18 March 2009 (retrieved 19 September 2012).

7. Christiansen C, Sandlow J. Testicular pain following vasectomy: a review of post vasectomy pain syndrome. *J Androl* 2003; 24(3): 293–8.

8. Vasectomy-information.com. Spontaneous recanalization of the vas deferens after vasectomy. http://www.vasectomy-information.com/ moreinfo/recanalisation.htm (accessed 1 March 2013).

Chapter 18

Emergency contraception

Anne Connolly and Lynne Garforth

Case scenario: Gemma

Gemma attends the morning surgery with her baby and toddler. Gemma is aged 25 and is anxious because the clinic appointment is delayed and she has to collect her 4-year-old child from the school nursery. She has run out of her contraceptive pills and was due to start her new pack four days ago, and so is keen to obtain a further supply as she knows she would struggle to cope with another pregnancy at the moment. She also asks for the 'morning after pill' because she had unprotected sexual intercourse last night.

Introduction

Emergency contraception (post-coital contraception) (EC) continues to be an important aspect of contraceptive care in spite of the free access to a wide range of reliable contraceptives from a choice of providers. It is a means of reducing the risk of pregnancy after unprotected sexual intercourse (UPSI) has occurred, whether this has been because a contraceptive has not been used, including during sexual assault, or when the regular contraceptive method has failed.

There have been many methods of post-coital contraception used since it was understood that sperm caused a pregnancy to occur, and a variety of concoctions have been inserted into the vagina in an attempt to prevent passage of sperm over the years. An estimated 25% of women today still attempt to 'wash-out' the sperm by douching before attending for EC. Unfortunately none of these methods are effective because of the speed of sperm, which are found within the cervical mucus within 90 seconds after ejaculation.

According to the 2008–09 Omnibus survey from the Office for National Statistics, approximately 7% of women had used EC in the previous year with only 0.5% using the emergency copper-containing intrauterine device (Cu-IUD) [1].

Although some have ethical concerns about the action of certain methods of EC, the Judicial Review of Emergency Contraception in 2002 ruled that a pregnancy is not recognized to exist until implantation has occurred.

Emergency contraception options

There are three methods of EC currently available within the UK and it is important in cases such as this to understand their action, their efficacy and which choices are appropriate for each woman.

Contraception, eds Paula Briggs, Gabor Kovacs and John Guillebaud. Published by Cambridge University Press. © Cambridge University Press 2013.

Table 18.1 Emergency contraceptive options available in the UK.

Method	Product available	Indication for use	Action
Cu-IUD	Various products available for contraception	Within 5 days following first episode of UPSI or earliest estimated date of ovulation, whichever is longer	Prevents fertilization Prevents implantation if fertilization already occurred
UPA	EllaOne®	Within 120 hours of UPSI or contraceptive failure	Inhibits or delays ovulation and suppresses growth of lead follicles
LNG	Levonelle® 1500 Levonelle® One Step	Within 72 hours of UPSI or contraceptive failure	Inhibits or delays ovulation if given before the luteinizing hormone surge

Cu-IUD, copper-releasing intrauterine device; LNG, levonorgestrel; UPA, ulipristal acetate; UPSI, unprotected sexual intercourse.

The options available (Table 18.1) are:
- Copper-containing intrauterine device (Cu-IUD)
- Progesterone receptor modulator – ulipristal acetate (UPA) 30 mg
- Progestogen – levonorgestrel (LNG) 1.5 mg

To help determine which of the options could be used in Gemma's case, it's important that a careful menstrual and sexual history is taken. The important points to determine in this consultation are:

- What type of pill was she taking?
- Has she had UPSI since taking the last 'proper' pill in her pack? (exclude dummy pills if taking an everyday preparation)
- A sexual health risk assessment including ensuring that the UPSI was consensual.
- Is the user-dependent 'pill' the best method of contraception for Gemma with her busy life or would one of the long-acting reversible contraceptive (LARC) methods be a more appropriate choice in the future?

If Gemma had been less than 16 years old, then an assessment of her competency would be required using the Fraser guidelines and any concerns would need to be discussed with the local Safeguarding Children Lead.

In this scenario a contraceptive method was being used. If she had attended the surgery requesting EC without using another method then it is important to estimate the timing of ovulation by careful assessment of her menstrual cycle, to help determine her risk and the options available to her.

The menstrual cycle explained

This is covered in detail in Chapter 4, but the key points are outlined below.

During the first half of the menstrual cycle:

- Follicle stimulating hormone (FSH), a pituitary gland hormone, is released and stimulates follicular growth.
- A batch of follicles will grow and by day seven, a dominant follicle is established. This continues to grow and is destined to ovulate, whilst the others degenerate (atresia).

- Once the leading follicle reaches maturity, luteinizing hormone (LH) is produced by the pituitary gland, but only as a 24 hour peak, and instructs the follicle to ovulate – release the ovum.
- Oestrogen is secreted by the developing follicle. Levels increase as the follicle grows and the endometrium thickens.
- Oestrogen levels inhibit FSH secretion (negative feedback), so that only one follicle matures. The oestrogen triggers the LH surge (positive feedback).
- Approximately 36 hours after the start of the LH surge (24 hours after the peak), the follicle ruptures and ovulation occurs.
- If sperm are present at this point then fertilization occurs in the Fallopian tube, within 12 hours of release of the ovum.

During the second half of the menstrual cycle:

- LH signals the corpus luteum (the remains of the follicle from which the egg was released) to produce progesterone in addition to oestrogen.
- Consequently, the corpus luteum continues to produce progesterone and oestrogen in high quantities.
- If pregnancy has not occurred the corpus luteum succumbs, and levels of both oestrogen and progesterone decline.
- Thus, if no conception has occurred, then about 14 days after ovulation, menstruation starts.

The calculation of the fertile time and highest risk of conception in this 28 day cycle is between days 7 and 15, as sperm survival is estimated to be a maximum of 5 days after sexual intercourse and fertilization is required within 12 hours of release of the ovum (Figure 18.1).

In women with differing cycle lengths this calculation becomes less predictable as ovulation usually occurs about 14 days before the next menses, thus giving a wider range.

Advising on whether there is an indication for EC

As part of the consultation the date of her last normal menstrual period should be ascertained along with information about her normal cycle length. This allows for an estimation of where she is in her cycle and the likely risk of pregnancy from her episode(s) of UPSI. If she is unsure, then the presumption should be that she is within her fertile window.

It emerges during the consultation Gemma has consensually agreed to have sex with her regular partner on a couple of occasions since she took her last combined oral contraceptive pill. One of these episodes was last night and the other a few days ago, but she could not remember precisely when.

Gemma is at risk of pregnancy because the pill-free interval has been extended by more than two days and she has had UPSI since her last active pill. Emergency contraception is indicated (Table 18.2) and the choices should be discussed with her.

The choices about which of the methods are appropriate in each individual case are dependent on the history and the relevant points to determine are:

- Is there a possibility of an implanted pregnancy already?
- When did the episode/episodes of UPSI occur?

Menstrual cycle regulation

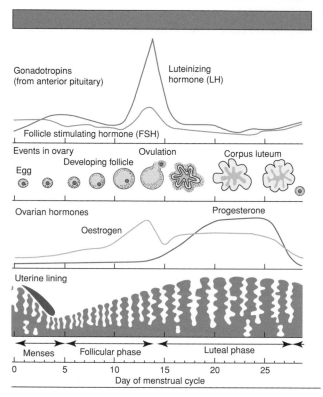

1. Hypothalamus releases GnRH, stimulating the pituitary

2. FSH secreted from pituitary stimulates follicle

3. Follicles produce oestrogen-negative feedback turning off FSH release

4. Critical level of E_2 stimulates-LH peak-positive feedback-ovulation

5. Corpus luteum secretes E_2 and P_4 life span 12–14 days

Figure 18.1 The menstrual cycle. (GnRH, gonadotrophin-releasing hormone.)

- When was the start of her last normal menstrual period or withdrawal bleed?
- What is her usual cycle length?
- Are there any potential drug interactions that might reduce the efficacy of any method [2]?
- Has EC been used previously during this cycle?
- Does she fit the UK Medical Eligibility Criteria (UKMEC) [3] for the different methods available?
- Individual preference.

Advising on EC options

It is difficult to calculate the efficacy of each of the methods of EC, as the exact risk of each episode of UPSI is dependent on the fertility of the woman and the timing of the UPSI in relation to ovulation. The majority of women presenting for EC will not be at risk of pregnancy, with the chance of conception after a single act of UPSI being estimated to be between 4 and 6%, increasing to between 20 and 30% at the most fertile time of the menstrual cycle [4].

Table 18.2 Indications for use of EC.

EC is required when there has been UPSI and:
No contraception was used
When taking combined oral contraceptive pills (except Qlaira®, see SPC for advice)
Two or more pills are missed
Or
The pill-free interval is extended by 2 or more days (either by missing pills from the last week of the previous pack or by delaying the start of the next pack)
More than 2 days late restarting other combined hormonal methods (patch or ring)
More than 3 hours late taking a progestogen-only pill (or more than 12 hours late taking the desogestrel-only pill)
IUD or IUS partially or completely expelled, or the threads are not visible and it is not clear if it is still in situ
The injectable DMPA is more than 2 weeks late
Non-perfect use of male or female barrier methods
Use of liver enzyme-inducing medication when using any combined hormonal contraceptive, progestogen-only pills or the progestogen-only subdermal contraceptive implant
The use of non-enzyme-inducing antibiotics does not reduce the efficacy of an oral contraceptive method and there is no requirement to consider emergency contraception for these women, unless the antibiotic has interfered with the absorption of the oral contraceptive by causing profuse diarrhoea

DMPA, depot-medroxyprogesterone acetate; EC, emergency contraception; IUD, intrauterine device; IUS, intrauterine system; SPC, summary of product characteristics; UPSI, unprotected sexual intercourse.

So which method should be offered to which woman?

The copper IUD (Cu-IUD)

The most effective method of EC is the Cu-IUD, which has a failure rate of less than 1% when used for EC. This should be offered to every woman, as recommended by the Faculty of Sexual and Reproductive Healthcare (FSRH), if the timing is appropriate [5].

The IUD is however not acceptable to every woman for many reasons, including the invasive nature of the fitting procedure and the perceived myths that she or her healthcare provider may have about this method. There may also be difficulties in accessing a service where this can be fitted without delay.

The use of this excellent method of EC is often not offered to nulliparous women because of the unfounded concern of problems with insertion. There is also the perceived risk of reducing future fertility in these women, which was dispelled by the study by Hubacher et al. [6], which confirmed that the use of a Cu-IUD is not associated with an increased risk of tubal infertility.

When used for EC the Cu-IUD has a mechanism of action both pre- and post-fertilization, which contribute to its efficacy. Copper is toxic to the ovum and sperm. However, if inserted after fertilization has occurred then provided the device is inserted within five days of the estimated day of ovulation the endometrial inflammatory reaction caused by the copper prevents implantation. It is essential therefore that a Cu-IUD must be inserted within five days following first UPSI or after the earliest anticipated day of ovulation, even if the woman had multiple acts of UPSI since her last menstrual period.

There are few contraindications to the use of a Cu-IUD and there are no interactions with other medications. This method cannot be used in women with a known copper allergy, or in women with current pelvic inflammatory disease. Reference to the UKMEC should be made if there are any concerns [3].

When using this method for EC, the woman can choose to have it removed after her next period or to leave the device in situ for ongoing contraception.

A careful menstrual and sexual history is obviously very important as part of any EC request, but is especially relevant prior to the insertion of a Cu-IUD both to ensure that insertion is correctly timed and also to make a sexually transmitted infection risk assessment. Testing for relevant pathogens is recommended prior to insertion. Chlamydia prophylaxis with a 1 g stat dose of azithromycin is recommended at the time of insertion if the risk of infection is deemed to be significant, without waiting for the test result.

Women fitted with an IUD should be taught to check for the threads of the device and to return to the clinic, or another healthcare provider, if they have any concerns. They should be counselled about the symptoms of a pelvic infection – offensive discharge; pelvic pain; raised body temperature – and also the need to perform a pregnancy test if their next period is delayed by more than a few days.

If an IUD fitting is not possible at the time of the consultation, either because of time or lack of skills required, then a streamlined pathway should be in place without unnecessary delay or barriers.

Gemma is an obvious candidate to consider using this method of contraception both for her long-term contraceptive needs and for the EC she requires today. Because of her need to collect her young child from nursery and other surgery commitments this procedure could not be performed immediately and she promises to attend an appointment at the local contraceptive clinic that evening.

In this instance it is advisable to also provide immediate oral EC, in case she changes her mind or other family commitments prevent this from happening. So an assessment for decision about the two available oral methods is required.

Oral EC

Ulipristal acetate

UPA works as a progesterone receptor modulator and has been available in the UK since 2009. The single dose of 30 mg provided in the EC regimen works by inhibiting or delaying ovulation, dependent on when it is taken during the menstrual cycle. There is also known to be an inhibitory effect on follicular rupture in some women even after the LH levels have started to rise. This action means that its effectiveness mid-cycle is better than that provided by LNG, which has no effect on ovulation prevention once the LH surge has started [7]. The effect on the endometrium is not fully understood and it is not known whether this adds to the efficacy of use.

UPA has a license for use as an EC until the fifth day after UPSI and is equally effective across the five days. This product is the only oral EC with a license for use on days 4 and 5 after UPSI.

Other points to consider when using UPA:

1. The current license for use is only once during the menstrual cycle.
2. It should not be used in women:

- who are pregnant.
- who are hypersensitive to any of the ingredients.
- who have severe asthma not controlled with oral steroids.
- who have severe hepatic or renal impairment.
- who have any of the rare hereditary disorders: galactose intolerance, Lapp lactase deficiency, glucose–galactose malabsorption.

UPA is metabolized by cytochrome P450, so it cannot be used in women using liver enzyme-inducing medication, e.g., rifampicin, phenytoin, phenobarbital, carbamazepine and St John's Wort as the plasma levels of UPA can be reduced thereby making it less effective. The dose should not be doubled for any reason at present.

Concomitant use of EC containing LNG and UPA is not recommended.

UPA is also not recommended for women who are breastfeeding.

As Gemma is on day 11 since taking her last active contraceptive pill she is at risk of ovulation. She stopped breastfeeding her baby three months previously. Using UPA was considered to be the best option for her. She was advised that if she vomits within three hours of taking this then she must return for a further consultation, if she doesn't attend her emergency IUD fitting.

Other side effects experienced by some women include menstrual irregularities. In phase III studies, 74.6% of women had their menstrual period at the expected time or within ± 7 days, whilst 6.8% experienced menses more than 7 days earlier than expected and 18.5% had a delay of more than 7 days beyond the anticipated onset. A delay of more than 20 days occurred in 4% of women [8].

Gemma is informed that she should perform a pregnancy test three weeks after the episode of UPSI if her next period is delayed or lighter than expected.

Levonorgestrel

The third and least effective method of EC is the progestogen-only 1.5 mg dose of levonorgestrel (LNG).

The precise mode of action of LNG is unknown, but it works primarily by inhibition of ovulation. If taken prior to the LH surge it can delay ovulation between five and seven days meaning that any sperm will be non-viable by the time the ovum is available for fertilization. LNG is no better than placebo, however, at suppressing ovulation if given after the LH surge has commenced, and has no effect once fertilization has occurred [7].

This method is licensed for use up to 72 hours post UPSI or contraceptive failure. A recent study combining data from four World Health Organization randomized controlled trials has shown action of LNG as an EC up to 96 hours and delay in treatment until this time did not alter efficacy [9].

It is a safe product. The UKMEC [3] does not identify any medical condition where LNG should not be used, other than it is not advised in a woman who is known to be pregnant, but there is no evidence that inadvertent use affects the pregnancy or the developing fetus.

Although outside of the product license, LNG can be given more than once per cycle. It can be used in a double dose (also off-license) in women who are taking or have taken enzyme-inducing drugs in the last 28 days.

As it is readily available from a number of providers including pharmacies, where it can be purchased without a prescription, LNG is currently the more commonly used method of EC. Some commissioners have developed local schemes to provide LNG via patient group directives (PGDs) from nurses in a variety of settings and pharmacists following recognized training. Ease of access to LNG may prevent some women from EC choice and delivery must be backed up by clear pathways to services where women can access all three EC options.

There are few side effects experienced in women taking LNG. Vomiting is a rare occurrence, but if this occurs within two hours of taking the dose, Gemma should be advised to return for a further consultation. She must also be warned that there may be some alteration to her next period and if this is delayed by more than one week after her expected date, or if she bleeds less than usual, she must perform a pregnancy test.

A further reason that UPA is recommended for Gemma is that she has a body mass index (BMI) of 34.

There is some evidence to suggest that UPA is more effective, not only in the fertile period of the cycle, but also in women who have a higher BMI. This evidence is the result of a meta-analysis of UPA and LNG studies, which demonstrate that in women who are obese (BMI > 30) using LNG is less effective at reducing pregnancy rates when compared to UPA. This difference is not seen in women with a BMI of less than 25 [10].

Future contraception

A further important aspect of an EC consultation is to offer advice on future, more effective contraceptive options, particularly in cases where the woman chooses not to consider a Cu-IUD.

Women who have taken oral EC methods should be advised about 'Quick Starting' an effective contraceptive method. There is a two to three times higher risk of pregnancy in women who continue to have UPSI during the same cycle compared to those who abstain [11].

The term 'Quick Starting' describes starting contraception at the time the woman presents for EC rather than the traditional way of waiting until her next period starts. This is outside the terms of the product license for hormonal contraception and needs to be considered on an individual basis. There are many advantages to 'Quick Starting'.

These include:

- Reducing the length of time a woman is at risk of pregnancy.
- Optimizing the opportunity to motivate her to use contraception while she is enthusiastic.
- Information given is more likely to be remembered.
- Further barriers to her accessing care are avoided.

This FSRH guidance [11] recommends that provided there is a reasonable estimation that the woman is not pregnant, then some contraceptive methods can be started immediately, along with abstinence from further acts of sexual intercourse or the use of condoms for a specified time period dependent on the oral EC method used. See the given guidance in Table 18.3.

A pregnancy test is recommended three weeks after 'Quick Starting' contraception to exclude a pregnancy resulting from failure of the EC.

Combined hormonal contraceptives, a progestogen-only oral method of contraception or the subdermal contraceptive implant can be used as 'Quick Starting' methods. The

Table 18.3 Summary of additional contraceptive requirements when 'Quick Starting' contraception following the administration of oral EC.

Method of ongoing contraception	Method of oral EC given	Requirements for additional contraception (condoms/abstinence)
Combined hormonal contraception (pill (excluding Qlaira®), transdermal patch or vaginal ring)	LNG UPA	7 days 14 days
Qlaira® combined oral contraceptive pill	LNG UPA	9 days 16 days
Progestogen-only pill (including desogestrel)	LNG UPA	2 days 9 days
Progestogen-only implant	LNG UPA	7 days 14 days
Progestogen-only injectable	LNG UPA	7 days 14 days
LNG-IUS	Not recommended as 'Quick Starting' method after oral EC	N/A
Cu-IUD	Oral EC not required if Cu-IUD used as method of EC	N/A

Cu-IUD, copper-releasing intrauterine device; EC, emergency contraception; IUD, intrauterine device; LNG, levonorgestrel; N/A, not applicable; UPA, ulipristal acetate.

progestogen-only contraceptive injections are not recommended as first line 'Quick Starting' methods, but can be used if none of the other methods are acceptable. The use of cyproteronel acetate (Dianette®) and the LNG-releasing intrauterine system (Mirena®) should not be used for this indication in view of their potential risk to the developing fetus.

There is no data on 'Quick Starting' after UPA, but as this is a progesterone receptor blocker, the time taken to achieve a contraceptive action is estimated to be seven days longer than the progestogen LNG and the woman must be informed of this.

An alternative way to commencing long-acting contraception at this time is to use a short-acting method, such as combined hormonal contraception or progestogen-only pill, as a **bridging method** until pregnancy can be excluded. A negative pregnancy test no sooner than three weeks after the last act of UPSI is sufficient and then the long-acting method can be provided.

As Gemma agrees to attend for a Cu-IUD insertion she is given information about timing of the clinic and the venue. She also chooses to take UPA as an extra precaution following the episode of UPSI four days ago in addition to last night.

Conclusion

There continue to be too many unintended and unwanted pregnancies and an ongoing need to improve contraceptive provision. There will always be times when contraception fails and women require EC. It is important that clinicians and other healthcare providers can

---

Box 18.1 Emergency contraception consultation points

- Sexual health risk assessment
- Was this a consensual act?
- Would she agree to have a Cu-IUD inserted?
- If oral EC is chosen, then the appropriate information about efficacy should be given to enable the woman to make an informed choice
- Following any of the options for EC, she must perform a pregnancy test if there is more than 7 days delay in her next period
- If oral EC is chosen, she should be informed that the next bleed could be earlier or later than usual
- Women should be warned regarding potential side effects of oral EC. These may include headaches, abdominal pain, breast tenderness, dizziness and fatigue, but usually last less than 24 hours
- Advise regarding future contraception requirements and 'Quick Starting' if possible
- Advise regarding safe sex and reducing risk of STIs

Cu-IUD, copper-releasing intrauterine device; EC, emergency contraception; STIs, sexually transmitted infections.

---

undertake the appropriate risk assessment during these consultations to ensure women are given the best information possible to make an informed choice about their options and ongoing contraception. This consultation (Box 18.1) must also include an assessment of their sexual health risk and appropriate investigations.

All women should be offered the option of a Cu-IUD. Improved access to IUD fitting services is essential and 'myths' must be dispelled. Streamlined, easily accessible referral pathways are vital in services where IUD fitting is not performed.

However, if an IUD is not acceptable, then an informed discussion about the appropriate use of oral EC is important. This will depend on time since UPSI, where she is in her menstrual cycle, other use during the current cycle, concomitant medication and choice. Women should be informed that UPA is more effective than LNG if used on day 4 or 5 following UPSI, at the fertile phase of the menstrual cycle, and in women who have a BMI > 30.

Ongoing information about sexual risk and future contraception should be included in the consultation in addition to 'Quick Starting' whenever appropriate, with follow-up arrangements.

Oral EC methods should not be used as a regular method of contraception because of the higher failure rate compared with other methods.

References

1. Lader D. Opinions Survey Report No. 41. *Contraception and Sexual Health. 2008/09.* Office for National Statistics, 2009. http://www.ons.gov.uk/ (accessed 4 March 2013).
2. Faculty of Sexual and Reproductive Healthcare. *Clinical Guidance. Drug Interactions with Hormonal Contraception,* January 2011 (updated January 2012). http://www.fsrh.org/pdfs/ CEUguidancedruginteractionshormonal.pdf (accessed 4 March 2013).
3. Faculty of Sexual and Reproductive Healthcare. *UK Medical Eligibility Criteria for Contraceptive Use, 2009.* http://www.fsrh.org/pdfs/UKMEC2009.pdf (accessed 4 March 2013).
4. Wilcox AJ, Dunson D, Baird DD. The timing of the 'fertile window' in the

menstrual cycle: day specific estimates from a prospective study. *BMJ* 2000; 321(7271): 1259–62.

5. Faculty of Sexual and Reproductive Healthcare. *Clinical Guidance. Emergency Contraception*, August 2011 (updated January 2012). http://www.fsrh.org/pdfs/CEUguidanceEmergencyContraception11.pdf (accessed 4 March 2013).

6. Hubacher D, Lara-Ricalde R, Taylor DJ, Guerra-Infante F, Guzmán-Rodriquez R. Use of copper intrauterine devices and the risk of tubal infertility among nulligravid women. *N Engl J Med* 2001; 345(8): 561–7.

7. Croxatto HB, Brache V, Pavez M, *et al.* Pituitary–ovarian function following the standard levonorgestrel emergency contraceptive dose or a single 0.75-mg dose given on the days preceding ovulation. *Contraception* 2004; 70: 442–50.

8. EMC+. EllaOne 30 mg. HRA Pharma UK and Ireland Ltd. http://www.medicines.org.uk/emc/medicine/22280/SPC/ellaOne+30+mg (accessed 4 March 2013).

9. Piaggio G, Kapp N, von Hertzen H. Effect on pregnancy rates of the delay in administration of levonorgestrel for emergency contraception: a combined analysis of four WHO trials. *Contraception* 2011; 84: 35–9.

10. Glasier AF, Cameron ST, Logan SJS, *et al.* Ulipristal acetate versus levonorgestrel for emergency contraception: a randomised non-inferiority trial and meta-analysis. *Lancet* 2010; 375: 555–62.

11. Faculty of Sexual and Reproductive Healthcare. *Clinical Guidance. Quick Starting Contraception*, September 2010. http://www.fsrh.org/pdfs/CEUGuidanceQuickStartingContraception.pdf (accessed 4 March 2013).

Chapter 19

Sexually transmissible infections and pelvic pain: what you really need to know

Mike Abbott

Case scenario: Nicola

Nicola is 27 years old. She has 3 children, only one of whom (aged 4) lives with her. She has a 20-year-old boyfriend. She has had an intrauterine device (IUD) for several years. She attended a department of genitourinary medicine recently and was diagnosed with gonorrhoea. This was treated with intramuscular antibiotics and her IUD left in situ.

She attends a community sexual health service with a request for her IUD to be removed. Her IUD threads are missing. She had her last menstrual period two weeks ago and last had sex two days before her current presentation. She is complaining of pelvic pain. How would you manage this situation?

Introduction

This case scenario requires the busy clinician to quickly consider several serious pathologies, most of which are not mutually exclusive.

For the sake of brevity, let us assume that the seemingly ubiquitous 'irritable bowel syndrome' (IBS) has been dismissed as unlikely in Nicola's presentation by virtue of the absence of associated features such as abdominal distension or temporal association of symptoms, or their relief, with eating, defecation or the passing of flatus. IBS or serious bowel pathology such as inflammatory bowel disease, particularly Crohn's disease may cause diagnostic confusion with gynaecological pathology, or even accompany it and should always be considered in the differential diagnosis of women presenting with abdominal pain.

Having considered IBS and inflammatory bowel disease, we can get down to the serious business in the remaining minutes of the consultation to consider an approach to sexually transmissible infections and, in particular, the presentation of abdominal pain in a sexually active woman. We shall need to tread carefully in order to avoid a number of pitfalls and will return to Nicola's management intermittently, during our short journey through this hazardous clinical landscape. Clinical intuition, developed with individual experience, will assist us but the reader is unapologetically directed to evidence-based guidelines.

Sexually transmissible infections

In order to get off to a good start, we should choose our words with care. 'Sexually transmitted infection' can be a pejorative misnomer and is not a term I use; the term sexually **transmissible** infection (STI) is preferable. Globally, many people with an STI acquired it vertically during pregnancy or the puerperium, others by blood products or injecting drug use but, nevertheless, may transmit the infection sexually. Hepatitis B provides a particularly good example of an STI that is frequently transmitted vertically, is transmissible to sexual partners and may also infect non-sexual contacts including household and healthcare-associated contacts.

Regardless of when or how an STI has been acquired, it remains the case that it may be transmitted by the sexual route. STIs share some important characteristics with which the clinician should be familiar.

Core STI principles

- STIs frequently co-exist; the presence of one STI increases the likelihood of others being present, including human immunodeficiency virus (HIV).
- All individuals with a diagnosed STI should be recommended to undergo an HIV test [1].
- STIs, particularly the more serious infections, are usually asymptomatic or cause mild symptoms frequently dismissed by patients or their clinicians. Many people who transmit STIs to others are unaware of the fact that they are themselves infected.
- STIs are **communicable diseases** and therefore require a public health perspective for their management; namely, the tracing and appropriate management of **all** others linked to the index case over the relevant time frame. The appropriate management of an STI does not stop with the index patient, because others are at risk. The management does not end with the 'sexual partner' either, rather, for certain conditions, with all contactable persons at risk within a specified time frame defined in the relevant guidelines. The more serious the STI, the more harm can be caused by failing to ensure that contacts at risk are traced.
- Efforts to prevent re-infection are required; in particular, the avoidance of any form of sexual contact until such time as the patient and her/his partner(s) have completed treatment. In the case of infections that cannot be eradicated, the duty to advise patients on how to minimize risk to others, remains.
- A test of cure is required following treatment of certain STIs in some situations.

The sexual history

There are two further important principles to consider when undertaking a sexual history, bearing in mind that it's perfectly clear how most people acquire STIs.

1. Many people who know they are infected or believe they are at risk of STI have reason to be 'economical with the truth', particularly when there is a lot to lose, such as a marriage, a house or a career. In any event, it is unsurprising that such persons may not share sensitive information if they do not trust the health professional, the clinical team or the health system with their personal, sometimes incriminating, information.
2. We can only know our own sexual history for certain. Patients are frequently unaware of the sexual histories of their partners and, therefore, their own risk of STI.

The sexual history should be appropriate, rather than exhaustive, but structured. It is best undertaken where the conditions are most likely to support the patient in being truthful in her/his responses. The patient should appreciate the need to be asked certain personal questions and should receive appropriate, but not absolute, reassurances around confidentiality,

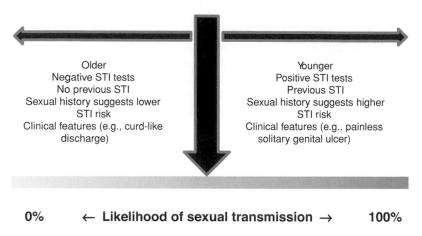

Older	Younger
Negative STI tests	Positive STI tests
No previous STI	Previous STI
Sexual history suggests lower STI risk	Sexual history suggests higher STI risk
Clinical features (e.g., curd-like discharge)	Clinical features (e.g., painless solitary genital ulcer)

0%   ← Likelihood of sexual transmission →   100%

Figure 19.1 Risk assessment for sexually transmissible infections (STIs).

which is limited by, for example, safeguarding concerns. The British Association for Sexual Health and HIV (BASHH) provides guidance on undertaking consultations requiring sexual history-taking. These guidelines, and many others, are available from the guidelines section of the BASHH website [2], to which the reader is referred frequently in the remaining pages of this chapter.

In Nicola's case, it would be necessary to establish, based on the sexual history, whether she was at risk of re-infection with *Neisseria gonorrhoeae*. In particular, it would be important to establish that her sexual contact(s) had been treated appropriately, without risk of re-infection. In addition, in line with the BASHH UK national guideline for the management of gonorrhoea, a test of cure for *Neisseria gonorrhoeae* is indicated. Failure of initial treatment, as opposed to re-infection, is also possible but less likely. Nevertheless, antibiotic resistance in strains of *Neisseria gonorrhoeae* continues to spread so one might expect initial failure of treatment to become more common in future years.

The sexually transmitted sliding scale

This is a model devised for this chapter, to aid the approach to clinical scenarios that may be due to STI (Figure 19.1). It is based on the certainty of sexual as opposed to non-sexual transmission of the causative agent. A score of 100% would imply exclusively sexual transmission. On such a scale, a penile chancre due to *Treponema pallidum* would score very highly, whereas vulvovaginitis due to *Candida albicans* would achieve a very low score.

The reason for highlighting the model is that many conditions, including pelvic inflammatory disease (PID), would have a score somewhere in the middle, and awareness of this informs the approach to the management of such conditions. In short, STIs frequently cause PID, particularly in younger women with STI risk factors. If such women are not treated with the possibility of STI in mind, they may be badly let down and they very frequently are by those clinicians who fail to appreciate this risk. Conversely, implying that PID is a 'sexually transmitted disease' is neither correct nor helpful.

On this sliding scale model, a woman with PID might score around 25% but a young woman with PID and recent gonorrhoea might score well above 50% and many of these women will also test positive for chlamydia. On the same sliding scale, men with epididymo-orchitis might score 30% but younger, sexually active men with recent gonorrhoea who present with epididymo-orchitis would certainly score above 50%.

This simple observation, and the core STI principles referred to above, have implications for how PID, epididymo-orchitis and many other presentations that may have been caused by STI should be managed. It is important to at least consider the possibility of STI in all women presenting with symptoms or signs consistent with PID and in all men with symptoms or signs consistent with epididymo-orchitis.

The likelihood of a clinical scenario being caused by an STI is related to several factors including causative organism or organisms, clinical features, age, sexual history, presence of other STIs, etc. For example, a 19-year-old woman who presents with features suggestive of PID and who also complains of vaginal discharge, has had numerous episodes of unprotected sex with casual male partners, is a contact of gonorrhoea and has a previous history of chlamydia, clearly has a higher probability that her presumed PID is related to STI than the 39-year-old woman with no previous history of STI in an apparently monogamous long-term relationship. This does not imply that women or men stop acquiring STIs as they get older, but the likelihood that these conditions are due to STI will fall. An appropriately conducted sexual history, mindful of the caveats indicated in the sexual history section above, will assist in assessing risk.

Predictive values of tests for STIs

An organism may be known to be the sole cause of a clinical scenario, e.g., *Neisseria gonorrhoeae* causing urethral gonorrhoea. However, the extent to which a single test or a group of tests confirm or exclude the presence of the said pathogen is affected by several factors. An understanding of the predictive values of diagnostic test results is needed, particularly when unexpected results are received.

The wise and experienced clinician considers laboratory results in the clinical context and also appreciates the limitations of diagnostic tests [3, 4]. It is particularly important to ensure that unexpected results relate to your patient (i.e., that they do not belong to another patient) before considering other potential causes of an unexpected result. Failure to do so may result in needless trauma to your patient and possibly, therefore, to yourself.

Presentation of STIs

Broadly speaking, there are two approaches to this topic. One is to classify according to the aetiological agent and then work through the viruses, bacteria, and fungi, etc., mapped to the possible clinical manifestations of the various organisms. The second approach is to classify according to clinical scenarios, mindful of the fact that the pathological mechanisms and causative organisms may be multiple, unrelated or unknown. Our only realistic option, in the pages that follow, is a brief account using this second approach. I have chosen those clinical scenarios that I believe to be particularly relevant for clinicians working in primary care settings and sexual health services.

Genital ulcer disease

Multiple, painful superficial ulcers

The majority of genital or ano-genital ulcer disease caused by STIs and presenting in primary care will be due to herpes simplex virus (HSV), either type 1 or type 2. The ulcers of primary genital herpes are characteristically multiple, painful and superficial and often associated with tender inguinal lymphadenopathy. The misdiagnosis of primary genital herpes as vulval candidiasis is usually due to a clinician failing to examine the vulva in women complaining of vulval soreness or severe thrush or urinary tract infection (UTI).

A woman with primary genital herpes will, if asked, usually report *superficial* dysuria, i.e., discomfort caused by urine passing over ulcers and, in contrast to women with UTI, an absence of frequency. These are important clues that should always prompt examination of the vulva and perineum. Laboratory confirmation of the clinical diagnosis is generally by viral culture or an appropriate nucleic acid amplification test (NAAT) after a correctly taken swab from one of the ulcers.

Delays in diagnosis of primary genital herpes lead to more severe disease and sometimes secondary bacterial infection. Primary genital herpes is occasionally further complicated by autonomic neuropathy affecting bladder and bowel function, other neurological manifestations or disseminated infection.

Recurrences, milder than the primary episode, are one of the hallmarks of ano-genital herpes and are more frequent in HSV-2 infection compared with HSV-1. Another hallmark is asymptomatic shedding of virus and, therefore, the very real possibility of sexual transmission when no lesions are clinically apparent. Management is as per the UK national guideline for the management of genital herpes, available from the guidelines section of the BASHH website [2].

Unilateral vulval ulceration should prompt the clinician to consider shingles, due to varicella-zoster virus (VZV), in the differential diagnosis. This condition requires higher doses of aciclovir than those used for HSV infections.

Solitary, painless ulcer

The likely diagnosis is primary syphilis and the lesion is the chancre. The chancre indicates infection with the causative organism, *Treponema pallidum*, in the previous 90 days. The ulcer is frequently slightly firm, conspicuously painless and often associated with painless inguinal lymphadenopathy.

The chancre is frequently not noticed by the patient, particularly if it is not visible or at an inaccessible site such as the cervix or rectum. Left untreated, the infection passes through to the secondary stage, which resembles glandular fever or primary HIV infection, discussed later in this chapter. A significant proportion of those infected but untreated may present many years later with one or more of the complications of late syphilis including neurological, cardiovascular, dermatological and soft tissue manifestations.

The clinical challenge with syphilis is to ensure that the diagnosis is never missed; it is not known as the 'great imitator' for nothing. The wary clinician considers syphilis whenever an undiagnosed ulcer, rash or neurological problem presents. Anyone with any doubts as to the effects of leaving this infection untreated should read one or more of the authoritative accounts of the notorious Tuskegee Syphilis Study (also known as the Tuskegee Study of Untreated Syphilis in the Negro Male). President Clinton, on behalf of the US Government, apologized very movingly to the surviving victims of this 40 year experiment on 16 May 1997 [5]. The reader, or any clinician in any specialty, is encouraged to watch this apology in the 32 minute video released by the US Presidential Libraries [6]. The detailed management of syphilis is as per the UK national guidelines, available from the guidelines section of the BASHH website [2].

The suspicion or demonstration of one STI should prompt the exclusion of others. Nicola was identified as having gonorrhoea; her management is not complete without excluding other STIs such as chlamydia, syphilis and HIV. This includes re-testing at appropriate times to cover relevant incubation periods.

Undiagnosed genital ulceration

The cause of ano-genital ulceration should be investigated in order to confirm or exclude important known causes. The use of correctly taken samples and serological tests at the appropriate times is required. In the case of suspected genital herpes, this may involve further swabs in the event of a recurrence if the diagnosis is not confirmed at initial presentation. For the exclusion of syphilis, if initial testing from the lesion has revealed negative results, serological follow-up is always required. The patient with a recent label of 'undiagnosed genital ulceration' may be incubating a serious STI and, if so, may be at significant risk of transmitting the infection to others.

For safe clinical practice, therefore, it is very reasonable to use the term 'undiagnosed genital ulceration' as this alludes to the essential management plan. The plan consists of: (i) appropriately advising patients of the diagnostic possibilities and implications including measures to prevent ongoing infection; (ii) having arrangements in place to confirm HSV on recurrence; (iii) reliably excluding treponemal and HIV infection using follow-up serology for an appropriate period.

Tropical ulcers

Less commonly, but where relevant, as directed by the sexual history and clinical features, the exclusion of tropical STIs may be important. Sexual history taking includes a geographical perspective, which is particularly relevant in the case of undiagnosed genital ulceration. Although your patient may not have had unprotected sex in an exotic part of the world, the same may not be true of her/his sexual partner(s) or, indeed, theirs.

Vaginal symptoms and balanitis

The three prominent vaginal symptoms in relation to STIs are the presence of vaginal discharge, itch and odour. These three symptoms give a reasonable impression of the likely cause and awareness of the nature of any discharge, and vaginal pH provides useful further information. The joint Faculty of Sexual and Reproductive Healthcare (FSRH) and BASHH management of vaginal discharge in non-genitourinary medicine settings guidelines are recommended [7].

Candidal vulvovaginitis

The discharge is variable. Itch, without odour, is the prominent symptom. Itch or soreness is present but odour is generally absent. Vaginal pH is normal. For further detailed guidance see BASHH UK national guideline on the management of vulvovaginal candidiasis, available from the guidelines section of the BASHH website [2].

Bacterial vaginosis

Odour, usually fishy, is the prominent symptom/sign. The discharge, if present, is generally homogenous, sometimes watery or frothy. Vaginal pH is elevated. For further detailed guidance see current UK national guideline for the management of bacterial vaginosis, available from the guidelines section of the BASHH website [2].

Trichomoniasis

The discharge is similar to bacterial vaginosis. However, itch, soreness or vaginal inflammation may be present. Odour may be a prominent symptom although this is slightly different in character to the odour of bacterial vaginosis. Again, the pH is elevated. Trichomonal vaginitis can, therefore, present rather like a combination of thrush and bacterial vaginosis but it scores considerably higher on the sexually transmitted sliding scale. Globally, *Trichomonas vaginalis* is very prevalent in some countries and may be an important facilitator of HIV transmission. For further detailed guidance see current UK national guideline for the management of *Trichomonas vaginalis*, available from the guidelines section of the BASHH website [2].

Nicola may have one or more of these causes of vaginal discharge.

Balanitis

Balanitis, inflammation affecting the penile glans, or balanoposthitis, where the foreskin is also involved, are usually caused by *Candida* spp., or mixed anaerobic flora. Candidal balanitis should prompt testing for glycosuria as diabetes mellitus is a common predisposing factor for fungal balanitis and it is not unusual for diabetes to first present as a balanitis or balanoposthitis.

Various infections, generalized dermatological conditions or specific genital dermatoses, malignancies and other pathologies can be associated with a balanitis/balanoposthitis. One catch for the unwary is balanitis caused by secondary syphilis. The complaint of a genital rash should always make the clinician consider STI. Detailed guidance is available from the BASHH UK national guideline on the management of balanoposthitis, available from the guidelines section of the BASHH website [2].

Upper genital tract symptoms

The striking characteristic of infection with oculogenital strains of *Chlamydia trachomatis* is their ability to cause damage in the relative absence of symptoms, so infection is usually clinically silent, particularly in women. *Neisseria gonorrhoeae*, in contrast, generates more clinical noise, particularly in male urethral infection and is associated with considerable inflammation and pus. However, asymptomatic infection remains the general rule in the endocervix, throat and rectum.

Endocervical infection with either organism not infrequently results in an endometritis or salpingitis and, more frequently than commonly realized, perihepatitis. Ascending infection from the male urethra may result in epididymo-orchitis. Several systemic manifestations occur in both sexes.

Nicola had gonorrhoea and may still have it. Her risk of co-existing chlamydial infection is high and the presence of both *Chlamydia trachomatis* and *Neisseria gonorrhoeae* would not exclude the presence of other organisms suspected as having a causative role in PID. Her pain, therefore, may be related to infection with *Neisseria gonorrhoeae*, *Chlamydia trachomatis*, *Gardnerella vaginalis*, various anaerobes and *Mycoplasma genitalium* may also be involved. Management of suspected PID should be in line with the BASHH UK national guideline for the management of pelvic inflammatory disease, available from the guidelines section of the BASHH website [2].

Lumps and rashes

Many ano-genital lumps are unrelated to STI or normal variants and may be mistaken by patients or their clinicians as ano-genital warts. However, some ano-genital lumps are due to STI and the commonest of these are genital warts.

Genital warts

Certain strains of the seemingly ubiquitous human papillomavirus (HPV) cause ano-genital warts. The aim of treatment is cosmetic improvement and the appearance of wart clearance, as opposed to viral eradication, which is not realistic. Treatments are generally unsatisfactory and recurrence after treatment is common. Ano-genital warts are often disabling psychologically. Management along the lines of the BASHH UK national guideline on the management of ano-genital warts is recommended, available from the guidelines section of the BASHH website [2].

The National Health Service Cervical Screening Programme recommends that no changes are required to screening intervals in women with ano-genital warts.

Molluscum contagiosum

Molluscum contagiosum are small, harmless umbilicated papules caused by a pox virus. Various treatment options are available. Management should be along the lines of the BASHH UK national guideline on the management of molluscum, available from the guidelines section of the BASHH website [2]. Large facial lesions in adults should alert the clinician to the possibility of underlying HIV disease.

Pediculosis pubis and scabies

Habitat destruction, thanks to the 'Brazilian' has contributed to the demise of *Phthirus pubis* infestation as a clinical problem. Management should be along the lines of the BASHH UK national guideline on the management of *Phthirus pubis* infestation, available from the guidelines section of the BASHH website [2].

The characteristic symptom of scabies is nocturnal itch, which should prompt clinicians to search for evidence of infestation with *Sarcoptes scabiei*. Sexual and household contacts require treatment. Management should be along the lines of the BASHH UK national guideline on the management of scabies infestation, available from the guidelines section of the BASHH website [2].

Glandular fever-like illness

Glandular fever is a very common clinical entity. However, presentations with clinical features suggestive of glandular fever may also be due to two serious STIs. In both cases, the illness indicates relatively recent acquisition of the infection and, compared with later stages of the infections, relatively high infectivity. In general terms, it is often the case that those who are incubating infection or who do not realize that they are infected, are most likely to transmit to others as they are less likely to take preventive measures such as avoiding or reducing sexual encounters or consistent safer sex.

A glandular fever-like illness should, therefore, always prompt the clinician to consider HIV and syphilis.

Primary HIV infection

Primary HIV Infection (PHI) is also known as the HIV sero-conversion illness and occurs two to six weeks following infection. A practical approach to the management of primary HIV infection is available from *HIV in Primary Care* produced by the Medical Foundation for AIDS and Sexual Health [8].

Secondary syphilis

This multisystem illness, often associated with rash, occurs within the first two years of infection. The diagnosis is confirmed with positive treponemal serology. Detailed management is as per the BASHH UK national guideline on the management of syphilis, available from the guidelines section of the BASHH website [2].

No symptoms

In many ways, the most characteristic and disturbing feature of STIs is the extent to which they may cause serious disease and be transmitted to others despite the absence of symptoms. If present, STI symptoms and certain physical signs are often mild or non-specific and easily attributable to other unrelated pathologies. In any case, other unrelated pathologies frequently co-exist with STIs.

The clinical rationale, therefore, is to *screen* those at risk of infection in the light of the sexual history, regardless of the presence or otherwise of symptoms; and at the same time, to ensure that those with particular symptoms or signs are appropriately *clinically tested*, in line with the relevant published guidance, where additional tests may be required.

Returning to Nicola

Her management should involve consideration of the following:

- She may have one or more STIs, including HIV, unrelated to her current presentation. The sexual history should be retaken to establish risk and the need for further STI testing. She should, at the very least, be tested for chlamydia, gonorrhoea, trichomonas, syphilis and HIV.
- She certainly had gonorrhoea and may still have it by virtue of either failure of treatment or re-infection either from an untreated sexual partner or another sexual contact.
- Another STI causing these symptoms such as *Chlamydia trachomatis* would be quite likely.
- She may be infected with *Mycoplasma genitalium* and/or have non-STI causes of PID.
- Management of suspected PID should be in line with published guidance.
- Her sexual partner(s) will need epidemiological treatment or re-treatment for gonorrhoea or other STIs if identified in Nicola. Equally, the presence of STI in a sexual partner may impact on Nicola's care.
- She may be incubating infection (including syphilis or HIV) and regardless of the outcome of her IUD deliberations, she requires serological follow-up to exclude these infections.
- The IUD threads are missing; the IUD may be displaced or missing (if so, unprotected sexual intercourse (UPSI) was only two days previously and she may need post-coital contraception).
- Pelvic actinomycosis is a possibility.

- She may be pregnant and, if so, her pregnancy may be ectopic.
- She may be having ovulation pain.
- She may have endometriosis, ovarian cyst or other gynaecological causes of abdominal pain.
- Some of her pain may be due to bowel (IBS, constipation, Crohn's disease) or from other non-gynaecological sources.

The suggested management plan for Nicola is outlined below.

- Sexual history to clarify STI risks.
- Investigations for STI exclusion as above or liaise with the relevant genitourinary medicine clinic that saw her, including antibiotic sensitivities of the *Neisseria gonorrhoeae* previously isolated.
- Pregnancy test.
- Pelvic examination to clarify symptoms.
- Transvaginal pelvic ultrasound scan to ascertain presence of the IUD, or its position, pregnancy (including ectopic), abscesses, pelvic cysts and collections or pelvic mass. If pelvic actinomycosis is considered a diagnostic possibility, liaise with local microbiologist.
- If not currently pregnant, commence a new means of contraception prior to removal of IUD.
- Removal of the IUD once protected from pregnancy by another method.
- Antibiotic treatment for PID according to BASHH guidelines, preferably in the light of known sensitivities of the recent isolate of *Neisseria gonorrhoeae*.
- Ensure partner/s is/are seen and in a timely fashion.
- Review progress in clinic and confirm adherence to treatment regimen, satisfactory clinical response (including test of cure for gonorrhoea if initially present), appropriate partner treatment and absence of risk of re-infection.

References

1. British HIV Association, British Association for Sexual Health and HIV, British Infection Society. *UK National Guidelines for HIV Testing 2008*. http://www.bhiva.org/documents/Guidelines/Testing/GlinesHIVTest08.pdf (accessed 4 March 2013).
2. British Association for Sexual Health and HIV. *BASHH Clinical Effectiveness Group Guidelines*. http://www.bashh.org/guidelines (accessed 4 March 2013).
3. Vecchio TJ. Predictive value of a single diagnostic test in unselected populations. *N Engl J Med* 1966; 26: 1171–3.
4. Lewis J. Selection and evaluation of diagnostic tests. In Morse SA, Ballard RC, Homes KK, Moreland AA. (eds) *Atlas of Sexually Transmitted Diseases and AIDS*, 3rd edn. New York, NY: Mosby, 2003: pp. 375–80.
5. The White House, Office of the Press Secretary. *Remarks by the President in Apology for Study Done in Tuskegee, 16 May, 1997*. http://www.cdc.gov/tuskegee/clintonp.htm (accessed 4 March 2013).
6. Presidential Libraries Master Tape Nos 06941–06942. Apology to Survivors of the Tuskegee Syphilis Experiment. Courtesy William J Clinton Presidential Library. http://www.youtube.com/watch?v=F8Kr-0ZE1XY (accessed 4 March 2013).
7. Faculty of Sexual and Reproductive Healthcare and the British Association for Sexual Health and HIV. *Clinical Guidance. Management of Vaginal Discharge in*

Non-Genitourinary Medicine Settings, February 2012. http://www.fsrh.org/pdfs/CEUGuidanceVaginalDischarge.pdf (accessed 4 March 2013).

8. Madge S, Matthews P, Singh S, Theobald N. *HIV in Primary Care*, 2nd edn. Medical Foundation for AIDS and Sexual Health, 2011. http://www.medfash.org.uk/uploads/files/p17abjng1g9t9193h1rsl75uuk53.pdf (accessed 4 March 2013).

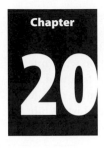

Chapter 20

Medical termination of pregnancy

Kristina Gemzell-Danielsson

Case scenario: Lisbeth

Lisbeth, a 20-year-old Swedish medical student, has become pregnant whilst taking the combined oral contraceptive pill. She is a good pill taker and has not missed any pills. She is distraught. She does not feel able to continue with the pregnancy and is afraid of having an abortion as she had a reaction to the anaesthetic when she had her wisdom teeth removed.

Introduction

Lisbeth has the option of a safe and efficient medical abortion without surgery or an anaesthetic. Today, medical abortion services can be offered or improved by minor changes in existing healthcare facilities. An important aspect of medical abortion during early pregnancy is the simplicity of the treatment. The similarities with miscarriage mean that the clinical events are well known, not only to the healthcare provider but also to the woman herself. Medical abortion has the potential to expand access to safe abortion care provided not only by specially trained clinicians but also by other healthcare providers who may or may not have training in surgical methods of abortion. Medical abortion is safe, effective and acceptable to women, and no doubt Lisbeth would find it less frightening. It can replace surgical abortion (if needed) and can be used for all gestational lengths if the regimen is modified. This chapter aims to provide basic information on regimens recommended for early medical abortion up to 63 days of gestation.

Development of medical abortion

In the first half of the twentieth century only surgical abortion methods such as dilatation and curettage (D&C) and hysterotomy were available for induced abortion. The identification of natural prostaglandins (PGs) by Professor Sune Bergström and his team at Karolinska Institute in the 1960s and its introduction in abortion care in 1971, followed by development of PG analogues, were the first steps of the development of medical abortion. The next step was taken by the French scientist, Professor Étienne-Émile Baulieu and co-workers in the early 1980s with the synthesis of the anti-progestin mifepristone. The significant breakthrough in the development of medical abortion was the finding by Professor Marc Bygdeman and his team at Karolinska Institutet that treatment with mifepristone increased the sensitivity of the myometrium to PG. The combined regimen was shown to be a highly effective and safe method for termination of pregnancy [1].

Medical abortion was first approved in France in 1988 (up to 49 days of amenorrhoea) followed by approvals in UK (1991) and Sweden (1992) (up to 63 days of amenorrhoea and combined with vaginal administration of a PG analogue in both the countries). However, it was only in 1999/2000 that both early first and second-trimester medical abortion with mifepristone and misoprostol were approved in several other European countries followed by the USA. In 2005, the World Health Organization (WHO) included the combination of mifepristone and misoprostol for use in medical abortion in its Essential Medicine List. While the access to mifepristone is still limited to a little more than 50 countries, the PG analogue of choice, misoprostol, is widely available worldwide [2].

Overview of the legal situation in Europe

Abortion laws vary widely in Europe. There are still several European countries where abortion is, in practice, not accessible on request in the first trimester (Andorra, Ireland, Liechtenstein, Malta, Monaco, Poland and parts of the UK (Northern Ireland, Isle of Man) and of Denmark (Faroe Islands)). Therefore many women are forced to travel for their abortion or turn to illegal and sometimes unsafe procedures. Examples of countries that receive women travelling from other countries for an induced abortion are the UK, the Netherlands, Austria and Sweden. Although legal in most countries, legal barriers may remain such as waiting periods of various length, obligatory counselling, signature of two doctors, written statement by the woman that she is in distress ... etc.). None of these restrictions have been shown to be of any benefit for the health of the woman with an unwanted pregnancy, but they may risk delaying the induced abortion. An informed consent may also have to be signed prior to the abortion treatment. Local guidelines should be consulted in regard to these regulations. Lisbeth is fortunate as in Sweden medical abortion is easily accessible.

Introduction of medical abortion in Europe

Introduction of medical abortion has been slow in most European countries, although it is the preferred method of many women if they have the choice [3]. The use of medical abortion, when available, shows a wide variation. However, the proportion of medical abortions is increasing in most European countries. According to National Official Statistics medical abortion is currently the most common method of abortion in the Scandinavian countries (i.e., Sweden 90%), Portugal (65%), Spain (63%) and Switzerland (62%). It is commonly used in France (54%) and the UK (Northern Ireland excluded, 53%), but still not so common in the Netherlands (20%), Belgium (17%) and Germany (15%), and rarely used in Italy (4%). In recent years, there has been a significant trend in most countries for abortions to be performed earlier, as shown, for example, in Sweden [4] (Figure 20.1). Medical abortion which can be performed in very early pregnancy, even before a visible intrauterine pregnancy, has contributed significantly to this trend.

Medical abortion regimens

Mifepristone followed by misoprostol has been shown to be safe and as effective as vacuum aspiration for termination of pregnancy up to 63 days of amenorrhoea [5]. The combination of mifepristone and misoprostol has synergistic effects and simulates expulsion of the pregnancy. The evidence-based regimen recommended by WHO is:

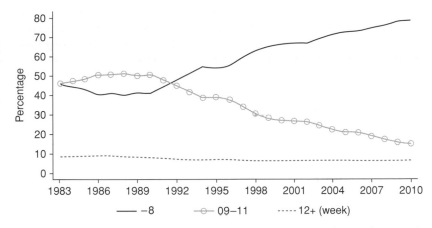

Figure 20.1 Impact of the introduction of medical abortion on gestational age at abortion in Sweden [4].

- Mifepristone, 200 mg, taken first and followed by:
- Misoprostol, 800 μg, administered vaginally, sublingually or buccally, 24–48 hours later. Vaginal misoprostol can be administered either by the woman herself or by a clinician according to the preference of the woman. Sublingual tablets are placed under the tongue and any remnants swallowed after 30 minutes. Buccally, tablets are placed between the cheek and gums and swallowed after 30 minutes if not dissolved.
- If indicated a second dose of 400 μg misoprostol could be administered if bleeding has not started within 3–4 hours following the initial dose of misoprostol.
- Analgesics should be offered to all women when required.
- Antibiotic prophylaxis is not recommended for medical abortion but this should be adjusted to the local prevalence of sexually transmitted infections (STIs). In the UK, the Royal College of Obstetricians and Gynaecologists (RCOG) clinical practice guidelines recommend antibiotic prophylaxis for medical abortion. If routine antibiotics are not provided, screening and treatment of STIs should be offered.
- Contraceptive counselling and provision should be part of the abortion care.
- Routine ultrasound following medical abortion is not required.

Mifepristone

Mifepristone is the only anti-progestin approved for the induction of abortion. It is a 19-norsteroid, which binds with high affinity to the progesterone receptor, thus inhibiting the effect of progesterone. Progesterone is a key hormone in maintaining the pregnancy by keeping the uterus in a quiescent state. It prevents softening and dilatation of the cervix, reduces PG output from the decidua and suppresses uterine contractions. Thus mifepristone blockage of progesterone receptors results in vascular damage, decidual necrosis and bleeding, which leads to cervical softening, increased uterine sensitivity to PGs and conversion of the quiet pregnant uterus into an organ of spontaneous activity with maximal effect on uterine contractility seen at 36–48 hours [1].

When administered orally, mifepristone reaches peak serum concentrations in pregnant and non-pregnant women within two hours regardless of dose. The pharmacokinetics of mifepristone differ for daily doses less than 100 mg than for higher doses; at a dose of 100 mg or more, serum levels are similar with similar peak serum concentrations of 2.0–2.5 μg/ml. The non-linear pharmacokinetics may be due to saturation of a specific transport protein for mifepristone, serum α1-acid glycoprotein; this protein is saturated at doses of 100 mg or more. These data indicate that single doses above 100 mg are likely to be equally efficacious to 600 mg. The half-life of mifepristone is approximately 24–29 hours [1, 5].

Misoprostol

Misoprostol is a synthetic PGE 1 analogue that induces cervical ripening as well as uterine contractions, thus resulting in expulsion of the pregnancy. PGs play an important role in the regulation of uterine contractility during pregnancy. The receptors are present throughout the pregnancy. Misoprostol has been shown to have several advantages over other PG analogues; it is widely available, usually cheap, stable at room temperature and can be stored for a long time if appropriately packaged. Misoprostol is equally or more effective compared with the PG analogue gemeprost. The oral tablet is effective in different routes of administration. In contrast to other PGs misoprostol has limited effect in the bronchi or blood vessels. Side effects are dose dependent, usually mild and self limiting [6].

A disadvantage may be that misoprostol until recently has not been approved for the indication of medical abortion, and thus has been used off-label. However, as long as clinical guidelines are followed this is usually not a problem. Treatment and prevention of gastric ulcer is still the only licensed indication for misoprostol, with the exception of GyMiso® in France (200 μg tablets for abortion) and Medabon® (combi pack with mifepristone 200 mg and misoprostol 800 μg for vaginal administration) recently approved by the European Medicines Agency in 2012.

Misoprostol is recommended in evidence-based clinical guidelines: it is widely used in practice in early medical abortion and for the treatment of incomplete abortion, as well as for other indications in obstetrics and gynaecology [7]. Misoprostol can be administered via the oral route in pregnancy up to seven weeks of amenorrhoea, or via vaginal, sublingual, or buccal route in pregnancy up to and beyond nine weeks of amenorrhoea. The peak plasma level of the active metabolite (misoprostol free acid) is seen at less than 30 minutes when administered orally. Absorption after vaginal administration is slower with lower peak plasma levels but a more prolonged elevation in plasma levels resulting in significantly greater bioavailability after vaginal than after oral administration. Following buccal administration, the shape of the absorption curve is similar to that of the vaginal route, although the serum drug levels attained are lower and the bioavailability for buccal administration is only half that seen after vaginal administration. The peak plasma levels, as well as the bioavailability of misoprostol, are the highest after sublingual administration. However, measures of uterine contractility comparing buccal, sublingual and vaginal administration are quite similar and significantly different from that of oral administration [6].

It should be noted that while the dose of mifepristone does not change, the dose of misoprostol needs to be modified according to gestational age. A higher total dose is often needed in late first trimester compared to early first trimester. During the second trimester, due to increased sensitivity of the uterine muscles to PGs, lower doses are sufficient.

If mifepristone is not available, misoprostol alone can be effective to induce abortion. However, it has been well proven that pre-treatment with mifepristone 24–48 hours before PG administration increases the success rate, shortens the induction-to-abortion interval and reduces the amount of PGs required. Therefore the combined regimen should always be used if possible [5].

Interval mifepristone–misoprostol

Although maximal priming effect on the myometrium is achieved 36–48 hours after pre-treatment with mifepristone, no difference was seen in induction-to-abortion time with mifepristone administered 24, 36 or 48 hours before PG administration [5].

Contraindications

Absolute contraindications

There are very few absolute contraindications to medical abortion. When using a combination of mifepristone and misoprostol they include:

- Known or suspected ectopic pregnancy
- Previous allergic reaction to one of the drugs
- Inherited porphyria
- Chronic adrenal failure
- Coagulation disorder/treatment

Relative contraindications

Caution is required if the woman:

- Is on corticosteroid therapy
- Has severe anaemia
- Has pre-existing heart disease or cardiovascular risk factors
- Has an intrauterine device (IUD) in situ

For further details see mifepristone labelling information [8].

Theoretically, medications that decrease the serum level of mifepristone may decrease the efficacy of medical abortion: phenytoin, phenobarbital or carbamazepine. Conversely, mifepristone reduces the activity of rifampicin, dexamethasone and St John's wort (*Hypericum perforatum*).

It should be noted that the following situations are not contraindications for medical abortion: young age, multiple pregnancy, obesity, previous Caesarean section, smoking, uterine malformation and previous cervical surgery.

Medical abortion and breastfeeding

The levels of mifepristone found in breast milk from lactating women following the intake of a single dose of 200 mg are low or immeasurable. The level of the active metabolite misoprostol free acid is low in breast milk and rapidly declines after single dose administration. Thus, based on available evidence, the doses of mifepristone and misoprostol used in medical abortion allow breastfeeding to be safely continued without interruption [9].

Efficacy

The combined regimen of mifepristone and misoprostol has success rates, measured as complete abortion without the need for surgical intervention or additional drug administration, of 95–99%. Between 2 and 5% of women will require further medical treatment or surgery for incomplete abortion, to terminate a continuing pregnancy or to control bleeding. In 0.5–1.0% of women the medical treatment fails and the pregnancy continues. Furthermore, 1–3% of treatments result in an incomplete abortion. Surgical evacuation of the uterus after a medical abortion is only indicated if there is a clinical indication such as heavy or prolonged bleeding, ongoing pregnancy and/or if the woman wishes for an intervention.

Thus, if Lisbeth chose medical abortion, there is less than 5% risk that she would need an anaesthetic.

The effect of misoprostol is dependent on the route of administration. Vaginal misoprostol although more effective and with less side effects is less acceptable to some women or healthcare providers. Therefore the sublingual and buccal routes have been investigated and shown to be convenient and acceptable although associated with more side effects [1, 5, 6].

Expected effects, side effects and complications

The side effects of medical abortion are similar to those experienced with miscarriage, with the most frequently reported adverse events being pain (caused by uterine contractions) and vaginal bleeding. To reduce side effects and the risk of complications abortion should be performed as early as possible without unnecessary delay.

An uncomplicated medical abortion has no effect on future fertility. Although the unwanted pregnancy may be a crisis situation and arouse paradoxical feelings, the abortion treatment itself has no negative impact on mental health. Furthermore, abortion does not increase the risk of breast cancer [10].

Pain

Lower abdominal pain (uterine cramps) is one of the most common adverse effects of medical abortion. Pain is most likely to be felt in the first few hours of PG analogue administration. Therefore, adequate pain treatment should be offered to all women prior to, or at the time of, misoprostol administration.

Bleeding

Prolonged or heavier than menstrual bleeding is an expected effect of medical abortion. Slightly more than 50% of women rate the bleeding as heavier than their normal menses. Bleeding continues for about 12–14 days on average but may continue up to the next menses. The mean blood loss is similar to that of a heavy menstrual period (80 ml). Bleeding duration and volume increase with pregnancy duration. Excessive bleeding is considered as soaking more than two or three sanitary pads per hour for more than two or three hours.

The need for surgery due to prolonged or heavy bleeding occurs in 0.3–2.0% of women. Blood transfusion is uncommon in early medical abortion (<1 per 1000 treatments). Women should be advised to seek immediate medical attention if they experience prolonged heavy vaginal bleeding, as it may be a sign of incomplete abortion or other complications and medical or surgical intervention may be needed.

Gastrointestinal side effects

Side effects may also include gastrointestinal side effects such as nausea, stomach cramps, vomiting and diarrhoea. Gastrointestinal side effects are transient and dose related. They usually occur within the hour following administration and last for one to two hours. In case of severe symptoms, anti-emetic treatments should be provided.

Shivering, increased body temperature

Transient (1–3 hours) rise in body temperature and shivering may occur after PG administration. If continuing for more than a few hours, an infection should be suspected.

Infection

Endometritis or pelvic inflammatory disease (PID) is a rare complication but depends on individual risk factors. While the risk in medical abortion is lower than in surgical abortion, it still exists and is similar to that found in spontaneous abortion. In large trials including 1000 participants or more, infection rates typically vary from 0.1 to 0.9%. Fatal infections with clostridium species (most commonly *C. Sordellii*) or Group A streptococcus have been reported following medical abortion. Severe constant pain still felt several days after administration of the abortion drugs requires careful attention, irrespective of fever being present or not, as it may be related to infection.

Failed treatment

Medical abortion fails in approximately 0.5–1.0% of cases. If the pregnancy is continuing, mifepristone and misoprostol can be administered again or surgical termination can be conducted.

In rare cases, the woman may change her mind and wish to continue the pregnancy after the start of the treatment or in case of an ongoing pregnancy found at follow-up. Mifepristone has no teratogenic effects in animals except in rabbits, where isolated cases of severe abnormalities were observed. Misoprostol has no direct teratogenic effects but has been reported to be associated with malformation, including cranial nerve defects and Mobius syndrome (limb defects) However, due to lack of data the possible associations are difficult to evaluate [5, 6].

The abortion procedure

Treatment with mifepristone and misoprostol typically involves one or two visits to the clinic by the woman. A follow-up visit may be offered in addition.

First visit

The first visit involves counselling (on abortion method(s) and contraception), determination of gestational age and treatment.

Counselling

Both counselling (information) and abortion should be provided without undue delay. Women should be free to choose to be counselled alone or with a partner, parent or a friend. Pre-abortion counselling should also include contraceptive counselling and prescription, making it possible to begin the chosen method of contraception immediately after the abortion.

Clinical assessment and laboratory investigations

A clinical history should be obtained to identify contraindications and risk factors for contraceptive – and abortion – method. History of a patient should include personal and family history of relevant diseases; current use of any medications, allergies; obstetric and gynaecological history; any anticoagulation disorder or treatment; and history of STIs. The local STI prevalence rates should be taken into account. If clinical signs indicate infection, the woman must be treated with antibiotics immediately. However, this should not delay the medical abortion treatment. The clinician should be alert to the possibility of violence or coercion in the context of the unwanted pregnancy.

There is no evidence to support the routine determination of blood group and Rhesus (Rh) typing in early medical abortion, but it may be needed based on local guidelines which may require that Rh-negative women should receive anti-D prophylaxis. In that case, it is recommended to administer a dose of 50 μg (250 IU) anti-D immunoglobulin G (IgG). The Rh-immunoglobulin can be given on the same day that mifepristone or misoprostol is administered [5, 11].

There is no indication for haemoglobin and haematocrit assays in the absence of clinical signs of anaemia.

Physical examination

In most cases, pregnancy is confirmed by urinary human chorionic gonadotrophin (hCG) and its length estimated on the basis of the woman's history and physical examination, which commonly but not necessarily includes an ultrasound scan. Ultrasound may also be used to diagnose pathologies such as ectopic pregnancy or missed abortion. Any genital infection should be excluded or treatment initiated (including partner(s)) prior to the abortion.

Treatment

A single 200 mg tablet of mifepristone is taken orally. The woman is advised to return after 24–48 hours for day-care admission to complete the abortion procedure with misoprostol. Rarely women abort following mifepristone but before the administration of misoprostol (0.2–0.4%). If legally permitted and chosen by the woman she can be provided with misoprostol and pain management to administer at home. At discharge from the clinic women should be given clear verbal and written information regarding expected effects and possible side effects or complications, if any. They should be informed on how to reach a healthcare provider in case of abnormal bleeding, suspected infection or other adverse events.

Second visit or home administration

During the second visit the woman is admitted to the clinic for misoprostol administration. Alternatively, if legally permitted, she could chose to administer the second course of tablets at home or in another place of her choice. This is the situation in Sweden, so Lisbeth could choose to do the treatment at home or to come back to the clinic for misoprostol administration. A few countries have a legal requirement for misoprostol to be administered in the clinic under supervision. Women may still choose to go home soon after misoprostol administration and expel the pregnancy at home. If a woman chooses to stay in the healthcare facility, she will usually remain for a few hours during which abortion occurs in around 70% of cases. Most women will start bleeding shortly after misoprostol intake and expel the pregnancy within a few hours. However, there are huge individual variations: A small proportion of women expel the gestational sac more than 24 hours after misoprostol intake.

An initial dose of 800 μg of misoprostol is administered vaginally (sublingually or buccally). This can be followed by a second dose of 400 μg of misoprostol (by the preferred route) if bleeding has not started within three to four hours or is scarce. Appropriate pain relief should be given during the abortion.

Pain management

The perception of pain and request for pain relief has wide individual and cultural variations. Studies have shown that analgesic requirement and the perception of pain are significantly higher in younger women, higher gestational age, those with longer induction-to-abortion interval and with increased number of misoprostol doses, whereas it is less in older, parous women and those at shorter gestations [12]. Non-steroid anti-inflammatory drugs (NSAIDs) are the first line treatment. They inhibit the production of endogenous PGs, which are important messengers responsible for uterine contractions, cramps and pain sensation. NSAIDs do not interfere with the action of misoprostol and/or mifepristone on inducing cervical ripening, uterine contractility or the time to abortion and expulsion of the products of conception [13]. Abdominal massage, a hot-water bottle or heating pad, warm shower and support from a partner, friend and/or family member can all help to relieve pain.

Follow-up

A follow-up visit is frequently offered at one to three weeks after the abortion treatment. However, there is no unequivocal protocol for the follow-up after medical abortion. Complications such as pain, bleeding and fever prompt women to seek health care, especially if appropriately counselled. Thus the only reason for a follow-up visit is to exclude a continuing pregnancy, if this has not been confirmed in the healthcare facility. Women's self-assessment has varying sensitivity to diagnose ongoing pregnancy [5]. Serum (s-) hCG has been found to be an accurate modality to detect ongoing pregnancy but adds both visits and costs to the medical abortion. Urine hCG has been shown to correlate well with serum levels. Verification of successful expulsion can be done in the facility, using ultrasound or hCG testing, or by the woman herself using a low-sensitivity hCG urinary test in combination with assessment of bleeding and the absence of pregnancy symptoms. This may or may not be evaluated in a telephone follow-up [14].

When ultrasound is carried out routinely after medical abortion, blood clots or thick endometrium are common findings. They are not an indication for evacuation of the uterus. The decision to perform an evacuation of the uterus should only be undertaken on the basis of clinical signs or symptoms and **not** on ultrasound findings alone.

Post-abortion contraception

Medical abortion has no adverse impact on future fertility. Ovulation may occur as early as 8–10 days after the treatment. Therefore, it is recommended to start contraception as early as possible and within one week of the abortion treatment [5]. Women may start hormonal contraception on the day of, or the day after, misoprostol administration. Combined hormonal pills do not affect the number of days of bleeding or measured blood loss after medical abortion. Intrauterine contraception (IUC) can be inserted when expulsion has been confirmed. Early insertion of the copper intrauterine device or the levonorgestrel-releasing intrauterine system (IUS) is safe, well tolerated and not associated with an increased risk of expulsion or complication. Women who choose to have an IUS after abortion have significantly fewer days of heavy bleeding after the procedure. Women are more likely to return for IUC fitting and less likely to have had prior unprotected intercourse if insertion is scheduled soon after the abortion.

Postponing contraception is associated with the highest rate of repeat abortion. Women who start using IUC or implants immediately after their abortion have a significantly lower rate of repeat abortions [5, 15].Therefore early fitting (within one week after the treatment) should be routinely suggested for women undergoing first-trimester medical abortion. If insertion of an IUC has to be delayed, the woman should be provided with an interim method of contraception to use after the abortion, until the IUC can be inserted. Barrier methods can be used as soon as sexual intercourse is resumed, while methods based on fertility awareness has to be delayed until regular menstrual cycles have resumed.

The future – towards increased access to safe abortion services

Without access to safe abortion services, women risk their health and their lives to obtain clandestine abortions. Globally, approximately 13% of all maternal deaths are due to complications of unsafe abortion and the proportion of unsafe abortion increases. Possible approaches to increase access to medical abortion worldwide include the option to allow task sharing with mid-level providers to allow these healthcare professionals to be more involved with the care of healthy women undergoing medical abortion. The provision of medical abortion by mid-level providers is as effective and safe as that provided by physicians [5]. This possibility would likely have a major impact on increasing access to safe induced abortion in countries where medical resources are scarce, where the number of physicians is limited or where physicians are unwilling to perform abortions. Another recently described alternative for women in countries where access to safe abortion is restricted, is use of the telemedicine service provided by 'Women on Web' [16]. Today, the Internet is a major source of information for people all over the world. On the 'wow' website, women can do an interactive web-based medical consultation. Women are closely guided in the process through an email or telephone helpdesk. Professional counselling is provided in different languages. The outcome of care is comparable to other medical abortion services provided in outpatient settings [17].

References

1. Fiala C, Gemzell-Danielsson K. Review on medical abortion using mifepristone in combination with a prostaglandin analogue. *Contraception* 2006; 74(1): 66–86.
2. Gynuity Health Projects. http://gynuity.org/ (accessed 19 March 2013).
3. Moreau C, Trussell J, Desfreres J, *et al.* Medical vs surgical abortion: the importance of women's choice. *Contraception* 2011; 84(3): 224–9.
4. The National Board of Health and Welfare. Official Statistics of Sweden: induced abortions [in Swedish]. http://www. socialstyrelsen.se/ (accessed 19 March 2013).

5. World Health Organization. *Safe Abortion: technical and policy guidance for health systems*. Geneva, Switzerland: WHO, 2012.

6. Tang OS, Gemzell-Danielsson K, Ho PC. Misoprostol: pharmacokinetic profiles, effects on the uterus and side effects. *Int J Gynaecol Obstet* 2007; 99 (Suppl 2): 160–7.

7. International Federation of Gynecology and Obstetrics. http://www.figo.org (accessed 19 March 2013).

8. European Medicines Agency. http://www.ema.europa.eu/ema/ (accessed 19 March 2013).

9. Sääv I, Fiala C, Hämäläinen JM, *et al.* Medical abortion in lactating women – low levels of mifepristone in breast milk. *Acta Obstet Gynecol Scand* 2010; 89(5): 618–22.

10. Rowlands S. Misinformation on abortion. *Eur J Contracept Reprod Health Care* 2011; 16(4): 233–40.

11. Fiala C, Fux M, Gemzell Danielsson K. Rh-prophylaxis in early abortion. *Acta Obstet Gynecol Scand* 2003; 82(10): 892–903.

12. Hamoda H, Ashok PW, Flett GM, *et al.* Analgesia requirements and predictors of analgesia use for women undergoing medical abortion up to 22 weeks of gestation. *BJOG* 2004; 111(9): 996–1000.

13. Fiala C, Swahn ML, Stephansson O, *et al.* The effect of non-steroidal anti-inflammatory drugs (NSAIDs) on medical abortion with mifepristone and misoprostol. *Hum Reprod* 2005; 20(11): 3072–7.

14. Cameron ST, Glasier A, Dewart H, *et al.* Telephone follow-up and self-performed urine pregnancy testing after early medical abortion: a service evaluation. *Contraception* 2012; 86(1): 67–73.

15. Sääv I, Stephansson O, Gemzell-Damielsson K. Early versus delayed insertion of intrauterine contraception after medical abortion – a randomized controlled trial. *PLosOne* 2012; 7(11): e48948.

16. Women on Web. https://www.womenonweb.org/ (accessed 19 March 2013).

17. Gomperts RJ, Jelinska K, Davies S, *et al.* Using telemedicine for termination of pregnancy with mifepristone and misoprostol in settings where there is no access to safe services. *BJOG* 2008; 115(9): 1171–5.

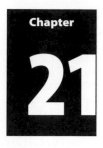

Chapter

21

Surgical termination of pregnancy

Kate Guthrie

Introduction

Abortion is a common procedure; the total number performed in England and Wales in 2011 was 189 931, of which 36% were in women who had experienced an abortion previously [1]. Fifty three per cent of the total number of abortions performed used a surgical method. Research has shown that what is important to women is that they have choice. However, the acceptability of medical termination declines with increasing gestation [2, 3]. Their choice of procedure will be influenced by what is available, their personal fears and experiences, what friends say and what they read in the media and information provided by their health carers.

What do primary care clinicians and women need to know about this very common procedure?

In the event of an unplanned pregnancy, a woman should have the choice of a surgical or medical method at any gestation and be counselled on the procedure itself, possible risks and expected care. In terms of surgery, the woman should know, tailored to the care she is to receive, what to expect during the course of her care such as:

- Her right to confidentiality
- Where to access support and counselling services, including leaflets, web addresses and helpline numbers for support organizations.
- What happens during pre-assessment
- Her right to delay or cancel the procedure
- For the procedure: routine medication; the procedure itself, potential length and extent of pain and/or bleeding; and possible side effects.
- Taking the drug misoprostol for cervical preparation should be seen as 'a point of no return' due to the potential for it causing fetal abnormality at least as published in one case report [4].
- What will happen to the fetal tissue?
- Information about post-operative care and what to expect during the recovery period – for example, amount and length of bleeding, when it is possible to resume work, exercise and sexual activity, contraception and how she will feel emotionally.
- Who to contact, at any given stage, if she has a problem, physical, emotional or social.
- Information about the likely impact of her treatment on her future health and wellbeing.

Contraception, eds Paula Briggs, Gabor Kovacs and John Guillebaud. Published by Cambridge University Press. © Cambridge University Press 2013.

A benefit of a surgical procedure is that any method of contraception can be provided in conjunction with the procedure (in the case of long-acting reversible contraception (LARC)) or post procedure (all other reversible methods). Sterilization should be tempered by the increased risk of regret and failure [5].

Method

This varies by gestation and is summarized in a table published by the Royal College of Obstetricians and Gynaecologists in their evidence-based guidelines. In all cases, even first trimester cases, the cervix is passively dilated pre-procedure to minimize the risk of trauma, bleeding, retained tissue and infection [6]. There will also be a local regime for infection reduction. Women should be warned that cramping abdominal pain, bleeding and sometimes loss of pregnancy tissue can occur between taking the drugs for cervical preparation and surgery, and it is not abnormal or dangerous.

Up to 14 weeks gestation, either electric or manual vacuum aspiration (MVA) techniques are used. MVA employs a handheld syringe and is ideal for procedures delivered in an outpatient setting. For cervical preparation, most commonly the synthetic prostaglandin analogue misoprostol is used (off-license), 400 μg delivered vaginally 3 hours or sublingually 2–3 hours pre-procedure. Mifepristone can also be used if given orally 48 hours pre-procedure but is more expensive [7]. Whichever equipment is used, pregnancy tissue is removed by a hollow tube inserted into the uterus through the open cervix. Mechanical dilation is only used if a wider canal is required to remove larger products at higher gestations.

Pain relief for the procedure can be local anaesthesia, conscious sedation or general anaesthesia, augmented with oral analgesia. The method of pain relief may dictate the setting within which the procedure takes place.

Local anaesthesia is delivered by injecting anaesthetic into the cervix/paracervical tissue, blocking the nerves from the cervix so that pain signals cannot reach the brain. The patient will still feel some pressure or movement, and a cramping feeling as the uterus empties. This can be reduced by adding an oral non-steroidal analgesic and having Entonox® available per procedure to be used if required 'on demand'. Listening to music decreased pre-procedure pain [8]. Fear increases pain, so addressing anxiety and providing psychological support reduces pain. The anxieties of both the patient and the assistants must be addressed; there is no place for the glib reassurances of untrained staff. It is widely acknowledged that the support of a skilled personal carer with 'vocal local' skills is greatly beneficial.

Conscious sedation is a combination of medicines to help relax (a sedative) and to block pain (an anaesthetic) during the procedure and is delivered intravenously by an anaesthetist. The patient will technically stay awake during the procedure, may chat or may sleep but, if required, will respond to verbal cues. She will probably have no memory of the procedure afterwards.

Both local anaesthesia and conscious sedation enables quick recovery and return to everyday activities soon after the procedure.

General anaesthesia makes the patient completely lose consciousness so that surgery can be carried out without causing any pain or discomfort. It is given in an operating theatre by an anaesthetist, either intravenously or by gas, and then intravenously. There is no memory of the procedure, it has a slower recovery time and may be associated with minor side effects such as shivering, nausea or vomiting.

All methods require post-operative analgesia for uterine cramps. Review of randomized controlled trials (RCTs) comparing methods of pain control in first trimester abortions showed premedication with ibuprofen or naproxen reduced post-operative pain after local anaesthetic procedures as did lornoxicam and diclofenac orally as a premedication. Again, the support of a skilled personal carer is greatly beneficial.

From 14 completed weeks' gestation, dilatation and evacuation (D&E) is the usual method of choice, although from 14–16 weeks gestation vacuum aspiration can be utilized with the appropriate equipment and training. From 15–19 weeks, 76% of abortion procedures are performed surgically and 67% at 20 weeks and over. General anaesthesia increasingly becomes the method of choice as gestation increases. The procedure usually includes a combination of vacuum aspiration, dilatation of the cervix and aspiration curettage and the use of surgical instruments (such as forceps), and it is commonly performed under ultrasound guidance to reduce the risk of surgical complications such as perforation of the uterus and retained products. At later gestations, an overnight stay or attending on two consecutive days may be required to ensure adequate cervical preparation pre-procedure, usually with osmotic dilators augmented with misoprostol for cervical softening and dilatation.

The pre-assessment consultation

Pre-assessment consultation is undertaken to assess gestation, identify multiple pregnancy and make an individual risk assessment for physical and mental health issues for any given individual. It is also important to identify and act upon any child or adult safeguarding concerns. Routine screening for blood group and Rhesus factor and also screening for chlamydia and gonorrhoea as well as a venous thromboembolism risk assessment [9] should be offered to everyone. For those women identified to be at risk of sexually transmitted infections, human immunodeficiency virus (HIV) testing should be offered. For women with haematological disorders, a haemoglobin estimation and haemoglobinopathy screening should be undertaken. Opportunistic cervical screening can be offered. A multidisciplinary team approach should be taken for women with complex medical conditions. Support and counselling should be available and offered to all, and in women identified with risk factors for mental health problems, specialist referral for mental health support should be undertaken. The issue of post-procedure contraception, specifically the provision of LARC should be addressed.

Risks (and myths of risks)

Specifically, the following risks and the steps taken within the service to minimize these risks must be discussed in a manner understandable by the woman for an informed decision regarding treatment. Risks can be summarized on a pre-printed consent form and supplemented by written and verbal information enabling discussion.

Haemorrhage (blood loss > 500 ml or bleeding requiring transfusion)

Less than 1% of procedures are complicated by haemorrhage [10] and even less require transfusion. The risk is lower at earlier gestations (0.88 per 1000 under 13 weeks vs 4 per 1000 over 20 weeks). Blood loss is less with local anaesthesia and conscious sedation compared to inhalational anaesthesia as the latter effects uterine contractility after emptying the uterus.

Injury to the cervix

Injury to the cervix is thought to occur in less than 0.2% of cases due to the current practice of cervical preparation, and if minor will not be relevant to future reproductive health. A large series on cervical injury requiring stitching [11] reported that cervical preparation, operator experience and local anaesthesia were protective.

Uterine perforation

A recent large study reported a perforation rate of 2.3 per 1000 [12]. The risks are increased in higher parity and higher gestation and, as with cervical injury, are lowered by cervical preparation and increasing operator experience [13]. Should one of the above complications occur, there is a small chance of blood transfusion, laparoscopy or laparotomy to diagnose/treat the complication.

Continuing pregnancy

This risk has been quoted as 2.3 per 1000 [14] and is greatest in very early procedures (gestation under 7 weeks), higher parity, multiple pregnancy, uterine abnormality, the use of narrow cannulae relative to gestational age and operator inexperience. However, using strict protocols that employ ultrasound pre-assessment of gestation, visual checking of uterine aspirates and utilizing quantitative serum, beta human chorionic gonadotrophin (β-hCG) and transvaginal ultrasound where required [15], a failure rate of 1.3 per 1000 in gestations under 7 weeks was reported, the same as gestations of 7–12 weeks [16].

Retained products

This can be tissue or blood clot. The incidence of this for first trimester procedures has been reported at 1.8%, less than for medical procedures at the same gestation [17]. A Cochrane review of first trimester procedures found the type of procedure had no effect [18].

Upper genital tract infection

Upper genital tract infection is a common recognized complication of abortion (10% of cases) and is associated with the presence of organisms in the genital tract, both sexually transmitted (e.g., chlamydia and gonorrhoea) and otherwise (e.g., bacterial vaginosis). Post-abortion infection can lead to immediate morbidity (pain, fever, discharge and bleeding) and in the long-term tubal subfertility and ectopic pregnancy. A Cochrane review of antibiotic prophylaxis for first trimester-induced abortion [18] showed overall the risk of post-abortal upper genital tract infection in women receiving antibiotics was 59% that of women who received placebo, and noted that if the infection is caused by a sexually transmitted organism, antibiotic prophylaxis will not protect the woman from becoming re-infected if her sexual partner has not been treated. Services have strategies for infection reduction including universal prophylaxis, 'screen and treat', and a combination of both. The last two enable partner notification and breaking the chain of infection if a sexually transmitted infection is detected. The evidence-based prophylactic regimes recommended by the Royal College of Obstetricians and Gynaecologists [5] are:

*   Azithromycin 1 g orally on the day of abortion **plus** metronidazole 1 g rectally **or** 800 mg orally prior to **or at** the time of abortion; **or**

- Doxycycline 100 mg orally twice daily for 7 days starting on the day of abortion, **plus** metronidazole 1 g rectally **or** 800 mg orally prior to or at the time of abortion; *or*
- Metronidazole 1 g rectally or 800 mg orally prior to or at the time of abortion for women who have tested negative for *Chlamydia trachomatis* infection.

Future reproductive health

A systematic review of women who had undergone abortion, reported an increased risk of preterm birth post-surgical abortion, increasing for repeated abortions [19]. Infection and mechanical trauma are suspected mechanisms for this. However, not all studies reviewed took account of confounding variables such as socioeconomic status. There may be similar risks with surgical management of miscarriage, for the same reasons.

Mental health

The majority of women undergoing an abortion by any method have short-term emotional distress tempered with feelings of relief, but there has been much debate about long-term mental health injury. The National Collaborating Centre for Mental Health in the UK undertook a systematic review of the mental health outcomes of induced abortion, including their prevalence and associated factors to clarify the relationship between induced abortion and mental health problems [20]. The review concluded that a pregnancy being unwanted was associated with an increased risk of mental health problems, irrespective of whether the woman had an abortion or gave birth, and that the most reliable predictor of post-abortion mental health problems was having a history of mental health problems before the abortion. The factors associated with increased rates of mental health problems for women in the general population following birth and following abortion were similar, but there were some additional factors associated with an increased risk of mental health problems specifically related to abortion, such as pressure from a partner to have an abortion, and negative attitudes towards abortions in general and towards a woman's personal experience of the abortion. They recommended that if a woman has a negative attitude towards abortion, shows a negative emotional reaction to the abortion, or is experiencing stressful life events, health and social care professionals should consider offering support. If any of the above risk factors are identified, appropriate referral, with the woman's consent, through her general practitioner should be forthcoming.

Other outcomes

There is no proven association between the following outcomes and surgical termination: breast cancer, placenta praevia, subfertility, ectopic pregnancy or miscarriage [5].

Post-procedure care

Rhesus-negative women should be given anti-D [21]. All women should leave the Unit with the most effective contraceptive of her choice and knowledge of her local sexual health services, a summary of how they should expect to feel and symptoms which would necessitate emergency care. She should be given a 24 hour helpline number and a letter summarizing the clinical episode to enable the provision of emergency care should it be needed [5]. She should also be aware of the signs and symptoms of ongoing pregnancy, be offered the option of a follow-up appointment and be aware of how to seek help if she feels the need for support or counselling.

Life returning to normal

Uterine cramps will usually settle within 24 hours. Bleeding will settle, and can last from a day to a few weeks, but will be influenced by the method of contraception used. Limitation on exercise and return to work will be dictated by the type of anaesthesia and personal preference. Emotions will be a mix of regret and relief, depending on circumstances and social support, and should settle progressively over the next few weeks.

What signs and symptoms should women be looking out for?

If the procedure has been straightforward and all prophylactic measures taken, the majority of women should have an uneventful course. They should, however, seek advice if they have any worries and particularly if they experience fever, heavy bleeding, dizziness or tachycardia or experience severe pain, as those symptoms may indicate infection or retained products of conception. Anxiety or depression, which do not resolve, should prompt a mental health referral.

Summary

Women can be reassured that annual statistics (Department of Health Abortion Statistics, England and Wales, National Health Service National Services Scotland Information Services Division and The Confidential Enquiry into Maternal and Child Health) backed by national and international audit and research reassure that surgical abortion, whilst never undertaken lightly, is a safe procedure following which major complications and mortality are rare.

References

1. Department of Health. *Abortion Statistics, England and Wales: 2011*. London: HMSO, 2012.
2. Robson SC, Kelly T, Howel D, *et al.* Randomised preference trial of medical versus surgical termination of pregnancy less than 14 weeks' gestation (TOPS). *Health Technol Assess* 2009; 13(53): 1–148.
3. Kelly T, Suddes J, Howel D, Hewison J, Robson S. Comparing medical versus surgical termination of pregnancy at 13–20 weeks of gestation: a randomised controlled trial. *BJOG* 2010; 117: 1512–20.
4. Dubrey S, Patel W, Malik O. Moebius–Poland syndrome and drug associations. BMJ Case Reports 2009; 10.11136/09.2008.0953.
5. Royal College of Obstetricians and Gynaecologists. *The Care of Women Requesting Induced Abortion. Evidence-based Clinical Guideline No. 7*. London: RCOG Press, 2011.

http://www.rcog.org.uk/files/rcog-corp/Abortion%20guideline_web_1.pdf (accessed 4 March 2013).
6. Meirik O, My Huong NT, Piaggio G, Bergel E, von Hertzen H. Complications of first-trimester abortion by vacuum aspiration after cervical preparation with and without misoprostol: a multicentre randomised trial. *Lancet* 2012; 378: 1817–24.
7. Ashok PW, Flett GM, Templeton A. Mifepristone versus vaginally administered misoprostol for cervical priming before first-trimester termination of pregnancy: a randomized, controlled study *Am J Obstet Gynecol* 2000; 183: 998–1002.
8. Renner RM, Jensen JT, Nichols MD, Edelman AB. Pain control in first-trimester surgical abortion: a systematic review of randomized controlled trials. *Contraception* 2010; 81: 372–88.
9. National Institute for Health and Clinical Excellence. 2010, Clinical Guideline 92,

Venous thromboembolism: reducing the risk: http://publications.nice.org.uk/venous-thromboembolism-reducing-the-risk-cg92 (accessed 4 June 2013).

10. Kerns J, Steinauer J. Management of postabortion hemorrhage: release date November 2012 SFP Guideline #20131. *Contraception* 2013; 87(3): 331–42.

11. Schulz KF, Grimes DA, Cates W, Jr. Measures to prevent cervical injury during suction curettage abortion. *Lancet* 1983; 1(8335): 1182–5.

12. Zhou W, Nielsen GL, Møller M, Olsen J. Short-term complications after surgically induced abortions: a register-based study of 56 117 abortions. *Acta Obstet Gynecol Scand* 2002; 81: 331–6.

13. Grimes DA, Schulz KF, Cates WJ, Jr. Prevention of uterine perforation during curettage abortion. *JAMA* 1984; 251: 2108–11.

14. Kaunitz AM, Rovira EZ, Grimes DA, Schulz KF. Abortions that fail. *Obstet Gynecol* 1985; 66: 533–7.

15. Creinin MD, Edwards J. Early abortion: surgical and medical options. *Curr Probl Obstet, Gynecol Fertil* 1997; 20: 6–32.

16. Niinimäki M, Pouta A, Bloigu A, *et al.* Immediate complications after medical compared with surgical termination of pregnancy. *Obstet Gynecol* 2009; 114: 795–804.

17. Kulier R, Cheng L, Fekih A, Hofmeyr GJ, Campana A. Surgical methods for first trimester termination of pregnancy. *Cochrane Database Syst Rev* 2001; 4: CD002900.

18. Low N, Mueller M, Van Vliet HAAM, Kapp N. Perioperative antibiotics to prevent infection after first-trimester abortion. *Cochrane Database Syst Rev* 2012; 3: CD005217.

19. Shah PS, Zao J; Knowledge Synthesis Group of Determinants of Preterm/LBW Births. Induced termination of pregnancy and low birthweight and preterm birth: a systematic review and meta-analyses. *BJOG* 2009; 116: 1425–42.

20. National Collaborating Centre for Mental Health. *Induced Abortion and Mental Health: a systematic review of the mental health outcomes of induced abortion, including their prevalence and associated factors.* London: Academy of Medical Royal Colleges, 2011.

21. Royal College of Obstetricians and Gynaecologists. *The Use of Anti-D Immunoglobulin for Rhesus D Prophylaxis. Green-top Guideline No. 22.* London: RCOG Press, 2011. http://www.rcog.org.uk/files/rcog-corp/GTG22AntiD.pdf (accessed 4 March 2013).

Chapter

22

Primary care treatment of subfertility and what every health professional needs to know about assisted reproductive technology

Gabor Kovacs

Case scenario: Maggie

Maggie (aged 34) and Brian (aged 36) have been living together for 3 years. They decided that they were ready to have a family, and stopped using contraception 12 months ago. Maggie's menarche was at 15, and her periods were irregular when she started the combined oral contraceptive pill (COC) at age 16 to regulate her menses, and also to help with her many pimples. She was given Dianette® (Bayer: ethinyl oestradiol 35 µg, cyproterone acetate 2 mg) which she continued taking until 12 months ago. Once stopping COCs her periods returned, but only about every six to eight weeks. They spoke to their general practitioner (GP) about 6 months ago about not conceiving but she said that nothing can be done till they have tried for 12 months.

Introduction

Approximately 25% of young couples will conceive within the first month, 60% within 6 months and 80% within 12 months of unprotected sexual intercourse. So when is a couple subfertile? Traditional advice was that a couple should try to conceive for 12 months, and if they do not succeed, then they should be investigated and treated. Today we are far more couple focused, and if the woman is older, or if there is an obvious problem (amenorrhoea or oligomenorrhoea suggesting anovulation) investigation and treatment should not be delayed. As Maggie has oligomenorrhoea, and she is unlikely to be ovulating regularly, delaying investigations and treatment was wrong and investigations should have commenced six months ago.

Subfertility is classified as 'Primary' if the woman has not been pregnant before and 'Secondary' if she has. This definition can be further divided into whether the couple have had a pregnancy together, or whether either partner has achieved a pregnancy in a previous relationship. These definitions are really just semantics, as the investigation and treatment is similar in all these situations.

The prevalence of subfertility is difficult to document, but it is estimated that approximately 15% of married couples in the developed world are subfertile. There is not good data on the incidence of subfertility, despite some suggestions that it has increased. What has changed are the expectations of couples with the availability of fertility hormones, in vitro fertilization (IVF), microsurgery, gamete and embryo donation as well as the more widely practised and accepted surrogacy; everyone presumes that they will succeed and nobody wants to wait.

Contraception, eds Paula Briggs, Gabor Kovacs and John Guillebaud. Published by Cambridge University Press. © Cambridge University Press 2013.

The care of the subfertile man or woman should commence with their GP or sexual health clinic. A family physician/GP can obtain an appropriate history and perform an adequate examination. They can also organize baseline investigations, such as investigating if ovulation is occurring, a semen analysis and confirming immunity to rubella and varicella, as well as an up to date cervical smear. If there is an obvious cause such as anovulation or irregular ovulation (with cycles longer than 32 days) then an experienced 'women's health doctor' can supervise ovulation induction with clomiphene citrate (see below). If male subfertility is involved, the male should be referred to an andrologist (an endocrinologist with special interest in males) or urologist.

Initial appointment

Ideally, it should involve both partners and focus on reviewing not only the medical but also the psychological, religious and social or cultural history. The content of the initial interview should consist of a discussion of the following topics:

- Duration of subfertility and results of any previous evaluation and treatment.
- Menstrual, gynaecological and obstetric history in the female. In Maggie's situation this points to the diagnosis of anovulation or at least irregular ovulation. Her other symptoms suggest that she may have polycystic ovary syndrome (PCOS) (late menarche, spottiness).
- Medical history including current systemic diseases, current use of medications, herbs or alternative therapies, allergies to medications and past medical history including any previous surgery.
- Reproductive history should include previous pregnancies, abortions, contraceptive methods, pelvic infections, abnormal cervical smears, exposure to sexually transmitted infections or sterilization.
- Family history of genetic disorders, birth defects and multiple miscarriages.
- Lifestyle, including diet, exercise, use of alcohol, tobacco or recreational drugs, exposure to environmental toxins or occupational factors.
- History in the male, including the results of all previous sperm analyses, current use of medication(s), alcohol, recreational drugs or alternative therapies, current illnesses or systemic diseases, surgery of the reproductive tract, including vasectomy, exposure to sexually transmitted infections and/or pregnancy with a different partner.
- Sexual practices and the frequency and timing of intercourse, as well as the presence of pain with intercourse, erectile dysfunction or retrograde ejaculation. A useful way of assessing the technique of intercourse is to ask four leading questions:

1. Asking the male if he has difficulty with erections.
2. Asking the female if she feels penetration is adequate.
3. Asking the male if he ejaculates.
4. Asking the female whether she can feel semen in the vagina after intercourse.

Following this detailed history, a physical examination of the female partner should be performed.

The examination of the female should include height, weight, a general physical assessment, blood pressure, hair distribution, breast development and abdominal and pelvic examinations.

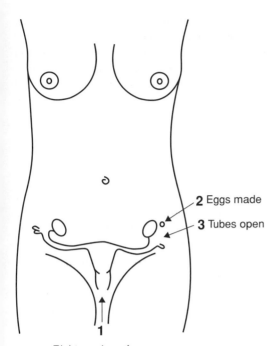

Figure 22.1 The three basic fertility parameters.

2 Eggs made

3 Tubes open

1

Right number of sperms
in the right place
at the right time

The male only needs to be examined if the semen analysis is abnormal or if the couple report a mechanical problem.

Many subfertile couples are concerned that their diet, exercise programme or other aspects of their lifestyle may be the cause of their problem. Excessive exercise (leading to minimal body fat) may impact on fertility in women, and this may be manifest by secondary amenorrhoea.

The approach to investigations revolves around the three baseline fertility parameters (Figure 22.1):

1. **Sperm** – the right number of fertile sperm have to be placed in the right place at the right time.
2. **Eggs** have to be matured and released.
3. **Tubes** – the female passages have to be normal to allow the eggs and sperm to be transported together, and for the embryo to form and be transported into the uterine cavity.

Fertility evaluation by the GP

The diagnostic evaluation is designed to identify the cause or causes of subfertility and determine the most effective and cost-efficient approach to therapy. In general, the least invasive, least expensive and least painful diagnostic tests are done first. Subfertility evaluation consists of some or all of the following tests: determination of ovulation, evaluation of the production and delivery of sperm, and ensuring the timing is appropriate. Once this has been shown to be normal, referral to a specialist unit is indicated, for determination of patency of the Fallopian tubes, size and shape of the uterine cavity and evaluation of the pelvic cavity with the exclusion of endometriosis or adhesions. In some situations, assessment of tubal patency can be undertaken by a sexual health doctor with expertise in in ultrasound, using the insufflation of contrast media under ultrasound control (HyCoSy). However the gold standard of pelvic assessment is diagnostic laparoscopy, with hydrotubation and hysteroscopy.

Sperm: evaluation of the production and delivery of sperm

It has been estimated that in 40–60% of all couples with subfertility the problem may be attributed to the male partner.

The standard test of male fertility is a semen analysis, which should be performed early in the course of the couple's evaluation. A minimum of two analyses should be performed several weeks apart in order to properly assess male fertility. It is important that clinicians use a laboratory capable of performing an appropriate semen analysis. Laboratories usually perform a semen analysis and report the results according to the recommendations of the World Health Organization (WHO) [1]. The semen should be examined for 'anti-sperm antibodies' [2].

Often general pathology laboratories may not utilize these standards, and consequently confidence in the results may be lacking – thereby misleading patients about their actual reproductive capabilities or problems. The semen analysis should be obtained through masturbation, after two or three days of abstinence into a clean container that does not contain soap residue or other substances that may be harmful to the sperm. For those men who have personal, cultural or religious objections to the collection of a sample in this way, special non-toxic condom-like devices (semen collection device: Hy-Gene® Seminal Fluid Collection Kit, Sepal Reproductive International) can/should be provided that facilitate collection of the sample during intercourse. Standard, over-the-counter condoms even if they don't contain spermicide are toxic to the sperm.

If there is a consistent abnormality in the quality or numbers of sperm seen on two or more occasions, an evaluation of the male by a urologist or andrologist is indicated. Physical examination of the male may detect systemic diseases, endocrine disorders, infections or developmental abnormalities of the male reproductive system, including congenital absence of the vas deferens (CBAVD). Because CBAVD may occur more often in men who carry a gene for cystic fibrosis, known as the cystic fibrosis transmembrane conductance regulator (CFTR), those in whom this abnormality is found should undergo genetic counselling (and testing of their partner) before the couple starts any fertility treatments. Men with CBAVD should also have an evaluation of their kidneys and ureters to look for congenital abnormalities. In addition, abnormalities of the urethra may lead to the abnormal deposition of sperm during intercourse. Finally, infertile men may also have a collection of varicose veins within the scrotum known as a varicocele. Large varicoceles may interfere with both the number and quality of sperm. Surgical correction of a varicocele may occasionally have a dramatic impact on the number and quality of sperm, although the role of varicocele ligation is still being debated [3].

The minimal hormone evaluation in the subfertile male should include the measurement of serum testosterone and follicle stimulating hormone (FSH) concentrations.

Finally, as many as 15% of men with significant oligospermia, have a missing fragment of their Y chromosome (micro-deletions) [4]. Genetic testing should be recommended to these men who have no evidence of an obstruction of their vas deferens or epididymis.

Men with azoospermia due to obstruction can be treated by fine needle aspiration (FNA) of testicular sperm, usually under local analgesia, and the sperm obtained can be used to fertilize their partner's oocytes, using intracytoplasmic sperm injection (ICSI) technique in an IVF programme. Even some men in whom the azoospermia is due to failure of sperm production may have some sperm collected by biopsying their testicles, either by needle biopsy, or sometimes by open testicular biopsy. The technique can be further improved by using the operating microscope to identify possible areas of sperm production, where even a few sperm can be recovered to enable ICSI [5]. However, there are some men where none of these treatments or therapies will restore fertility. The reality is that for these couples their only alternatives are the use of donor sperm, adoption or child-free living. As is the case with all couples considering third-party reproduction, these couples should be offered professional counselling in addition to medical care.

Eggs: detecting and evaluating ovulation

The menstrual history is a reliable indicator of the presence or absence of ovulation. A history of regular, cyclic and painful menstrual periods with premenstrual symptoms usually indicates that ovulation is occurring. However, the patient who is not ovulating may still have menstrual periods. An inexpensive, convenient, and non-invasive approach to the documentation of ovulation is to chart the basal body temperature (BBT) each day through one or two menstrual cycles. A woman who is ovulating will usually have an early morning temperature that is less than 98°F (36.6°C) during the first half of the menstrual cycle and higher than 98°F (36.6°C) during the second half of the menstrual cycle. The BBT gives an indication of which day ovulation occurred, but is not a good method for predicting which day ovulation will actually occur; thus it is a retrospective test. Also, as couples are often inaccurate in describing their timing of intercourse, a temperature chart with coital plotting enables the assessment of whether timing was appropriate. About the time of the ovulation, the ovary begins to produce progesterone, and as a result the BBT rises, and one can be reasonably certain that ovulation has occurred (see Chapter 4).

However, because some women find their BBT is not easily interpreted, the detection of progesterone within the blood during the mid-luteal phase should also be used to confirm that ovulation has occurred. A serum prolactin should also be measured, and some endocrinologists recommend routine screening of thyroid function via thyroid stimulating hormone (TSH) in all subfertile women. Serial ultrasound examinations of the ovaries is another way of assessing ovulation, but this approach is not always accurate and can be expensive, and so it is not recommended.

Over-the-counter ovulation predictor kits are often helpful in determining the day of ovulation in women with regular monthly periods. However, they are not a substitute for a BBT or blood progesterone test in women with irregular periods because they may occasionally produce false-positive or false-negative results. Nor do they provide proof of ovulation, as they detect the LH peak, which is the signal from the brain to the ovary, but is not a proof that the ovary responded. Also, they are an additional expense.

Tubes: evaluation of the pelvis and Fallopian tubes

A transvaginal ultrasound of the pelvis should probably be one of the first investigations of pelvic anatomy. Whilst this is not particularly effective at assessing tubal patency unless it is combined with the injection of positive contrast media (HyCoSy), it is good at imaging the uterus and the ovaries.

Polycystic ovaries (PCO) are present in about 20–25% of women, and this is a clear ultrasound diagnosis according to the European Society of Human Reproduction and Embryology (ESHRE)/American Society for Reproductive Medicine (ASRM) criteria, where '12 or more small (2–8 mm) peripheral follicles are present in one ovary' [6].

A woman has PCOS if, in addition to the ultrasound findings, she has symptoms related to hyperandrogenism (oligo/amenorrhoea, acne, obesity, hirsuitism). One in two women with PCO never experience symptoms and only find out that they have PCO when they have a pelvic ultrasound. Pelvic ultrasound is very good at diagnosing intrauterine abnormalities including septae, polyps and fibroids.

Another test which gives limited information is the hysterosalpingogram. This is a radiological examination, with radio-opaque contrast medium being injected through the cervix, with its passage through the tubes being monitored by X-rays. It does give some information on whether the tubes are patent or blocked, but it is a painful procedure and it does have false positives and false negatives.

The 'gold standard' in the twenty-first century for evaluating the 'tubes', and of course the rest of the pelvic organs, is diagnostic laparoscopy. Laparoscopy is an outpatient surgical procedure during which a telescope is placed through a small incision below the umbilicus. The pelvic cavity is then visualized and the various pelvic structures viewed. Laparoscopy is clearly indicated in women with subfertility and either moderate-to-severe pain with their periods or pain with intercourse. It is also indicated in women who have a history of pelvic surgery or pelvic infections and may have pelvic scar tissue. Finally, many women with otherwise unexplained subfertility are candidates for laparoscopy. However, laparoscopy is the most expensive of the diagnostic procedures, and many physicians are now delaying or omitting laparoscopy in women who have no significant history or symptoms and in whom a pelvic ultrasound with contrast medium studies is normal.

The evaluation of the couple is not complete until a laparoscopy has been performed, although many couples today bypass this test and head straight for IVF.

What if sperm, eggs and tubes appear 'OK' and there is still no pregnancy?

Couples who fulfill the three basic fertility parameters but still don't succeed are said to have 'unexplained subfertility'. Let us try and explain what this is. If we work through the steps of conception, after eggs, sperm and tubes there are three other possible factors:

1. **Transport.** Although the tubes may be open and look normal or fairly normal at laparoscopy, they may not be functioning normally and may not transport the sperm up (including up through the cervix – cervical factor) or may not pick up the egg from the surface of the ovary and transport it down. Performing IVF will place the egg and sperm together and eliminate this variable.
2. **Fertilization.** It is possible that in nature, the egg and sperm may not be combining – fertilization failure. In an IVF cycle this can be diagnosed and then treated in a subsequent cycle by ICSI.
3. **Implantation.** The final requirement is implantation. Using IVF technology, the embryo is introduced transcervically, and this may be an alternate approach, which is successful.

Treatment of anovulation

If it is determined that a woman is not ovulating, a search for specific causes of the ovulation disorder should be performed. Investigations should include measurement of the following hormones:

- Follicle stimulating hormone (FSH)
- Luteinizing hormone (LH)
- Prolactin
- Thyroid stimulating hormone (TSH)

A baseline ultrasound is probably indicated to exclude any gross abnormality and to diagnose PCO, although the treatment of anovulation is similar whether the ovaries are polycystic or not.

In rare situations, the process of ovarian ageing is accelerated, a condition called premature ovarian failure. This is diagnosed by amenorrhoea associated with an elevated FSH level in excess of 25 IU/ml on at least two occasions. Not all women who experience premature ovarian failure are menopausal, 5–10% have a chance of resuming spontaneous ovulation. However, the resumption of ovulation and return of fertility is unpredictable, and there is no test that can predict this. This condition is called 'resistant ovary syndrome' and is only a retrospective diagnosis if ovulation returns. Its mechanism is poorly understood, and it is explained as a temporary resistance of the FSH receptors.

For women with ovarian failure, there is no way of reversing this. For these women, their only options are using donated oocytes, embryos, adoption or child-free living.

For women who are not ovulating and do not have an elevated level of FSH, ovulation can almost always be restored. If that is the only cause of the couple's subfertility, ovulation induction should solve the problem.

The first question in a woman who is not ovulating is to check her prolactin hormone level. If this is elevated, a reason for this should be looked for – sometimes it can be due to medications or a pituitary tumour, often microscopic. If the raised prolactin level is the cause of the anovulation, this can be treated by normalizing the levels using 'bromocriptine' or 'cabergoline'. Once prolactin levels return to normal, ovulation usually resumes.

If the prolactin level is normal, one of two groups of hormones can be used to induce ovulation.

The first are termed *anti-oestrogens* and the most commonly used one clomiphene citrate. It is available in tablet form and is taken for five days during the early part of the menstrual cycle. Approximately one week after the last tablet is taken, ovulation will usually occur, and the couple should have intercourse regularly at least every second day during and around this time. These drugs may cause hot flushes and blurring of vision in higher doses, but are usually free of other side effects, except for a multiple pregnancy rate of approximately 3–4%. It is usual to commence women with oligomenorrhoea (cycles up to 42 days) with a dose of 25 mg (1/2 tablet) daily for 5 days from day 5 to day 9 of a cycle (where day 1 is the first morning of bleeding). If ovulation does not occur after this dose, the course of medication is usually repeated at a higher dosage (increasing stepwise to 50 mg, 100 mg to a maximum of 150 mg/day for 5 days).

For women who are amenorrhoeic, it is best to induce a withdrawal bleed. After checking the blood level of oestrogen and progesterone to exclude recent ovulation, either a two-week course of the combined hormonal contraceptive pill can be administered, or if there is a reasonable level of oestrogen, suggesting some follicular activity but anovulation, a five day course of progestogen (norethisterone 5 mg daily for 5 days or medroxyprogesterone 10 mg daily for 5 days) can be administered. This will result in a 'withdrawal bleed' and day 1 of the bleed is then used as day 1 of the treatment cycle. Clomiphene citrate is then administered either from day 5 to day 9, or some prescribers prefer from day 2 to day 6. There is little difference in the two regimens, and it is purely the practitioner's preference. Approximately 60–70% of women will ovulate on clomiphene citrate and 30–40% will conceive within 3–6 ovulations. The administration of clomiphene citrate is most cost effectively monitored by a BBT chart (see Figure 4.3, which shows a conceptual cycle on clomiphene citrate or use 'Fertilityfriend.com') and a mid-luteal (not necessarily day 21 but somewhere between days 19–23) blood test for oestradiol and progesterone. A rise in oestrogen indicates ovarian activity, whilst a rise in progesterone is biochemical circumstantial evidence of ovulation. If there is a clear indication that anovulation is causing the couple's fertility problem, it is not essential to complete tubal evaluation before commencing clomiphene. If, however, there is no conception after three good ovulations with well-timed intercourse with a fertile partner (as documented on a BBT) then assessment of tubal patency is mandatory. Because a semen analysis is easy and inexpensive, this should usually be performed before treatment.

Should a woman not respond to clomiphene citrate, she needs to be referred to a fertility centre for ovulation induction with *gonadotrophins*. These drugs are similar to the human hormones that are produced by the pituitary gland, and they are either extracted and purified from human urine or produced using recombinant DNA technology. They can be self administered by subcutaneous injection and tend to stimulate several follicles to grow and for several oocytes to ovulate. Of those who conceive on these medications, 15–20% will have a multiple pregnancy. Because of the potential for multiple follicular development and a condition called *ovarian hyperstimulation syndrome*, close monitoring in the form of blood hormone tests and pelvic ultrasound examinations is regularly performed, usually every three or four days. These medications are much more expensive and more potent than the anti-oestrogens, and therefore are much more time consuming. The chance of pregnancy in suitable women is about 20% per cycle. Because of the cost and complexity of FSH injections, the confirmation of tubal patency (and of course the fertility of the male partner) is strongly recommended.

Treatment of tubal abnormalities and endometriosis

Laparoscopy can identify pelvic abnormalities such as adhesions or endometriosis. With the exception of sterilization reversal, it is rare that tubal blockage can be successfully treated surgically. The tubes have a complicated function and intricate structure, and once damaged they often cannot be repaired. Laparoscopic surgery is limited to removing peritubal adhesions, if present, and to the surgical excision or destruction of endometriosis.

Abnormalities of the cavity of the uterus are uncommon but often very treatable causes of infertility. Submucosal fibroids, endometrial polyps and uterine septae are the most common abnormalities of the cavity that are treated by hysteroscopic surgery. Other less common abnormalities such as a bicornuate uterus are not generally remediable nor do they necessarily need treatment.

Treatment of endometriosis

Endometriosis is a common condition characterized by the presence of endometrium in locations outside the uterus. It is commonly found in and around the ovaries and Fallopian tubes and may cause pelvic pain and subfertility. It is found in 30–35% of women with subfertility. Exactly how endometriosis contributes to inability to conceive is unknown, although it can cause the formation of scar tissue. Fortunately not all women with endometriosis will be subfertile.

In cases of endometriosis, surgery and drug therapy have been used to improve pregnancy rates. Several medications are commonly used in the treatment of endometriosis, including contraceptive pills, progesterone or progestogens and gonadotrophin-releasing hormone (Gn-RH) agonists. These medications are most useful in treating the pain of endometriosis and, perhaps, preventing its recurrence, but less useful in treating subfertility. By themselves, they have not been shown to improve fertility. The most successful approach to the treatment of endometriosis appears to be surgery. The surgical removal of mild endometriosis may not only improve fertility, but can be useful in reducing pelvic pain. Surgical removal of extensive endometriosis and restoration of the normal anatomical relationships between the ovaries and the Fallopian tubes may dramatically improve fertility. While most surgery for endometriosis can be performed on an outpatient basis through the laparoscope, occasionally a laparotomy is required.

Treatment of male factor

A few infertile men may have a congenital or acquired deficiency in the secretion of the pituitary hormones, LH and FSH. In these cases there is inadequate stimulation of the testes and poor or no sperm production. Normal production of sperm and testosterone may be induced by administration of human chorionic gonadotrophin (hCG), which mimics the action of LH and, if that is unsuccessful, by FSH injections. Treatment often has to continue for several months.

There are numerous other hormonal therapies that have been studied and used in men who have a normal pituitary gland but produce sperm in reduced numbers. They include clomiphene, tamoxifen, low-dose testosterone, human menopausal gonadotropins, thyroid hormone, vitamins A, C and E and zinc. Unfortunately, while these treatments may benefit an occasional individual, none has been proven consistently successful in the treatment of low sperm production.

The surgical treatment of a varicocele is sometimes undertaken, but it is not currently possible to state that varicocele repair improves fertility due to the methodological limitations of the scientific studies that have been published [3].

Surgery may be helpful when there is obstruction or other abnormalities of the ejaculatory duct. Unfortunately, fertility is not always restored due to either scar tissue formation in the vas deferens or anti-sperm antibodies in the testes. However, up to 50% of men may father children after surgical repair of a previous vasectomy. If the vasectomy was performed more than seven years ago, then vasovasostomy is less likely to work.

When there is no treatment for or success after attempting treatment, IVF technology is used to take 'the mountain to Mohammed'. What this means is that if there are insufficient sperm produced to reach and fertilize the ovum the natural way, then the eggs can be surgically removed and either mixed with the sperm, or the micro-injection ICSI technique can be used to fertilize it. The embryo is then cultured in vitro for a few days, and is then transferred into the uterus.

Treatment of unexplained subfertility

As it can be used to further assess possible problems, or even overcome them without a diagnosis, IVF is indicated for the treatment of unexplained subfertility. It eliminates any problems of transport as the gametes are placed together, the fertilization rate can be assessed and, if low, ICSI introduced in the next cycle. It is hoped that the transcervical introduction of the embryo may result in better implantation.

Future implications

In 2013 we have reached a stage in the treatment of subfertility that means most couples can have a chance of conceiving. It has to be remembered that IVF does not work the first time for everyone, and several attempts may have to be undertaken to result in a realistic cumulative chance of pregnancy.

In vitro fertilization

While IVF was originally designed to overcome irreversible disorders of the Fallopian tubes, it has become the final treatment for virtually all forms of infertility in men and women.

IVF consists of five principal steps. The first step is the stimulation of the ovaries to produce multiple eggs or follicles. In response to FSH, most women will produce numerous follicles enabling the collection of several eggs.

The second step is 'monitoring'. During ovulation stimulation blood tests to measure the level of oestradiol, and pelvic ultrasound examinations are performed to monitor the response of the ovaries.

Once the eggs have reached an appropriate maturity, the third step is the collection of eggs, using a needle introduced into the pelvis through the vagina and guided by ultrasound. The follicles are aspirated and the fluid sent to the laboratory, where the oocytes are identified under the microscope.

The fourth step is that once the oocytes are identified, they are either mixed with 50 000–100 000 sperm or, alternatively, a single sperm may be injected into a single oocyte to achieve fertilization. Within 24 hours, evidence of fertilization can be observed through a microscope. The fertilized oocytes are allowed to divide into 2, then 4, then 6–8-celled embryos over the next 48–72 hours. The embryos are cultured from two to five days (see Figure 4.2).

Step five is embryo transfer. This is undertaken using a thin, soft catheter, which is passed painlessly through the cervix into the uterine cavity, preferably under ultrasound guidance.

The luteal phase is supported by the administration of progesterone supplements, usually by a vaginal cream or pessary. This is necessary to ensure the endometrium is secretory and receptive to the implanted embryo(s).

Finally any embryos that are left over are assessed and, if suitable, cryopreserved for future use.

Approximately two weeks later, blood pregnancy tests are done.

The success of IVF has recently improved, so that approximately one in every three IVF cycles will result in the birth of a baby.

Third-party reproduction

Many persons who cannot produce their own sperm or eggs wish to have children. While adoption is one alternative, some couples may choose to use sperm or eggs from a known or anonymous donor. In the case of a woman without a fertile male partner, specially prepared sperm from a donor can be inseminated into her cervix or uterus with a reasonable chance of success. Sperm is collected from donors who have been screened for genetic diseases, infections and other undesirable traits. The sperm is frozen and quarantined for six months and then thawed for insemination at the time of ovulation each month. If the woman has diseased or absent Fallopian tubes, donated sperm can also be used during an IVF cycle to inseminate her eggs in the laboratory.

In oocyte donation, a woman, referred to as an egg or oocyte donor, volunteers to receive fertility drugs and undergo the retrieval of her oocytes just as though she were undergoing IVF. Her eggs are then fertilized with sperm from the infertile woman's partner or donated sperm. The resulting embryo is then transferred into the uterus of the infertile woman so that she may carry and deliver the baby.

Finally, in the case of a woman who does not have a uterus but has functioning ovaries, surrogacy using a gestational carrier (surrogate) is an option. In gestational carrier pregnancies, the infertile woman receives fertility drugs and undergoes egg retrieval as though she was undergoing IVF. Her eggs are fertilized by her partner's sperm or donated sperm, but the resulting embryo(s) are transferred into the uterus of another woman, called a gestational carrier. After delivery of the baby, the infertile woman or couple become the legal parents of the baby via adoption.

Thus, women without a uterus or functioning ovaries or men without sperm can still participate actively in overcoming their childlessness, using the new reproductive technologies and/or a third party.

Consequently, the concept of infertility no longer exists.

Take-home messages

- Subfertility is defined as the inability to conceive during 12 months of unprotected sexual intercourse, but if there is an obvious cause or if the woman is older, investigate earlier.
- Approximately one in six couples will experience subfertility.
- Causes of subfertility include:
  - poor timing or technique of intercourse;
  - failure to deliver adequate sperm (quantity and quality) into the cervix/Fallopian tubes;
  - abnormality of the passages including endometriosis or adhesions involving the ovaries or Fallopian tubes;
  - failure to ovulate;
  - unexplained subfertility, which requires IVF.
- The medical work-up of the subfertile couple consists of:
  - determination of ovulation;
  - evaluation of the semen;
  - evaluation of the uterus and Fallopian tubes (pelvic organs) preferably by laparoscopy.
- Treatment options include:
  - hormones to induce ovulation;
  - surgery of the uterus or Fallopian tubes;
  - drug or hormone therapy to improve sperm production (rarely effective);

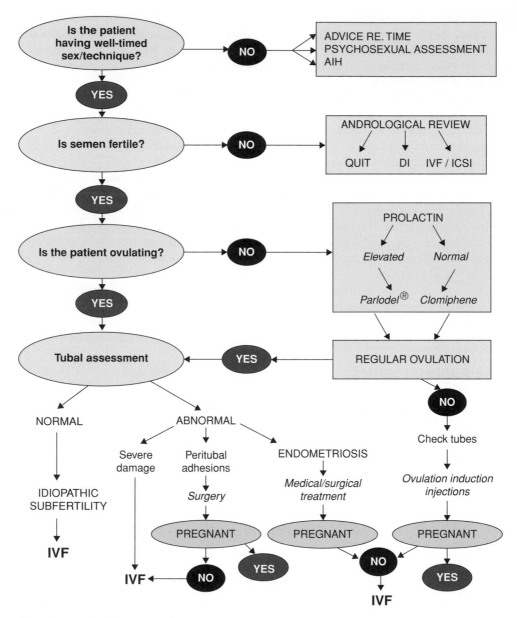

Figure 22.2 A flowchart approach to the subfertile couple. (AIH, artificial insemination by husband; DI, donor insemination; IVF, in vitro fertilization; ICSI, intracytoplasmic sperm insemination.)

- · surgery of the male reproductive tract to improve delivery of adequate numbers of sperm (rarely indicated);
- · assisted reproduction: IVF, ICSI.
- • The new reproductive technologies include fertility preservation by cryopreservation of ovaries or oocytes from women prior to chemotherapy for cancer.

A flowchart approach to diagnosis and treatment is summarized in Figure 22.2.

References

1. World Health Organization. *WHO Laboratory Manual for the Examination of Human Semen and Sperm – Cervical Mucus Interaction*, 3rd edn. Cambridge, UK: Press Syndicate of the University of Cambridge, 1992.

2. Check JH. Antisperm antibodies and human reproduction. *Clin Exp Obstet Gynecol* 2010; 37: 169–74.

3. McIntyre M, Hsieh TC, Lipshultz L. Varicocele repair in the era of modern assisted reproductive techniques. *Curr Opin Urol* 2012; 22(6): 517–20.

4. Najmabadi H, Huang V, Yen P, *et al.* Substantial prevalence of microdeletions of the Y-chromosome in infertile men with idiopathic azoospermia and oligospermia detected using a sequence-tagged site-based mapping strategy. *J Clin Endocrinol Metab* 1996; 81: 1347–52.

5. Ramasamy R, Lin K, Gosden LV, *et al.* High serum FSH levels in men with nonobstructive azoospermia does not affect success of microdissection testicular sperm extraction. *Fertil Steril* 2009; 92(2): 590–3.

6. Rotterdam European Society of Human Reproduction and Embryology (ESHRE)/American Society for Reproductive Medicine (ASRM) Sponsored PCOS Consensus Workshop Group. Revised 2003 consensus on diagnostic criteria and long-term health risks related to polycystic ovary syndrome. *Fertil Steril* 2004; 81: 19–25.

Chapter 23

Sexual assault

Catherine White

Case scenario 1: Caroline

Caroline, aged 29, attends her general practitioner (GP) surgery on a Friday afternoon. She is wearing dark glasses. She requests, 'the morning after pill'. You are running late, but recognize that she seems agitated and distracted. She has her two small children with her.

You decide to ask her if she is OK and she removes her dark glasses to reveal marked bruising and swelling to her face. She goes on to describe an assault the previous night by her husband, Philip, including sexual intercourse (vaginal and anal) without her consent.

Caroline has a good job and is the family breadwinner since her husband was made unemployed last year.

She does not wish to pursue the matter with the police as she feels partly responsible for him losing his temper and she is confident that it will not happen again. She is close to Philip's parents and says it would 'break their hearts' to have their son arrested for this. The children witnessed some of the violence, but she says he has never been violent towards them. At the time of the assault Caroline thought that he was going to kill her.

She becomes very distressed when you mention referring the case to social care … she is afraid that her children will be 'taken away'.

Points to consider

Therapeutic issues:

- Assessment and treatment of injuries sustained
- Risk assessment for emergency contraception
- Sexually transmitted infections (STIs)
- Self harm

Forensic issues:

- Documentation of history, injuries
- Collection of trace evidence

Psychological issues:

- Immediate and ongoing support for Caroline, her children and potentially her husband, if he is your patient
- Yourself

Contraception, eds Paula Briggs, Gabor Kovacs and John Guillebaud. Published by Cambridge University Press. © Cambridge University Press 2013.

- Consider support provided by other organizations: Woman's Aid, local Sexual Assault Referral Centre, Independent Domestic Violence Advisor (IDVA), Independent Sexual Violence Advisor (ISVA)

Safeguarding:

- Immediate risk assessment for safety of Caroline and the children, although Philip left the house, he is likely to return
- Ongoing risk assessment

Case scenario 2: Henry and Margo

Henry, 40 years old, and his wife Margo, 35 years old, come to see you to discuss a referral for a vasectomy. You know them both very well. They have no children and you know Margo has spoken in the past of her desire to have a family. Henry has suffered with depression for many years and you have tried him on a variety of anti-depressants none of which ever seem to work. He also tends to drink heavily and you have spoken to him about this several times over the years. He has always declined any further intervention including counselling saying that his wife Margo is supportive and he doesn't need anything else. You like Henry but find looking after him pretty frustrating.

Recently Henry's symptoms seem to have become worse. He's not sleeping well and his wife notes that he's irritable and weepy. He feels very anxious all the time. He admits to drinking more every day and has recently restarted smoking. You explore further about the decision not to have children together. Henry becomes upset and discloses that as a seven year old he was sexually abused by a male babysitter. He has never told anyone before except his wife. He attributes all his problems as an adult to this abuse. Recently there have been numerous news stories of child sexual abuse on the television and newspapers that have forced him to remember all of this. Henry feels that the world is too bad a place to inflict on any children of his own. Margo sits quietly resigned next to him holding his hand.

Points to consider

- Child sexual abuse as an entity
- Long-term health ramifications (physical and psychological) of sexual abuse.
- Immediate health needs of Henry, including suicide risk assessment.
- Possible future criminal proceedings
- Note keeping (medical records may be requested for disclosure as part of criminal justice process).
- Assessment of request for vasectomy: is Henry able to consent for this at the moment?
- Needs of Margo
- Reflection on approach to 'heartsink' patients.

Case scenario 3: Cassie

Cassie is a 15-year-old girl. She comes to see you asking for 'the rod in the arm' to stop her getting pregnant. Although it is a school day she is not in school uniform. You know that Cassie lives at home with her mum and three younger siblings and money has been tight recently for the family. Despite this Cassie is wearing expensive looking coat and boots and has the latest smartphone.

You ask Cassie about her boyfriend and whether or not she is already sexually active. Cassie starts to look less self assured. She tells you her boyfriend is 20 years old. They don't really do much together except meet up every few days when he gives her gifts and they have sex. He says he really loves her and they will see more of each other soon but he is really busy with work at the moment. It was his idea that she got protected regarding contraception.

Points to consider

- Child sexual exploitation
- Gillick competency and Fraser guidelines
- Child safeguarding
- Information sharing and links with school nurses
- Accessibility and confidentiality of services to young people

The statistics

- Of those aged 16–59 years, 2.5% of women and 0.5% of men had experienced a sexual assault (or attempted assault) in 2010–11 [1].
- It is estimated that of the people who have experienced rape, only 1 in 5 will go to the police and around 40% will choose not to report it [1].
- In 2011–12 the police recorded 14 767 rapes of women and 1274 rapes of men (UK Office for National Statistics, July 2012 [1]).
- The number of recorded rapes had risen by 1% in women but dropped 2% in men (UK Office of National Statistics, July 2012 [1]).
- Around 400 000 women are sexually assaulted and 80 000 women are raped each year (British Crime Survey, 2011 [1]).
- Nearly a quarter of young adults aged between 18 and 24 (24.1%) experienced sexual abuse (including contact and non-contact) by an adult or by a peer during childhood (NSPCC, 2011 [1]).
- Just under 50% of women Mental Health Service users have been subject to sexual abuse and around 50% to physical abuse in childhood, notwithstanding adult abuse which they may also be surviving [2].
- Of women who have experienced domestic violence, 40–50% are raped within their physically abusive relationship [3].
- Most victims will know their assailant.

The law

The Sexual Offences Act 2003 is the basis of the legal terms relating to sexual assault referred to in this book. This would apply to offences committed after 1 May 2004. Prior to that, the Sexual Offences Act 1956 would apply.

Sexual Offences Act 2003

Section 1 (Statutory definition of rape)

1. A person (A) commits an offence if:

   a. he intentionally penetrates the vagina, anus or mouth of another person (B) with his penis.
   b. B does not consent to the penetration, and
   c. A does not reasonably believe that B consents.

2. Whether a belief is reasonable is to be determined having regard to all the circumstances, including any steps A has taken to ascertain whether B consents.

Section 5 (Statutory definition of rape of a child under 13 years)

1. A person commits an offence if:

    a. he intentionally penetrates the vagina, anus or mouth of another person with his penis, and

    b. the other person is under 13 years.

Disclosure of sexual assault

As has been noted above most victims of sexual violence do not disclose the assault immediately if at all.

Clinicians require a high degree of suspicion and alertness as to the possibility that sexual violence may be the cause for the patient's presentation if they are to be able to help the patient in a timely manner.

Anyone of any age can become a victim of sexual violence, even an alpha male rugby player or top female businesswoman. That said, as with many crimes, assailants are more likely to target the vulnerable. This will include those with learning difficulties, communication difficulties, the young, the old and those with poor support systems. The doctor needs to be a champion for these groups, both in protecting them and also considering if they are victims of abuse.

Acute assault

*   Direct disclosure
*   No direct disclosure but health advice sought for:

    emergency contraception;
    STI screening;
    human immunodeficiency virus (HIV) post-exposure prophylaxis (PEP);
    injuries;
    victim of violence including domestic violence.

Historic and or chronic abuse

*   Direct disclosure
*   No direct disclosure but health advice sought for:

    unwanted pregnancy;
    STIs;
    pelvic pain;
    irritable bowel syndrome;
    mental health problems including but not exclusively: anxiety, depression, dyspareunia, drug and alcohol misuse, self harm, suicide.

Initial response

In eliciting a history of sexual assault, the doctor should listen to what the patient doesn't say as much as to what they do say.

Once a disclosure is made the doctor must consider the possible options (Table 23.1). These will be dictated in part by:

Table 23.1 Things to consider when someone discloses rape.

Immediate safety	• Are they safe? • Are there any third parties to consider, e.g., children, other dependants? • Are any safeguarding referrals required? • Are you safe?
Medical needs	• Injuries, assessment and treatment • Emergency contraception • HIV PEPSE • Hepatitis B PEPSE • Screening for sexually transmitted infections • Pregnancy testing
Forensic needs	• Preservation of evidence • Documentation of injuries including photography where necessary • Documentation of allegations • All to be done in a manner that makes evidence admissible to court
Psychological needs	• Of the complainant (including risk of self harm, suicide) • Of other witnesses • Of you

HIV, human immunodeficiency virus; PEPSE, post-exposure prophylaxis after sexual exposure.

Urgency:

• Is this an acute or historic assault?

Patient choice:

• What are the ideas, concerns and expectations of the patient?

Doctors' legal obligations:

• Are there safeguarding issues that the doctor must act on?
• Are there matters of Public Interest that may override any decision by the patient?

Resources available:

• What support is in place for the patient?
• Is there a Sexual Assault Referral Centre (SARC) available?

The doctor must:

• Treat the patient with respect.
• Not be judgemental in approach.
• Assess the needs and wants of the patient.
• Explain to the patient what their options are.
• Offer back choice and control to the patient as much as possible.
• Not make promises you are unable to keep, such as the promise of confidentiality.

Capacity, consent and confidentiality

When a patient discloses that they have been a victim, the doctor must consider what duty they have to maintain confidentiality balanced against any requirements to share information. The sharing of information may be in order to protect the patient from future abuse or to protect others; for example, the patient's children (see Case scenario 1: Caroline) or in a situation whereby the decision not to inform the police regarding information that may help identify a perpetrator allows this person to go on to abuse others.

To be able to do this the doctor must consider their legal obligations and also the ethical considerations (such as balancing the sometimes competing four bioethical principles as laid out by Beauchamp and Childress [4]):

1. Autonomy
2. Beneficence
3. Non-maleficence
4. Justice

The doctor, when eliciting the wishes of the patient, must put them into the context of the patient's capacity.

Capacity and the Mental Capacity Act

The definition of, assessment of and responsibilities in relation to capacity (also known as mental capacity) in England and Wales are laid out in the Mental Capacity Act (MCA) 2005.

- The MCA 2005 applies to all adults aged over 16.
- The MCA 2005 defines capacity as the ability to make a decision. It relates to the *process* of making a decision and not to the *outcome* of the decision. It is not limited to medical decisions, but can apply to any decision-making process; for example, financial or social choices.
- Capacity is task specific. A person may be capable of deciding one issue but not another.
- Capacity is also time specific. A person's capacity may alter with time.

The MCA 2005 defines the lack of capacity as:

If, at the time the decision needs to be made, patients are unable to make the decision because of an 'impairment of, or a disturbance in the functioning of, the mind or brain', they are deemed incapable.

The term 'capacity' was previously used interchangeably with the term 'competence'. Since the MCA 2005, 'capacity' is the preferred term.

The MCA 2005 lays out five statutory principles:

1. A person must be assumed to have capacity unless it is established that he/she lacks capacity.
2. A person is not to be treated as unable to make a decision unless all practicable steps to help him or her to do so have been taken without success. *(This includes communicating in an appropriate way. In forensic practice the clinician may need to arrange for interpreters or signers to be present or use visual aids.)*
3. A person is not to be treated as unable to make a decision merely because he/she makes an unwise decision.
4. An act done, or a decision made, under this Act for or on behalf of a person who lacks capacity must be done, or made, in his/her best interests.
5. Before the act is done, or the decision is made, regard must be had as to whether the purpose for which it is needed can be as effectively achieved in a way that is less restrictive of the person's rights and freedom of action.

Healthcare professionals are warned that a person cannot be judged to lack capacity simply because of age, appearance or behaviour.

Assessment of capacity

All adults are presumed to have capacity unless there is evidence to the contrary.

In order to assess someone's capacity to make a valid treatment decision, two criteria have to be considered:

1. Do they have an impairment of mind or brain (temporary or permanent)?
2. Does the impairment mean that the person is unable to make the decision in question at the time it needs to be made?

Confidentiality

The degree to which the allegations are kept confidential will be dependent upon:

- The wishes of the patient.
- The capacity of the patient.
- The legal obligations of the doctor.
- The ongoing risk to:
  - patient;
  - any children;
  - any vulnerable adults;
  - general public.

Where there is doubt seek advice from:

- Senior clinicians
- Local Safeguarding Team
- Medical defence organization
- Caldicott Guardian

Documentation

It is a given that medical notes should always be of a high standard. This is especially vital in situations such as disclosure of sexual violence, where the potential for legal scrutiny is high.

Therefore as a minimum the medical notes should be:

- Legible
- Clear as to who made them, be signed and dated.
- Clear as to who gave the information and who else was present when information given.
- Stored safely

History

The amount of history taken by the GP depends a lot upon any proposed further action.

So, for example, in a situation where a referral to police, social services, SARC, etc., is going to happen, then the history taking should be kept to a minimal level in order to ensure immediate needs are met. This is partly to avoid the patient having to recount their story any more than necessary but also to minimize the chance of contamination of evidence, such as asking leading questions.

Where the disclosure is from an adult with capacity who does not wish to engage with the criminal justice system at the present time, and does not wish to be referred to a SARC, then the GP should take a more detailed history, again bearing in mind that the records may be required by the courts in the future.

The history and note taking should be:

- Done in a private place with minimal chance of interruption.
- At the pace of the patient not the doctor.
- Intelligent and tailored to the circumstances of the patient.
- Accurate.
- Comprehensive and comprehensible.
- Objective.

Examination

The extent of the examination after disclosure of sexual violence will depend upon several considerations including:

- Consent of the patient.
- Immediate needs of the patient.
- Time elapsed since the assault.
- Whether or not an examination by a Forensic Physician is planned.
- Nature of the allegation.
- Activities of the patient since the assault.

For example, let us return to the case scenarios, below.

Case scenario 1: Caroline

Whether or not Caroline is seen by a forensic doctor, with her consent the GP should document the injuries he/she has seen to her face.

A full body examination should be conducted. This may be done by a forensic doctor. The GP should be satisfied that Caroline has no life-threatening condition in the meantime.

The GP should also advise Caroline on the preservation of forensic evidence (e.g., avoid washing, showering, etc., prior to the forensic examination).

Case scenario 2: Henry

Given the time elapsed between the assaults on Henry as a 7 year old and his presenting now 33 years later, unless the allegations were of such an extreme nature that there may be scarring, then physical examination of Henry is unlikely to be productive (although some patients are reassured by a 'normal' examination).

Case scenario 3: Cassie

It would appear that Cassie has been a victim of child sexual exploitation. An immediate examination by the GP does not appear to be necessary. A forensic examination may be of value if the last sexual intercourse was recent and trace material such as DNA might be secured. In addition, when recording examination findings it is important to:

- Describe the extent of the examination.
- Keep objective findings clearly separated from subjective opinion.
- Record negative findings as well as any positive findings.

Injuries

Contrary to popular belief most victims of sexual violence will not have many, if any, injuries. However, should the GP find any it is important that they are classified and recorded correctly.

Types of injuries

The classification of injuries is as follows:

- Bruise
- Abrasion
- Laceration
- Incision
- Burn

Bruises
- Due to blunt force causing blood to escape from vessels
- May not appear immediately
- Under force of gravity may appear at a site distant to site of original trauma
- May also be known as contusions or ecchymoses
- A large collection of blood may be known as a haematoma
- Petechial haemorrhages are defined as bruises of less than 2 mm diameter. Sometimes seen in strangulation, or suction of the skin, blunt trauma through woven fabric, medical conditions, e.g., vasculitis

Age of bruises
- It is very difficult to age a bruise. As the red blood cells are destroyed, the bruise will undergo a colour change.
- However it important to note:

    1. Different bruises, sustained simultaneously by a person, may undergo colour changes at a different rate: i.e., one bruise may still be red in colour whilst the other is purple and yellow, yet they are the same age.
    2. Bruises do not all go through every colour change.
    3. In adults a bruise that contains yellow must be at least 18 hours old. The converse is not true: i.e., a bruise that does not contain yellow may still be older than 18 hours old [5].
    4. In darker skins it may be more difficult to see colour changes within a bruise.
    5. Some people detect the colour yellow less well than others making observer factors an issue.

Abrasions

- Abrasions are defined as a superficial disruption of the surface epithelium (epidermis) caused by trauma.
- Non-medical terms are scratch or graze.
- They are usually due to movement of a rough surface over the skin or vice versa.
- They may bleed due to the corrugations of the dermal papillae.
- Trace material may be found in abrasions.
- Unlike some bruises, they do not extend or gravitate.
- In sexual assaults, crescentic abrasions due to fingernails may sometimes be seen.
- Skin piling at one end of an abrasion may assist in determining the mechanism of causation.
- Abrasions will exude serum which goes on to form a scab.

Lacerations

Here the full thickness of the skin is split by blunt force.

Typical features of a laceration are:

- Irregular edges and irregular division of tissue planes
- Tissue bridges including blood vessels or nerves may be seen.
- May have abraded and/or bruised margins
- May contain debris
- The shape may replicate the object responsible.
- When over a bony surface, may initially look like an incision.
- Often bleed
- Rarely self inflicted

However the genital lacerations that may be seen in sexual assault tend, especially those seen on the external genitalia, to be very superficial and without many of the features noted above. They tend to be due to a tearing and overstretching of the tissues, usually as penetration is attempted. The posterior fourchette is the site most often injured in this manner.

Incisions

- These are due to sharp objects breaching the epithelium.
- They are sometimes known as cuts.
- The edges tend to be straight without associated abrasions or bruising.
- Tissues are cut in the same plane. Blood vessels and nerves are cleanly divided.
- May bleed profusely.
- An incision that is wider than it is deep may be described as a slash injury.
- If it is deeper than it is wide, it may be termed a stab injury.

Key points to note for any injury

The following information should be noted by the clinician whenever an injury is found. Remember good note keeping will include negative findings as well as positive findings where relevant.

- Type of injury
- Size

- Shape
- Depth (if possible, e.g., laceration)
- Edges (e.g., abrasion – is skin at one end?)
- Laceration – is there debris or a foreign body contained in it?
- Colour (red, purple, does it blanche with pressure etc. If a bruise, is there any yellow?)
- Surface covering (dry or wet blood, scab, dirt?)
- Swelling
- Tenderness
- Distance from fixed anatomical point
- Explanation, noted verbatim, if offered

Absences of injuries

In dealing with sexual assault cases it is probably worth noting that most complainants will have few if any injuries. Any injuries present are likely to be of a minor nature that will heal rapidly leaving no trace.

The presence of injuries in sexual assault cases varies hugely. It is a common misconception, held among clinicians, police, lawyers and also the public who make up juries, that all victims of sexual violence will have injuries to back up their claim [6].

This is often not the case and an important role of the forensic clinician is to work towards dispelling that myth. Not withstanding this, some complainants will have multiple severe injuries.

Forensic samples

In acute cases of rape or sexual assault forensic evidence in the form of trace evidence may be available.

Any forensic samples required should ideally be taken by someone with the knowledge, experience and training to do so. The Faculty of Forensic and Legal Medicine produces a guide, which is reviewed every six months, on how to take forensic samples [7].

For the GP to whom the patient first discloses it is important to minimize the risk of destroying evidence or making its subsequent interpretation difficult. That said, care of the patient's immediate health risks will always take precedence over forensic issues.

Advising the patient on not washing, eating, drinking, throwing away sanitary wear, etc., prior to examination by a forensic physician is essential. If in doubt the GP should seek advice from the forensic physician or the local SARC.

Chain of evidence

Should any samples be obtained by the GP, then the chain of evidence must be clear. This is the documentation that follows any piece of evidence, from its initial retrieval up to its use in a court case. It should say what the evidence is, its source, the time and date it was taken, by whom and where and how it has been stored since.

The Faculty of Forensic and Legal Medicine has produced guidance on the correct labelling of samples [7].

Statements

The GP may be asked to provide a statement for the courts. This is an opportunity to communicate information. The doctor should remember who the statement is intended for. In criminal cases this will ultimately be the jury.

The key to writing a good statement is:

- Good contemporaneous records
- Clear simple language
- Logical approach

The statement should include, for example:

- The qualifications and experience of the doctor
- The circumstances in which the patient was seen
- How the disclosure came about
- What the details given were, who gave them, who else was present
- The extent and findings of any examination
- Outline any care given

Safeguarding

Safeguarding is the duty of all healthcare workers.

In the case of sexual violence the doctor should risk assess the safeguarding issues of the victim, any dependants they may have and other potential victims.

Male rape

Male rape and sexual abuse (boys and adult males) is not uncommon although it often goes unreported.

Often men will worry that their sexuality will be questioned should they disclose. As with female victims the vast majority of assailants are male.

Child sexual exploitation

The standard definition of child sexual exploitation, based on 2009 UK government guidance [8] is as follows:

Sexual exploitation of children and young people under 18 involves exploitative situations, contexts and relationships where young people (or a third person or persons) receive 'something' (e.g., food, accommodation, drugs, alcohol, cigarettes, affection, gifts, money) as a result of then performing, and/or another or others performing on them sexual activities.

Child sexual exploitation can occur through the use of technology without the child's immediate recognition; for example, being persuaded to post sexual images on the Internet/mobile phones without immediate payment or gain. In all cases, those exploiting the child/young person have power over them by virtue of their age, gender, intellect, physical strength and/or economic or other resources. Violence, coercion and intimidation are common, involvement in exploitation being characterized in the main by the child or young person's limited availability of choices resulting from their social/economic and/or emotional vulnerability.

Services available

Sexual Assault Referral Centre

SARCs are one-stop centres for victims of sexual violence.

The delivery aim of the SARC is to provide clients with:

1. Acute healthcare and support.
2. Comprehensive forensic medical examination.
3. Follow-up services which address the client's medical, psychosocial and ongoing needs.
4. Direct access or referral to an ISVA.

Most SARCs will see victims even if the victim does not wish to proceed down the criminal justice process by involving the police. (Remember for children there will be a need to share information with social services/police).

Third sector

Some patients will benefit from the support of specialist organizations, be that from a SARC or a third sector/voluntary group such as Rape Crisis.

The GP should have knowledge of these groups or at least know where to look for their contact details.

Vicarious trauma

Dealing with victims, hearing their accounts and the ramifications of the assaults can be harrowing. Doctors should be mindful of the effect this can have on them. Sometimes the effects may not be immediately obvious.

Good self awareness is essential, be kind to yourself. No one expects you to be superhuman.

Prevention

Sexual violence has been an unfortunate feature of human relationships from time immemorial. There are many anthropological and social theories around this.

There has been work done to look at reducing the rate of sexual violence, including awareness raising projects, school-based projects, etc. [9, 10].

References

1. Home Office. *British Crime Survey 2010/11.* http://www.homeoffice.gov.uk/publications/science-research-statistics/research-statistics/crime-research/hosb1011/ (accessed 15 March 2013).
2. Department of Health. *Mainstreaming Gender and Women's Mental Health,* September 2003. http://www.dh.gov.uk/prod_consum_dh/groups/dh_digitalassets/@dh/@en/documents/digitalasset/dh_4072069.pdf (accessed 4 March 2013).
3. Martin EK, Taft CT, Resick PA. A review of marital rape. *Aggress Violent Behav* 2007; 12(3): 329–47.
4. Beauchamp TL, Childress JF. *Principles of Biomedical Ethics,* 5th ed. New York, NY: Oxford University Press, 2001.
5. Langlois NE, Gresham GA. The ageing of bruises: a review and study of the colour changes with time. *Forensic Sci Int* 1991: 50: 227–38.

6. White C. Genital injuries in adults. *Best Pract Res Clin Obstet Gynaecol* 2013; 27(1): 113–30.

7. Faculty of Forensic and Legal Medicine. *Recommendations for the Collection of Forensic Specimens from Complainants and Suspects*. http://fflm.ac.uk/upload/documents/1309786594.pdf (accessed 4 March 2013).

8. Department for Children, Schools and Family. *Safeguarding Children and Young People from Sexual Exploitation*, August 2009. https://www.education.gov.uk/publications/eOrderingDownload/00689-2009BKT-EN.pdf (accessed 4 March 2013).

9. World Health Organization and London School of Hygiene and Tropical Medicine. *Preventing Intimate Partner and Sexual Violence Against Women: taking action and generating evidence*, 2010. http://www.who.int/reproductivehealth/publications/violence/9789241564007/en/index.html (accessed 4 March 2013).

10. Centers for Disease Control and Prevention National Center for Injury Prevention and Control (NCIPC) http://www.cdc.gov/ViolencePrevention/index.html (accessed 4 March 2013).

Chapter 24

Future developments in contraception

Jean-Jacques Amy

This topic was not chosen by the author, who is very much aware of the truth of the saying 'Prediction is difficult, especially about the future' – variously attributed to, among others, Niels Bohr, Sam Goldwyn, Mark Twain, Confucius, but, most probably first divulged by some Cro-Magnon humourist. The said author makes no claim to have succeeded in disproving the aphorism, or to provide in this chapter a comprehensive overview of methods presently being developed or belonging to a – by definition – hypothetical future.

Allow me to illustrate my point. Some 13 years ago, David Baird and Anna Glasier, two undisputed authorities in the domain of family planning, predicted that within 10 years from then three methods such as (i) a 'once-a-month' pill capable of inhibiting implantation; (ii) anti-progestogens released from an oestrogen-free oral contraceptive to be taken daily; and (iii) orally active, non-peptide antagonists of gonadotrophin-releasing hormone (GnRH) that could be administered to both women and men, would become available [1]. None of these predicted developments have materialized so far and, likely, the second one never will because of endometrial safety being threatened by long-term use of selective progesterone receptor modulators (SPRMs).

To meet the existing needs and barriers confronting birth control, targets involved in highly specific phases of reproductive processes in women and men must be identified, and innovative approaches developed. Progress in genomics and proteomics will be critical in this regard. Many approaches that may be safer, more efficacious and better tolerated, are currently being explored [2]. An interesting list of desirable characteristics for contraceptive targets, even though already eight years old, is to be found elsewhere [3].

Genomics research has already led to the identification of a multitude of genes, which in the reproductive tract of one or the other gender, are expressed solely in certain cells and tissues, not in any other structure of the body. Based upon these findings, attempts are being made to develop contraceptives that will each specifically interfere with a particular step in the reproductive process and which, because of that specificity, will elicit only minimal or no unwanted side effects [3]. One of the molecules under investigation is leptin, a cytokine receptor which plays an important role in implantation [2].

Also, innovative and more acceptable drug delivery systems must be devised. Finally, there is an urgent need for a contraceptive (method) that also protects against sexually transmitted infections (STIs), including that caused by the human immunodeficiency virus (HIV) [3].

Contraception, eds Paula Briggs, Gabor Kovacs and John Guillebaud. Published by Cambridge University Press. © Cambridge University Press 2013.

Contraception in women

Combined oral contraceptives

The evolution that combined oral contraceptives (COCs) have undergone over the past five decades has consisted chiefly of (i) the lowering of the oestrogen dose; (ii) the introduction of new progestins differing in potency, androgenicity, affinity for steroid receptors and interactions with oestrogens; (iii) variations in regimens of administration; and (iv), most recently, the replacement of ethinyl oestradiol (EE) with the natural oestrogen 17β-oestradiol (E_2) or its valerate. The efficacy of the pill is high in the case of perfect use, but that observed in association with typical use is considerably lower, due to poor compliance. Another major problem encountered is the high discontinuation rate of this contraceptive method caused by alleged, associated side effects. In the future, during counselling of women desirous of starting contraception, more emphasis will need to be placed on the non-contraceptive beneficial effects of COCs, and on the fact that, except for chloasma and spotting, the frequency of symptoms perceived as side effects of the method actually is *not* notably higher than among women of the same age not using hormonal contraceptives.

The dose of EE in COCs has already been lowered to the clinically acceptable minimum of 20 µg. The use of pills containing only 15 µg of this oestrogen is associated with a notable increase in the occurrence of spotting. Consequently, no further lowering of the amount of EE in COCs is to be expected. Future changes related to the oestrogen contained in COCs will pertain to the nature of this component. It is hoped that the frequency of certain complications seen among users of COCs containing EE will be lower in women taking a pill containing E_2 or E_2-valerate.

After oral intake, unlike E_2, EE is not actively metabolized at its first and subsequent passages through the liver, which results in its prolonged circulation. Further, compared to the natural oestrogen, a much lower fraction of EE binds to sex hormone-binding globulin (SHBG), so that most of it circulates free; it also binds with much greater affinity to beta-receptors than oestradiol does. Last, the very potent synthetic EE stimulates, to a considerably greater extent than does E_2, the synthesis in the liver of proteins such as angiotensin, lipoproteins and coagulation factors. These proteins augment the risks of cardiovascular events of either venous or arterial nature. Epidemiological studies conducted in some 10 years from now should reveal whether COCs containing E_2 or E_2-valerate will indeed have met the presently entertained expectation of their greater safety [4].

A four-phasic COC containing E_2-valerate and dienogest (Qlaira®) has been on the market for a few years. Its perfect use appears to be associated with an efficacy and acceptability which are comparable to those of low-dose pills containing EE. In the opinion of the author, the major shortcoming of this new pill is its polyphasic concept: as for other non-monophasic COCs, cycle length cannot be extended to more than 28 days, thus precluding delaying (as in extended regimens) or avoidance (as in a continuous regimen) of withdrawal bleeding (see Chapter 12). Also, women desirous of postponing the occurrence of such bleeds for social, professional or other reasons will not be able to tailor the length of their pill-driven cycle.

The other available COC containing a natural oestrogen is a monophasic preparation (Zoely®) combining in each pill 1.5 mg micronized E_2 and 2.5 mg nomegestrol acetate (NOMAC). This recently developed, highly selective progestin behaves as a complete agonist at the progesterone receptor site, with absent or negligible binding to other steroid receptors, including the oestrogen, androgen and glucocorticoid receptors. It has no effect on carbohydrate and lipid metabolisms. 'Active' pills are taken for 24 days, followed by placebo for 4 days. Compared with a pill combining drospirenone and EE, the NOMAC/EE COC appeared to be associated with more acne, and shorter, lighter or absent withdrawal bleeding.

A COC containing a progestin and the natural oestrogen oestetrol (E_4) is currently being investigated. E_4 is a natural oestrogen with remarkable properties, whose synthesis from E_2 and oestriol (E_3), in the human fetal liver, is regulated by the enzymes 15α and 16α-hydroxylase. In the newborn, the liver promptly loses its capacity to synthesize E_4 because these enzymes are no longer expressed. E_4 is a selective oestrogen receptor modulator (SERM): it acts as an *agonist* on the vaginal wall, endometrium, bone and the brain, but it *antagonizes* E_2 in the breast as potently as tamoxifen does. E_4 suppresses ovulation. It binds highly selectively to the oestrogen receptors, mainly – unlike EE and E_2 – to the alpha-receptors. Also, in contrast with EE and especially with E_2, E_4 does not bind to SHBG and does not stimulate the production of SHBG in vitro. It causes fewer side effects and its use is associated with less risk than EE: it does not induce liver enzymes to the same extent, and should protect against breast cancer.

Progestin-only pills

The short-term use of an SPRM can be contemplated for treatment of episodes of breakthrough bleeding that are frequently encountered during use of these and other progestin-only contraceptive methods.

Oral contraceptives with a non-steroid substance added

The rationale for adding iron, folic acid or dehydroepiandrosterone sulphate (DHEAS) to the active or placebo-tablets of oral contraceptives has been questioned, and the health benefit of these and similar innovations must still be demonstrated.

Contraceptive gel to be applied on the skin

A contraceptive gel whose active components are absorbed through the skin is being tested. The gel contains E_2 and the novel progestin Nestorone®. This steroid, which is 100 times more potent than progesterone and 10 times more than levonorgestrel (LNG), is very effective at suppressing ovulation at a low dose when applied topically, for instance by means of a transdermal gel. It is not active when given orally. It is devoid of androgenic effects.

Previous research has shown that a transdermal formulation combining E_2 and Nestorone® causes fewer side effects than do many currently available combined hormonal contraceptive methods. The lowest effective doses of the oestrogen and progestin, also capable of maintaining normal bleeding patterns, have been determined.

The Nestorone®/E_2 gel represents an attractive contraceptive alternative. The formulation, the nature of its active compounds, and the drug-delivery system have all been designed to diminish the frequency and severity of side effects (e.g., acne, weight gain, altered cholesterol levels) and thus to optimize users' ability and willingness to continue using the method [5].

Spray-on contraceptive

The Population Council, in collaboration with the pharmaceutical firm Acrux Ltd, is developing a transdermal spray delivery system for Nestorone®. After the product has been sprayed a depot forms within the skin from which the progestin, over a certain time, is gradually released into the circulation. A Phase 1 study of a spray delivering Nestorone® was recently completed. The results of this trial may eventually lead to a contraceptive formulation delivering a combination of E_2 and Nestorone®. The parenteral route has the advantage of substantially lowering the risk of venous thromboembolism that is associated with the oral administration of E_2. In addition, the spray technology concerned is relatively low cost [6].

Implants
Because Nestorone® is not absorbed orally by the breastfed infant, implants delivering this progestin are appropriate for use by lactating women. Implants releasing 150 μg Nestorone® per day have a duration of action of 2.0–2.5 years.

Progestin-only vaginal rings
Rings releasing either nomegestrol acetate or Nestorone® are being assessed. Another ring releasing natural progesterone, Silesia®, is intended for use during the breastfeeding period.

Vaginal rings releasing a combination of an oestrogen and a progestin
The ring containing Nestorone® and EE remains sufficiently active for one year. It is to be left in the vagina for three weeks, removed for one week and then reinserted.

Injectables
Population Council scientists are also exploring ways to inject contraceptive steroids in innovative microspheres with different formulations.

Copper-intrauterine devices
As stated by two acknowledged experts, the best copper-intrauterine devices (IUDs) currently in use have (i) an efficacy which is comparable to that of sterilization; (ii) an exceptionally long duration of action; and (iii) the greatest cost-effectiveness of all reversible methods. Further improvement, therefore, seems difficult to achieve. In China, IUD research still aims at enhancing efficacy and at reducing adverse effects. In the Western world, research focuses less on device development but more on methods aiming at increasing acceptance of these contraceptives, both among users (regardless of parity) and providers, and on the study of the non-contraceptive benefits of IUDs [7].

Nanotechnology is presently being investigated by a number of Chinese companies and university researchers with a view to (i) achieve greater effective release of copper from the IUD; and (ii) reduce the size of the devices. The potential effects of this approach on essential aspects such as efficacy, safety, acceptability and continuation have yet to be determined.

Also in China, copper-IUDs releasing indometacin, a potent inhibitor of prostaglandin synthesis, are the object of much research whose ultimate purpose consists in reducing bleeding problems encountered with regular copper-IUDs and the related discontinuation of use [7]. It remains that, in such women, a progestin-releasing intrauterine system (IUS) may seem a more logical choice.

Progestin-releasing IUS

All current intrauterine delivery systems release LNG. Smaller LNG-IUSs are about to be made commercially available. One such device is the 'levonorgestrel contraceptive system', which releases 15 µg LNG per day and has a duration of activity of 3 years. It is intended for use by nulliparous women, or other women with a smaller uterine cavity. Also, frameless IUSs (e.g., the Fibroplant®-LNG, with a structure derived from that of the frameless copper-IUD GyneFix®) can be better tolerated by such women [8].

Some women object to the discrete bleeding or spotting which may supervene during the first months of IUS use, and some more develop persistent acne, mood changes or are affected by other adverse effects. Alternative progestins, capable of preventing metrorrhagia and uterine disease, should therefore be assessed for this application [9].

It is not known whether these progestins, like LNG, should have a mild androgenic profile or be more 'neutral' in that respect. The original Progestasert (Alza, Palo Alto, CA, USA), that is no longer marketed, released progesterone; it caused much more troublesome and erratic breakthrough bleeding than the Mirena® LNG-IUS. Possibly stimulation of endometrial androgen receptors is required to maximally suppress endometrial proliferation, to interfere with angiogenesis and to elicit amenorrhoea [9].

Anti-progestin-releasing IUSs

Earlier animal experiments had shown that IUSs releasing an anti-progestin over time suppressed endometrial glandular and arterial proliferation; it was therefore thought that these devices might offer an alternative for intrauterine contraception that would be accompanied by minimal breakthrough bleeding. Yet, as mentioned earlier, long-term exposure of the endometrium to the action of SPRMs may lead to cytological anomalies.

Female condoms

Currently available female condoms (FCs) are made of natural rubber latex (NRL), synthetic latex (nitrile) or polyurethane. FC2, which became available in 2005, is made of nitrile. The latter, which is also used for manufacturing surgical gloves, has no particular storage requirements. A thin layer of this material conducts heat well and preserves sensation [10]. Several new, innovative models are in various stages of development, but progress in this domain is hindered by the fact that funding allocated to condom technology is grossly insufficient. In Europe, female and male condoms belong to the same class (Class IIb), with regard to European Conformity (CE: 'Conformité Européenne'). There is a harmonized European standard (EN/ISO 4074) for male condoms but none for FCs. Consequently, for the latter, more clinical evidence must be provided to obtain CE Mark clearance. As for other contraceptives, there are few manufacturers willing to confront the financial burden and the obstacle course separating product design from final approval. In spite of these barriers to marketing new FCs, there is a resurgence of interest in FC technology. Augmenting FC use would indeed be of great benefit as a cost-effective way for preventing HIV transmission. Prerequisites are that new FCs be cheaper, easier, more comfortable, more pleasurable to use and more widely accessible [10, 11].

Single-size diaphragm

The SILCS diaphragm is a 'one-size-fits-most' diaphragm made of silicone and fitted with a non-metallic spring, which has been developed in the USA. Silicone is more durable than latex, and holds up to extreme temperatures and poor storage conditions. The device is easy to insert. As it does not need prior fitting like its traditional latex counterparts do, the SILCS diaphragm requires less intervention on the part of health personnel, and hence seems to be particularly suitable for use in developing countries where resources and access to health-care facilities are limited. It evidently could be employed for delivery of a microbicide gel, conferring protection against HIV and other STIs to the women.

Spermicides and microbicides

The detergent nonoxynol-9 (N-9), which for many years was employed as a spermicide, appears to increase the risk of transmission of agents of STIs. It acts as an irritant on the vaginal epithelium and can cause erosions which facilitate penetration of infective micro-organisms, including HIV. With a view to replacing N-9, non-detergent molecules (e.g., ACIDFORM; Ushercell™; acid buffering gel, BufferGel® Duet) and natural products are currently being investigated, the latter particularly in India [10, 12].

Microbicides are substances which, once in the vagina, are capable of inactivating micro-organisms responsible for STIs. The outcomes of some recent trials, especially those with microbicides (e.g., Carraguard®), have been unfavourable; thus creating new challenges in this field of research [10, 12].

Contraceptive vaccines for women

A method of female immunocontraception, targeting the C-peptide terminal of the β-chain of human chorionic gonadotropin (hCG), has reached phase 2 of its clinical assessment. Its advantage relates to the fact that it neutralizes a hormone which is produced solely during pregnancy. Its efficacy in the majority of women thus treated must still be established [8].

Fertility awareness methods

There is presently a resurgence of interest in natural family planning. Methods of sufficient reliability, when properly employed, have been devised. Among these, the symptothermal method is probably best. It combines monitoring and recording of changes in cervical mucus characteristics *and* variations in basal body temperature (BBT, recorded on awakening) (see Chapter 4). Other signs indicating the imminence or the occurrence of ovulation, such as the position of the cervix, breast tenderness, low-back pain, mittelschmerz (lower abdominal and pelvic pain occurring mid-cycle) or light intermenstrual spotting, are all useful as well for determining the likelihood of fecundability at the time. To identify the beginning of the fertile 'window', copious, clear and highly stretchable cervical mucus manifests itself. One may consider that ovulation is likely to have occurred and that the fertile period has ended when the BBT has remained high for three days and thickening of the mucus is observed [13].

Be that as it may, having an instrument that more objectively identifies physiological changes occurring during the ovulatory cycle should add to the accuracy of the determination of beginning and end of the fertile phase. Several such instruments are already marketed; they monitor changes in BBT, urinary luteinizing hormone (LH) and urinary oestrone-3-glucuronide concentrations. Other monitors measure the content of certain electrolytes or sodium chloride in saliva and cervical-vaginal secretions. Other devices still integrate BBT measurements during the current cycle and data from the menstrual calendar during the previous months. In all likelihood these diagnostic methods for home use will be further refined [13].

Tubal occlusion methods

The availability of sophisticated instruments for hysteroscopic surgery has paved the way for ambulatory transcervical sterilization methods, necessitating little or no anaesthesia (see Chapter 16). The methods currently in use need to be further refined: (i) the hysteroscopic procedures are rather lengthy (median times of 12 and 13 minutes have been reported for Adiana® and Essure®, respectively) and thus cause discomfort; (ii) occlusion of the lumen of the Fallopian tubes must be confirmed by hysterosalpingography or a three-dimensional ultrasound three months post-operatively; and (iii) the long-term safety and efficacy of these methods needs to be further assessed, in particular for those, like Essure®, requiring insertion of a microcoil of nickel (a potential allergen) and titanium in the proximal part of the tube. Even if future techniques of female sterilization would combine the greatest ease of performance with the optimal outcomes, it remains that reversibility of the thus created infertility would, as in the past, require some intervention such as suppression of the mechanical obstacle or a cumbersome in vitro fertilization procedure. In all likelihood, the gradual decrease in incidence of tubal sterilization observed in industrialized countries will continue, women resorting increasingly to long-acting reversible contraceptive methods.

Emergency contraception

There is a great need for developing pharmacological products considerably more effective than LNG and ulipristal, whose success rates are far lower than that of copper-IUDs. It has been shown that meloxicam, an inhibitor of cyclo-oxygenase (COX)-2, can delay rupture of the leading follicle, even after initiation of ovulation. Possibly adding this COX-2 inhibitor to LNG may increase the efficacy of this progestin in the application concerned [8].

In all likelihood the development of a compound with anti-nidatory activity would give rise to some heated ethical debates.

Contraception in men

Representative surveys conducted in industrialized nations have brought to light that a sizeable proportion of the population would be interested in using a pharmacological male contraceptive. The latter might also come in useful for developing countries, assisting these in controlling their explosive population growth. Finally, male contraception constitutes an important issue in the political process that will eventually lead to gender equity [14].

Periodic abstinence, withdrawal and condoms are associated with relatively frequent contraceptive failures, and each interferes somehow with normal sexual activity. Vasectomy, on the contrary, is a highly effective surgical method, but it has the disadvantage of not being easily reversible: a surgical re-anastomosis of the vasa deferentia or sperm extraction from a testicular biopsy specimen and intracytoplasmic sperm injection into the ovum are required, with no guarantee that fatherhood will eventually be achieved [14]. None of the aforementioned methods can be considered as optimal. The search for an ideal male contraceptive method focused in the past decades on the development of a suitable hormonal preparation.

Indeed, of all male pharmacological contraceptive methods tested to date, combinations of an androgen with a progestin seem to best meet the requirements [14, 15].

Diverse other approaches, both hormonal and non-hormonal, are currently being assessed with regard to their contraceptive potential in men. The *former* comprise selective progesterone and androgen receptor modulators, and GnRH antagonists of long duration of action. Next to those targeting genes and proteins influencing spermatogenesis, *non-hormonal approaches* include – among other means – vaccines, antibodies against eppin, indenopyridines, sperm-specific Na^+/H^+ exchangers and substances impairing either certain cell junctions or DNA binding proteins in the testes [15].

Male hormonal contraception

The exogenous progestin and androgen (i) suppress the release of LH and follicle stimulating hormone (FSH) and, as a result thereof, (ii) inhibit *both* spermatogenesis *and* steroidogenesis in the testis; the androgen achieves substitution of the depressed testosterone production and thus maintains androgenicity [14, 15]. The observed effects are fully reversible on discontinuation of treatment. In spite of promising results, research in this domain has been characterized by misadventures and has nearly come to a standstill. The latter is due to the lack of public advocacy for male contraception, doubts about the wide acceptability of male hormonal contraceptives and the fact that the two pharmaceutical firms involved in assessing the very successful combination of etonogestrel implants and testosterone undecanoate injections, namely, Organon and Schering, were taken over by other companies which showed no interest in this application. Luckily, a number of institutions and organizations (e.g., the Population Council, World Health Organization) continue to actively investigate in this field [14].

A recent randomized controlled trial has demonstrated that application on the skin of a gel containing a combination of Nestorone® and testosterone effectively suppressed gonadotropins, justifying further assessment of this formulation for reversible suppression of spermatogenesis and contraception [16].

Novel androgens

The Population Council's Centre for Biomedical Research is currently investigating the contraceptive potential of subdermal implants releasing the synthetic steroid MENT®, which structurally resembles testosterone, but – unlike the latter – does not stimulate prostate growth.

Contraceptive vaccines: immunocontraception

One can resort to antigens or antibodies with a view to disrupting a given phase of gametogenesis (e.g., by targeting sperm antigens) and thus inducing infertility. Immunization of male monkeys with human recombinant epididymal protease inhibitor (EPPIN), a serine protease inhibitor expressed by the testis and epididymis, markedly reduces sperm progressive motility and induces reversible infertility. But, due to variations in host immune responses, contraceptive vaccines do not succeed in inducing long-term infertility in all subjects thus treated. The effect elicited must be restricted to a sperm-specific antigen (i.e., one that is not expressed by other cells in the body) located on the cell surface. Some genetically engineered antibodies seem promising in this respect [17].

Calcium channel blockers

Ca^{2+} is closely involved in sperm motility, capacitation and the acrosome reaction. A variety of Ca^{2+}-permeable channels are present in sperm, some of which, the so-called CATSPERS, are unique to these cells. HC-056456, a CATSPER channel blocker, abolishes hyperactivated motility in vitro. Acting on CATSPER function would likely elicit effects only on sperm, and this approach shows great promise with regard to the development of a modality of male contraception devoid of side effects [17].

Indenopyridines

The indenopyridine CDB-4022 has anti-spermatogenic effects that vary according to the species concerned. The compound targets the Sertoli cell, altering biochemical processes and leading to germ cell loss from the seminiferous epithelium. In the monkey, the *l*-isomer of this substance induces reversible oligospermia.

Adjudin

Adjudin (AF-2364), an analogue of indazole-3-carboxylic acid, disrupts the adhesion between the Sertoli cell and spermatogonia, leading to a sloughing and loss of the latter. It does not destroy spermatogonial stem cells and impairs neither the hypothalamic–pituitary–testicular axis nor testosterone production. Cell adhesion in other organs is unaffected. The testis being equipped with interconnected cell junctions, targeting of one particular junction type may affect the others; these cumulative effects could achieve the blocking of spermato-genesis. At 210 days after treatment discontinuation, normal spermatogenesis was restored in 95% of the seminiferous tubules of the rats. When given orally to adult rats, adjudin appears to have a very low bioavailability and its uptake by the testis is extremely low (: 0.05%), a greater proportion of the compound reaching other compartments such as the serum (3.5%), the muscle (0.8%), the liver (0.6%) and the small intestine (0.2%). Administration of 50 mg/kg for 29 days to these rodents resulted in muscle atrophy and liver inflammation in the male (but not the female) animals. In order to avoid the aforementioned adverse effects and to deliver the drug directly to the testis, it has been coupled to a 'carrier', namely, a mutant form of FSH whose hormonal activity, but not its capacity of binding to the FSH-receptors on Sertoli cells, was deleted. Parenteral (intraperitoneal) administration of 0.5 μg adjudin-FSH mutant to adult male rats was, in addition to being more selective, markedly more effective than administration of 50 mg/kg adjudin. The adjudin-FSH complex is injected or delivered from a gel or from an implant. Research conducted into this and related compounds may eventually lead to one being marketed in the future as a male contraceptive. But the pro-hibitive cost represented by the production of recombinant protein and the conjugation of adjudin to it constitute a formidable barrier to its being manufactured for this application [17, 18].

Intravasal devices

Alternatives to the various modalities of vasectomy, intended to be reversible, consist in placing either flexible silicone plugs or devices made of polyurethane into the vasa defer-entia. A disadvantage of these techniques is that, like after vasectomy, sperm antibodies may form.

Reversible inhibition of sperm under guidance

Reversible inhibition of sperm under guidance (RISUG) could be another alternative to vasectomy. It consists of injecting steric maleic anhydride (SMA) and dimethyl sulfoxide (DMSO) into the vas deferens with a view to partially obstructing this duct, and causing severe damage to the plasma and acrosomal membranes, midpieces and tails of passing sperm, thus causing infertility. Other products are currently being investigated for a similar application; some of these have more outspoken spermicidal effects than the original RISUG formulation. Phase 3 clinical trials of RISUG are currently in progress in India [17].

Concluding remarks

In addition to the aforementioned developments in contraceptive technology, and even more important than the latter, is the need for implementing worldwide gender equality, empowering women, and reducing infant mortality, all being prerequisites for successful family planning programmes. A cultural environment must be created in which contraception is considered to be not only acceptable but also highly valued. In such a setting, couples allowed to use the method best suiting them, even if the latter is not associated with the lowest overall failure rates, will most effectively control their fertility.

References

1. Baird DT, Glasier AF. Science medicine and the future: contraception. *BMJ* 1999; 319: 969–72.

2. Burkman R, Bell C, Serfaty D. The evolution of combined oral contraception: improving the risk-to-benefit ratio. *Contraception* 2011; 84: 19–34.

3. Institute of Medicine Committee on New Frontiers in Contraceptive Research. *New Frontiers in Contraceptive Research: a blueprint for action.* Report Brief, January 2004. http://www.iom.edu/(/media/Files/Report%20Files/2004/New-Frontiers-in-Contraceptive-Research-A-Blueprint-for-Action/ContraceptiveResearchpdfonly.pdf (accessed 29 November 2012).

4. Calaf i Alsina J. After 50 years of ethinylestradiol, another oestrogen in combined oral contraceptives. *Eur J Contracept Reprod Health Care* 2010; 15: 1–3.

5. Population Council. Transdermal delivery systems for women: contraceptive gel. http://www.populationcouncil.org/projects/44_TransdermalDeliveryContraceptiveGel.asp (accessed 1 November 2012).

6. Population Council. Transdermal delivery systems for women: spray-on contraceptive. http://www.popcouncil.org/projects/249_TransdermalWomenSpray.asp (accessed 1 November 2012).

7. Sivin I, Batár I. State-of-the-art of non-hormonal methods of contraception: III. Intrauterine devices. *Eur J Contracept Reprod Health Care* 2010; 15: 96–112.

8. Serfaty D, d'Arcangues C. Contraception du futur. In Serfaty D. (ed.) *Contraception*, 4th edn. Issy-les-Moulineaux, France: Elsevier Masson, 2011: pp. 516–48.

9. Fraser IS. The promise and reality of the intrauterine route for hormone delivery for prevention and therapy of gynecological disease. *Contraception* 2007; 75 (Suppl): S112–17.

10. Batár I, Sivin I. State-of-the-art of non-hormonal methods of contraception: I. Mechanical barrier contraception. *Eur J Contracept Reprod Health Care* 2010; 15: 67–88.

11. Beksinska M, Smit J, Joanis C, Usher-Patel M, Potter W. Female condom technology: new products and regulatory issues. *Contraception* 2011; 83: 316–21.

12. Batár I. State-of-the-art of non-hormonal methods of contraception: II. Chemical barrier contraceptives. *Eur J Contracept Reprod Health Care* 2010; 15: 89–95.

13. Freundl G, Sivin I, Batár I. State-of-the-art of non-hormonal methods of contraception: IV. Natural family planning methods. *Eur J Contracept Reprod Health Care* 2010; 15: 113–23.

14. Nieschlag E. Clinical trials in male hormonal contraception. *J Reproduktionsmed Endokrinol* 2011; 8 (Special issue 1): 227–38.

15. Mahmoud A, T'Sjoen G. Male hormonal contraception: where do we stand? *Eur J Contracept Reprod Health Care* 2012; 17: 179–86.

16. Mahabadi V, Amory JK, Swerdloff RS, *et al.* Combined transdermal testosterone gel and the progestin nestorone suppresses serum gonadotropins in men. *J Clin Endocrinol Metab* 2009; 94: 2313–20.

17. Cheng CY, Mruk DD. New frontiers in nonhormonal male contraception. *Contraception* 2010; 82: 476–82.

18. Lee NP, Wong EW, Mruk DD, Cheng CY. Testicular cell junction: a novel target for male contraception. *Curr Med Chem* 2009; 16: 906–15.

Index